# Nutrients in Cancer Prevention and Treatment

# Experimental Biology and Medicine

# Nutrients in Cancer Prevention and Treatment

Edited by

## Kedar N. Prasad, PhD

*University of Colorado Health Sciences Center, Denver, CO*

## Leonida Santamaria, MD

*University of Pavia, Italy*

## R. Michael Williams, MD, PhD

*Cancer Treatment Center of America, Des Moines, IA*

 Humana Press • Totowa, New Jersey

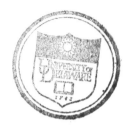

© 1995 Humana Press Inc.
999 Riverview Drive, Suite 208
Totowa, New Jersey 07512

This publication is printed on acid-free paper. ∞
ANSI Z39.48-1984 (American National Standards Institute) Permanence of Paper for Printed Library Materials.

**Photocopy Authorization Policy:**

Printed in the United States of America.  10  9  8  7  6  5  4  3  2  1

Library of Congress Cataloging in Publication Data

Nutrients in cancer prevention and treatment / edited by Kedar N.
  Prasad, Leonida Santamaria, R. Michael Williams.
      p.  cm. — (Experimental biology and medicine)
  Includes bibliographical references and index.
  ISBN 0-89603-318-X (alk. paper)
    1. Vitamins—Therapeutic use. 2. Cancer—Nutritional aspects.
  I. Prasad, Kedar N. II. Santamaria, Leonida. III. Williams, R.
  Michael. IV. Series: Experimental biology and medicine (Totowa, NJ)
    [DNLM: 1. Neoplasms—prevention & control. 2. Vitamins—
  therapeutic use. 3. Antioxidants—therapeutic use. QZ 200 N9757 1995]
  RC271.V58N88 1995
  616.99'40654—dc20
  DNLM/DLC
  for Library of Congress                                    95-15205
                                                                 CIP

# Preface

*Nutrients in Cancer Prevention and Treatment* contains articles that were presented by leading researchers and physicians in the field of nutritional oncology. Most of the previous conference proceedings on Nutrition and Cancer have dealt primarily with the issue of the role of nutrients in cancer prevention. This is logical because enormous quantities of laboratory and epidemiologic data have been published on the topic.

*Nutrients in Cancer Prevention and Treatment* also contains several studies on the role of diet and vitamins in cancer treatment. There are very few books that have reviewed laboratory and clinical studies and the role of vitamins in cancer treatment. There are preliminary data suggesting that daily supplementation with high doses of certain vitamins in combination with conventional therapeutic agents may enhance their growth inhibitory effects on tumor cells, and may protect normal tissues against some of their toxic effects. This book is unique in the sense that several articles have discussed the mechanisms of action of individual vitamins on cellular and molecular parameters. It is very exciting to note that some of the vitamins inhibit protein kinase C activity, increase the production of certain growth factors, and modulate the expression of a number of oncogenes. These studies, at least in part, offer rationales for the cancer protective effects of vitamins.

*Nutrients in Cancer Prevention and Treatment* contains an article showing that these vitamins not only have direct effects on differentiation and growth inhibitory effects of X-irradiation, chemotherapeutic agents, and hyperthermia. In addition to vitamins, there are also articles describing the roles of protease inhibitors, calories, exercise, and fat in the mechanisms of carcinogenesis. We believe that this book will serve as an excellent reference source for those who are involved in nutrition and cancer research, as well as those oncologists who are involved in the actual treatment and care of cancer patients. We hope that *Nutrients in Cancer Prevention and Treatment* will stimulate much new research in all the many promising areas of basic and clinical nutritional oncology.

*Kedar N. Prasad,* PhD
*Leonida Santamaria,* MD
*R. Michael Williams,* MD, PhD

# Preface

# PART I
# Carcinogenesis

# G protein Pathways and Regulation of Neoplastic Transformation

Jianghao Chen, Michael DeVivo
and Ravi Iyengar
Department of Pharmacology, Mount Sinai
School of Medicine, City University of New
York, NY 10029

The processes that underlie the conversion of a normal cell to a transformed phenotype are complex. Signal transduction pathways are thought to play important roles in regulating events that eventually result in the transformed phenotype. It is now well established that many oncogenes code for mutated proteins whose normal counterparts are components of cellular signaling systems (1). Cooperation between such oncogenes in regulating transformation is a well-established phenomenon (2). In normal physiological state signal transduction pathways are important for regulating cellular functions so that they are responsive to current environmental conditions. All cells possess several signaling pathways that are used to convey a variety of signals. Pathways that involve tyrosine kinases are used to produce long term responses such as regulation of proliferation. Many of the best known oncogenes such as v-erb-B, v-src, v-ras and v-raf are components of the tyrosine kinase signaling pathway. Other pathways, such as those that utilize heterotrimeric G protein as signal transducers, are largely used to evoke acute responses such as the activities of metabolic enzymes. Often cells receive

*3*

multiple signals that simultaneously activate different signaling pathways. The net amplitude and duration of the cellular response to these signals reflect a balance between the multiple signals that are received within a fixed period of time. The mechanisms by which multiple signals can be integrated and the loci at which such integration occurs is an important issue in regulatory biology. We have attempted to develop an understanding of how interactions between signaling pathways result in integrated biological responses. For this we have chosen to study interactions between heterotrimeric G protein pathways and growth factor receptor-tyrosine kinase signaling pathways in regulation of cell proliferation.

Signal transduction through G protein coupled pathways is a cell surface phenomenon. Hormone occupancy of the receptors results in activation of G proteins. G proteins are heterotrimers composed of $\alpha$-, $\beta$-, and $\gamma$- subunits. The $\alpha$-subunits bind and hydrolyze the GTP and share regions of homology with other GTPases. During the activation process, the hormone receptors promote the release of bound GDP and the binding of GTP. Binding of GTP leads to the dissociation of the $\beta\gamma$-subunit complex from $\alpha$-GTP (3). The $\alpha$-GTP is capable of regulating the activity of effectors. It is now known that free $\beta\gamma$-subunits also modulate the activity of effectors (4). Effectors includes enzymes such as adenylyl cyclase and phospholipase C that produce second messengers such as cAMP, inositol trisphosphate and diacylglycerol. Elevation of second messenger levels leads to the activation of protein kinases that regulate the activity of enzymes, ion channels and transcription factors by phosphorylation.

The signal transduction pathway utilized by many growth factors such as epidermal growth factor (EGF), fibroblast growth factor (FGF), and platelet derived growth factor (PDGF) are very similar and also involve

GTP binding proteins. However production of diffusible intracellular messengers is not required for signal transmission through this pathway. Rather signal is transmitted through a series of protein-protein interactions. Upon occupancy by growth factors, receptors with intrinsic tyrosine kinase activity undergo autophosphorylation. The autophosphorylated receptor is then capable of interacting with an adaptor protein called GRB2. This interaction occurs because the phosphotyrosine residue interacts with a defined region (the SH2 domain) of GRB2. Hence tyrosine autophosphorylation of the receptor is an obligatory step in signal transduction. The receptor-tethered GRB2 protein recruits another protein called SOS to the cell surface membrane. SOS is a guanine nucleotide exchange factor that can promote the dissociation of GDP from, and the binding of GTP to, the guanine nucleotide binding protein Ras. Also attached to the cell surface membrane, the Ras protein is a binary switch that is inactive in its GDP-bound form and active in its GTP-bound form. Upon recruitment to the membrane SOS activates Ras and thus the signal is transmitted from the receptor to Ras in a membrane delimited manner (5). Upon activation Ras serves as an anchor for Raf, a protein kinase that can phosphorylate substrates at ser-thr residues. GTP-bound Ras has been shown to recruit Raf to the cell surface. The interaction between Ras and Raf results in the autophosphorylation and activation of Raf which is part of a cascade of ser-thr protein kinases that transmits the signal from the cell surface to the nucleus (6). Raf phosphorylates and activates a cytoplasmic protein kinase called MEK. MEK in turn phosphorylates and activates MAP-kinase. MAP-kinase upon activation translocates from the cytoplasm to the nucleus and is capable of turning on several genes that are required for the initiation of proliferation (7,8).

Studies in our laboratory have focused on interactions between the receptor tyrosine kinase/ras/raf/MAP-kinase pathway and $G_q$/phospholipase C or $G_S$/adenylyl cyclase pathways in regulating the proliferation of NIH-3T3 cells. In this review we will describe our studies on interaction between G protein and receptor tyrosine kinase pathways in regulating MAP-kinase activities as well as proliferation. Depending on which G protein pathway is used such interactions can be result in both positive and negative regulation of proliferation.

### Activation of $G_S$ and inhibition of proliferation:

Generally hormonal stimulation of the $G_S$/cAMP pathway usually results in acute or short term physiological effects. A good example is the aerosol spray used for temporary relief of asthma attacks. It contains β-adrenergic receptor agonists that stimulate the production of cAMP. This results in the immediate relaxation of the airway passages. Stimulation of glucose production in liver and muscle is also regulated by cAMP dependent processes. In addition to these effects of the cAMP pathway that are evoked due to phosphorylation of ion channels or enzymes, expression of certain genes are regulated by transcription factors that are responsive to cAMP. Such regulation of gene expression allows cAMP to have long-term effects on cell function. One of the long-term effects of cAMP is its regulation of cell proliferation. Depending on the cell type cAMP can have varied effects on cell proliferation. Elevation of cAMP levels stimulate proliferation of a few types of cells such as thyroid and pituitary cells. Elevation of cAMP also stimulates hormone secretion from these cells. In contrast, in other cells, such as the RAT-1 cells, smooth muscle cells and lymphoid cells, raising cAMP levels inhibits proliferation and lowering of cAMP levels triggers proliferation. In the majority of tissues and cell types, alterations in cAMP levels by itself has little or no effect on cell proliferation. Even though alterations in cAMP by itself does not affect proliferation, recent studies from our laboratory have shown that the cAMP pathway can have a profound effect on proliferation stimulated by signaling through other pathways.

We constructed activated forms of $G\alpha_S$ by mutating Glu-227, a key residue within the GTPase hydrolysis domain. This results in inhibition of the intrinsic GTPase activity and the persistent activation of the G protein (9). Expression of activated $G\alpha_S$ results in suppression of transformation of NIH-3T3 cells by H-ras (10) and v-raf. The effects of activated $G\alpha_S$ are mediated through the cAMP pathway since dominant negative regulatory subunit of protein-kinase A can block the effects of the activated $G\alpha_S$. These observations indicated that even in NIH-3T3 cells the cAMP pathway may be a negative modulator of signaling through the MAP-kinase pathway.

The role of cAMP pathway as a negative modulator of proliferation in some systems has been known for some time now. However the biochemical basis for this inhibition was not known until recently. Studies from a number of groups including ours have provided information about how the cAMP pathway affects signal transmission through the MAP-kinase pathway. Elevation of intracellular cAMP by stimulation of $G_S$ coupled receptors or addition of 8-Br-cAMP, or forskolin, inhibits growth factor stimulated MAP-kinase activity (11-15). We have found that H-ras induced MAP-kinase activity can be inhibited by elevation of intracellular cAMP by expression of mutant activated $G\alpha_S$ (9). Individual steps of growth factor signaling pathway have been analyzed to determine

where signals from the cAMP pathway can regulate
signal transmission from the MAP-kinase pathway. It
has been shown that elevation of cAMP does not affect
growth factor stimulated activation of c-ras. (11).
However growth factor activation of raf, MEK and MAP-
kinases are inhibited by elevation of cAMP levels.
Sturgill and co-workers have shown that increased
concentrations of cAMP blocked EGF-induced activation
of Raf-1, in Rat fibroblasts. This was accompanied by
protein kinase A mediated phosphorylation of Raf on
Serine 43, which reduces the affinity of Raf to interact
with Ras (12). These observations suggest that protein
kinase A phosphorylation of Raf-1 in its regulatory
domain, and the resultant disruption between ras to raf
communication could be one mechanism by which the
cAMP pathway block signal transmission through the
growth factor signaling pathway. Recent and as yet
unpublished studies in our laboratory show that
expression of mutant activated $G\alpha_S$ can inhibit v-Raf-
induced activated MAP kinase activity. Since v-Raf is
constitutively active and does not require association
with activated Ras for signal transmission our
observations suggest that there may be additional
down-stream loci where protein kinase A can inhibit
signal transmission through the growth factor-MAP-
kinase pathway. The possible loci where the $G\alpha_S$
signaling pathway intersect with the growth factor-
receptor tyrosine kinase signaling pathway is shown in
Figure 1

While the finding that activated $G\alpha_S$ suppressed
transformation in RAT-1 fibroblasts were not
surprising since cAMP is antiproliferative in these
cells, the NIH-3T3 cells were far more interesting to
study. Elevation of cAMP levels by itself does not
affect the proliferation of NIH-3T3 cells under normal
culture conditions. However when there is a strong

proliferative signal such as H-ras, modest (less than two fold) elevation of cAMP is effective in almost completely blocking the expression of the transformed state. Thus in certain systems the cAMP pathway can function as a conditional brake, by allowing normal proliferation to continue while at the same time blocking abnormal proliferation. Since NIH-3T3 cells are known to be on the verge of transformation and sometimes even transform without the introduction of foreign oncogenes (16) our observations suggest that targeted expression of activated $G\alpha_s$ could be useful could be useful in devising therapeutic strategies for inhibiting abnormal cell growth and the conversion of benign growth into malignant tumors. cAMP analogs have also been shown to inhibit growth of transformed cells from several tissues (17). These cancer cell lines include breast, colon, lung and gastric carcinomas, fibrosarcomas, gliomas and leukemias. The growth inhibition effect of cAMP analogs appears to be selective for the transformed cells. With the availability of the cDNA for $G\alpha_s$ and the capability for introducing activating mutations in the cDNA it is now feasible to raise intracellular cAMP levels in a cell type specific manner. In developing the use of the cAMP pathway in the treatment of cancer the major concern remains as to how suppression of proliferation can be achieved without increasing cAMP to levels where it alters acute metabolic processes. Indeed it would not be useful if suppression of proliferation is accompanied by new pathophysiology due to malfunctioning metabolic processes.

**FIGURE 1.**

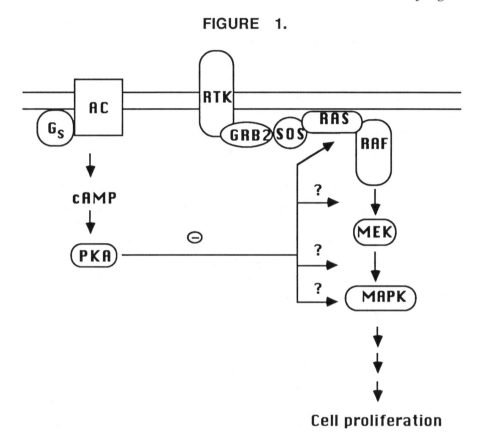

**Cell proliferation**

Interaction between the $G_S$/protein kinase A and receptor-tyrosine kinase/ras/MAP-kinase pathway. The schematic describes the transmittal of signal through the two pathways and the known and putative loci where protein kinase A can inhibit signal transmital in the receptor tyrosine kinase pathway. One known locus of protein kinase A action is on raf which disrupts interaction between ras and raf. Several additional loci are also possible and these are indicated with question marks. Abbreviations used are AC, adenylyl cyclase; cAMP, cyclic AMP; PKA, protein kinase A; RTK, receptor tyrosine kinases; MAPK, MAP-kinase.

Activation of Gq and potentiation of PDGF responses in confluent cultures:

Members of the $G_q$ family of G proteins including $G_{11}$, $G_{14}$ and $G_{16}$ couple receptors to phospholipase C-β. Many agonists that bind to receptors that couple to Gq and stimulate phospholipase C-β also stimulate proliferation. These include angiotensin-II and serotonin. It also has been shown that ectopic expression of receptors such as the serotonin 1C and muscarinic M1 and M3 result in transformation of NIH-3T3 cells (18,19). Thus it appeared likely that continuous activation of the $G_q$ pathway could lead to transformation. To test this hypothesis we studied the effects of mutant activated $G\alpha_q$ on transformation of NIH-3T3 cells. For this the $G\alpha_q$ subunit was mutated to convert the Glu-209 to a Leu. This mutation in $G\alpha_q$ is analogous to the one described above in $G_S$ and results in activation of the $G\alpha_q$ as assessed by the elevation of basal phospholipase C. Under these conditions we and others observed that expression of mutant activated $G\alpha_q$ results in transformation of NIH-3T3 cells (20,21). This effect was cell type specific. Under conditions where we were able to obtain transformation of NIH-3T3 cells, expression of mutant activated $G\alpha_q$ elevated phospholipase C activity but did not transform RAT-1 fibroblasts (20).

The biochemical events that underlie the $G_q$ promoted transformation of NIH-3T3 cells appear to be complex. Even though expression of mutant activated $G\alpha_q$ transforms NIH-3T3 cells as assessed by colony formation in soft agar, expression of mutant activated $G\alpha_q$ by itself does not stimulate proliferation in serum starved cells. Since the assays for transformation including the soft agar colony formation assay are conducted in the presence of serum we tested the interplay between the expression of mutant activated

G$\alpha_q$ and responses to serum. Initial observations indicated that expression of mutant activated G$\alpha_q$ greatly potentiated serum stimulated phospholipase C activity in NIH-3T3 cells. From further studies we were able to establish that mutant activated G$\alpha_q$ potentiated PDGF stimulation of phospholipase C. The role of phospholipase C activation in the communication of proliferation signals is still unclear. However PDGF exerts its effects by interaction with its receptor which is a tyrosine kinase. One of the pathways activated by the PDGF receptor is the ras/raf/MAP-kinase pathway. Since this pathway has been shown to transmit proliferation signals from growth factors we tested if there might be synergy between the G$_q$ and PDGF pathways that could be measured at the level of MAP-kinase activity. We found that interactions between the PDGF and G$_q$ pathways was observable only in a cell state-dependent manner. In pre-confluent cells, which are rapidly proliferating, PDGF greatly stimulates mitogenesis and activates both ERK1 and ERK2 isoforms of MAP-kinase. In confluent cultures that are contact-inhibited, PDGF stimulated mitogenesis poorly and only activates the ERK2 isoform. Upon expression of the mutant activated G$\alpha_q$ PDGF stimulates both the ERK1 and ERK2 activities and is able to stimulate mitogenesis again (22). Thus it appears that activation of the G$_q$ pathway selectively allows for ERK1 activation and restoration of the mitogenic potential PDGF. The molecular events by which G$_q$ facilitates PDGF activation of ERK2 is not yet known. The interactions between the G$_q$ and PDGF pathways are summarized in the schematic shown below.

## FIGURE 2

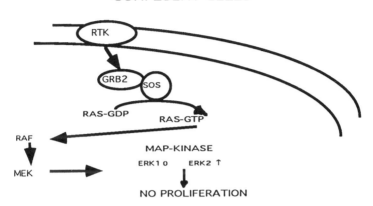

CONFLUENT CELLS

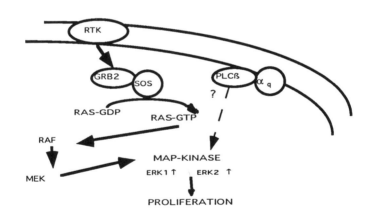

Our studies as well as those from other laboratories show that G protein pathways play an important role in regulating the events responsible for unregulated proliferation and transformation. However, although activation of G protein pathways by itself causes transformation in model systems such as NIH-3T3 cells, it is becoming increasingly clear that activation of G protein pathways is insufficient to induce transformation in most other cell types. Rather, it appears that cooperation between G protein and other signaling pathways may be crucial in triggering of the processes that result in transformation. The $G_q$/phospholipase C pathway appears to be in involved in triggering the transformation of NIH-3T3 cells. Both receptors that couple to $G\alpha_q$ and the mutant activated $G\alpha_q$ are capable of transforming NIH-3T3 cells in the presence of serum. This effect is in consonance with the long established role of protein kinase C as a target for tumor promoters. Protein kinase C is also activated by diacylglycerol, a second messenger produced by phospholipase C. Thus this pathway clearly plays an important role in oncogenesis. Recent studies also indicate that the point of convergence between the Gq/phospholipase C/protein kinase C and the growth factor/receptor tyrosine kinase pathway is at the level of MAP-kinases. Our data suggest that selective activation of the ERK1 isoform may be important. Irrespective of the details of which isoform of MAP-kinase is activated it appears fairly certain that activation of MAP-kinase is a necessary step for transformation of NIH-3T3 cells (23). The identification of a common locus at which extracellular signals can be integrated to regulate proliferation is likely to be very useful in identifying novel therapeutic strategies by which unregulated proliferation and transformation may be inhibited.

## Acknowledgments

Research in our laboratory is supported by NIH grants CA44998 and DK-38761 and a grant from the American Cancer Society. MDV is an Aaron Diamond Fellow.

### References
1 Bishop, J. M. (1991) Molecular Themes in Oncogenesis *Cell* **64**: 235-248

2 Hunter, T (1991) Co-operation between Oncogenes *Cell* **64**: 249-271

3 Iyengar, R. and Birnbaumer L.. (1987) Signal transduction by G-proteins, *ISI Atlas of Science:* **1**: 213-221.

4 Clapham D. E. and Neer E. J. (1993) New Roles for G protein βγ-dimers in transmembrane signaling *Nature* **365**: 403-406

5 Schlessinger, J. (1993) How receptor tyrosine kinases activate ras *Trends in Biochem Sci* **18**: 273-275

6 Hall, A. (1994) a biochemical function for Ras-At Last *Science* **264:** 1413-1414

7 Avruch, J., Zhang, X-f and Kyriakas, J. M. (1994) Raf meets Ras: Completing the framework of a signal transducing pathway *Trends in Biochem Sci* **19**: 279-284

8 Davis, R. J. (1993) The Mitogen Activated Protein kinase Signal Transduction Pathway *J. Biol Chem* **268**: 14553-14456

9  Bourne, H. R., Sanders, D. A. , McCormick, F. (1991) The GTPase superfamily : conserved structure and molecular mechanism  *Nature* **349**: 117-127

10  Chen, J., and Iyengar, R. (1994) Suppression of Ras-Induced Transformation of NIH-3T3 Cells by activated G$\alpha_S$. *Science*  **263**: 1278-1281

11  Burgering, B. M. Th, Pronl, G. J., van Weeren P. C et al ( 1993) cAMP antoagonizes p21$^{ras}$ -directed activation of extracellular signal -regulated kinase 2 and phosphorylation of mSos nucleotide exchange factor. *EMBO J* **12** : 4211-4220

12  Wu, J. , Dent, P, Jelink, T. et al (1993) Inhibition of the EGF-Activated MAP-kinase Signaling Pathway by Adenosine 3'5' monophosphate  *Science* **262**: 1065-1068

13  Cook, S. J. and McCormick, F. (1993) Inhibition by cAMP of Ras Dependent Activation of Raf *Science* **262**: 1069-1072

14  Graves, L. M., Bornfeldt, K. A., Raines, E. et al (1993) Protein kinase A antagonozes platelet-derived growth factor induced signaling by mitogen activated protein kinase in smooth muscle cells *Proc. Natl. Acad. Sci. USA* **90**: 10300- 10304

15  Sevetson, B, King, X, and Lawrence, J. C. (1993) Increasing cAMP attenuates activation of the mitogen activated protein kinase *Proc. Natl. Acad. Sci. USA* **90**: 10305- 10309

16  Grundel, R., and Rubun, H. (1991) Effect of interclonal heterogeneity on the Progressive, Confluence-mediated Acquisition of the Focus forming

phenotype in NIH-3T3 populations    *Cancer Res* **51**: 1003-1013

17   Cho-Chung Y. S. (1990) role of cAMP receptor proteins in growth, differentiation and Suppression of Malignancy: New Approaches to Therapy *Cancer Res* **50** : 7093-7100

18   Julius, D., Livelli, T. J., Jessell T. M. and Axel R. (1989) Ectopic Expression of the Triggering of Malignant Transformation *Science* **244**: 1057-1062

19  Gutkind, J. S., Novotny, E. A., Brann, M. R., and Robbins, K. C. (1991) Muscarinic acetyl choline receptor subtypes as agonist -dependent oncogenes *Proc. Natl. Acad. Sci USA* **88**: 4703-4707

20  De Vivo, M. , Chen, J., Codina , J. and Iyengar, R. (1992) Enhanced Stimulation of Phospholipase C Activity and Cell Transformation in NIH-3T3 Cells Expressing  Active Q209L G$_q$-$\alpha$ subunits  *J. Biol Chem* **267:** 18263-18266

21   Kaleinec,  G., Nazarali, A. J., Hermouet, S. , Xul N., Gutkind, J. S. (1992) Mutated $\alpha$-Subunit of the G$_q$ protein Induces Malignant Transformation of NIH-3T3 Cells *Mol Cell Biol* **12**: 4687-4693

22  De Vivo, M., and Iyengar R.(1994) Activated Gq-$\alpha$ potentiates PDGF-stimulated Mitogenesis in Confluent Cell Cultures  *J. Biol Chem* **269**: 1971-196674

23   Cowley, S. , Paterson, H., Kemp, P., and Marshall, C. J. (1994) Activation of MAP-kinase kinase is necessary and sufficient for PC12 differentiation

and for transformation of NIH-3T3 cells    *Cell* **77**: 841-852

# PART II

# Cancer Prevention Studies: Lab Studies

# VITAMIN E SUCCINATE INHIBITS PROTEIN KINASE C: CORRELATION WITH ITS UNIQUE INHIBITORY EFFECTS ON CELL GROWTH AND TRANSFORMATION

R. Gopalakrishna, U. Gundimeda, and Z. Chen

Department of Cell and Neurobiology,
School of Medicine, University of Southern California,
Los Angeles, CA 90033 USA

## ABSTRACT

Both succinate and phosphate esters of vitamin E (d-$\alpha$-tocopherol) at low (1-25 $\mu$M) concentrations either inactivated or activated protein kinase C (PKC) depending on the conditions. These esters, in the absence of cofactors (ATP, $Mg^{2+}$, and substrate protein), irreversibly inactivated PKC, while in their presence reversibly activated the enzyme. Nonetheless, at physiological ionic-strength the inhibition (inactivation) was favored even in the presence of protective cofactors. Furthermore, at this condition, vitamin E succinate completely abolished the diolein-sensitized arachidonic acid-mediated activation of PKC. Contrary, vitamin E, its charge-free esters acetate and nicotinate, and the water soluble analogue Trolox all failed to affect PKC activity even at a high (250 $\mu$M) concentration. In intact cells treated with vitamin E succinate, there was an initial inhibition of PKC activity as judged by *in vitro* protein phosphorylation, followed by an irreversible inactivation of the enzyme with a prolonged treatment. Among the various analogues of vitamin E tested, only vitamin E succinate inhibited growth and transformation of various cell types in culture. Vitamin E phosphate, although was very effective in inhibiting PKC activity in a test tube, did not inhibit cell growth and transformation probably due to its cell impermeability. Since orally administered vitamin E succinate is hydrolyzed, a topical administration could allow chemopreventive actions of this charged ester at sites such as oral cavity and skin. Taken together these results suggest that unhydrolyzed vitamin E succinate, having a negative charge, membrane permeability, and stability in intracellular compartments, inhibits cell growth and transformation, at least in part due to the inhibition of PKC.


## INTRODUCTION

The growth of a variety of cell types is inhibited by $d$-$\alpha$-tocopheryl acid succinate (vitamin E succinate) *in vitro* (1-3). This agent also induces differentiation in melanoma and neuroblastoma cell types (4). Either $d$-$\alpha$-tocopherol (vitamin E) or its analogues such as acetate and nicotinate esters, as well as the water soluble analogue Trolox, have very little effect on cell growth and differentiation *in vitro* (1-4). Therefore, vitamin E succinate may be a unique agent among the vitamin E analogues to influence growth and differentiation (1-4). Furthermore, vitamin E succinate was also shown to decrease cell transformation induced by radiation and chemicals in cell culture (5,6). This ester form of vitamin E was also shown to protect cells from toxicity induced by high oxygen tension and carcinogenic transition metals such as chromium, nickel, and cadmium (7-10). The mechanism of action of vitamin E succinate to inhibit growth and transformation or to induce differentiation and cytoprotection is not known.

Protein kinase C (PKC) may play a crucial role in growth regulation and in tumor promotion (11). PKC, besides being activated by transmembrane signals such as $Ca^{2+}$, diacylglycerol and arachidonic acid, is also activated by phorbol ester tumor promoters (11). Oxidant tumor promoters such as hydrogen peroxide and $m$-periodate also activate PKC under the conditions where a selective oxidative modification of the regulatory domain is achieved (12-13). Furthermore, another class of structurally unrelated tumor promoters, okadaic acid and calyculin-A, may also induce the translocation (activation) of PKC indirectly through the generation of second messengers (14). Since PKC may play an important role in growth and transformation of cells, the agents that inhibit this enzyme activity may affect these cellular processes. Consistent with this speculation, diverse agents that inhibit PKC, such as sphingosine, H-7, tamoxifen, staurosporine, and calphostin C all have been shown to inhibit cell growth (15-17). Moreover, agents such as sphingosine have been shown to decrease tumor promotion (18). Since vitamin E succinate inhibits both cell growth and transformation, we have determined whether this agent could affect PKC activity. In this study we show that both kinase activity and phorbol ester binding associated with PKC are inhibited by vitamin E succinate at the physiological ionic strength which correlated well with the unique growth inhibitory effects elicited by this vitamin E ester.

## MATERIALS AND METHODS

Materials: Vitamin E (*d*-α-tocopherol) and its succinate ester were obtained from Eastman Kodak. Acetate, nicotinate, and phosphate esters of vitamin E were purchased from the Sigma Chemical Company. Trolox was obtained from Aldrich. PKC from rabbit brain was purified to apparent homogeneity by using $Ca^{2+}$-dependent hydrophobic chromatography as described previously (12). Vitamin E analogues were initially dissolved in ethanol at a concentration of 100 mM and then diluted in 10% ethanol. Vitamin E phosphate was dissolved in 10% alcohol by sonication for 30 sec. The final concentration of alcohol in PKC assay and in cell culture was 0.5% which had no affect on PKC activity or cell growth. However, appropriate controls with the same amount of alcohol with or without sodium succinate or sodium phosphate were setup.

Treatment of PKC with various vitamin E analogues. The effect of various vitamin E analogues on purified PKC activity was determined in 96-well plates with fitted filtration discs made of a Durapore membrane (19). The order of addition of various components in the reaction mixture was very important to observe inhibition or activation of PKC induced by vitamin E succinate. The following order of addition lead to PKC inhibition. To 25 µl of diluted PKC preparation, where necessary, NaCl was added followed by the indicated concentrations of various analogues of vitamin E, and then the sonicated lipid mixture containing phosphatidylserine (20 µg/ml) and diolein (0.8 µg/ml) was added. After prewarming the PKC samples and the reaction mixture separately at 30°C for 3 min, the reaction was initiated by adding the reaction mixture to PKC samples containing both vitamin E and lipids. The $^{32}P$ incorporated into histone H1 was then determined by multiwell filtration assay (19). To observe the activation of PKC, to vitamin E

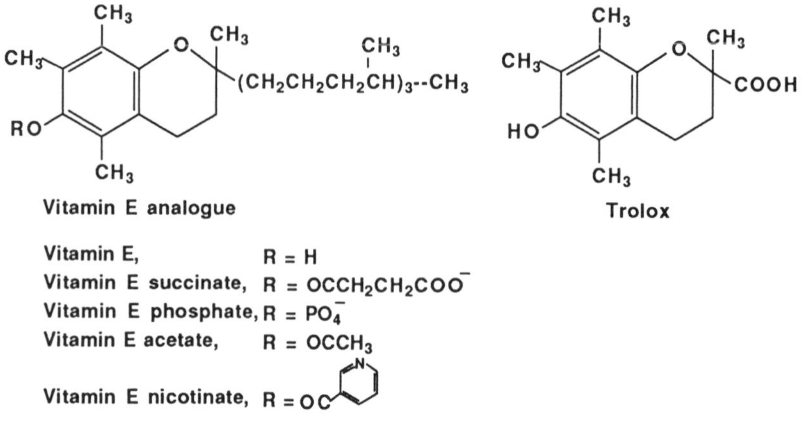

Fig. 1. Structures of various vitamin E analogues evaluated for the inhibition of PKC activity and cell growth.

succinate samples, the reaction mixture was added; then the reaction was initiated by the addition of PKC preparation. PKC activity was expressed as units, where one unit of enzyme transfers 1 nmol of phosphate to histone H1 per min at 30°C.

Phorbol ester binding was carried out using [³H]phorbol 12, 13-dibutyrate (PDBu) as the ligand. To PKC samples (25 µl) with various amounts of NaCl, indicated concentrations of vitamin E analogues were added followed by phosphatidylserine (20 µg/ml), and then the PDBu binding mixture was added. Then the samples were incubated and the amount of PKC associated PDBu binding was determined by multiwell filtration assay as described previously (19). This order of addition of various components for PDBu binding determination was maintained throughout these experiments.

## RESULTS

Vitamin E succinate can either inactivate or activate PKC depending on the order of addition of various components during incubation. Since the physiological ionic strength favors inhibition or inactivation of PKC by vitamin E succinate, the inactivation mechanism was discussed first.

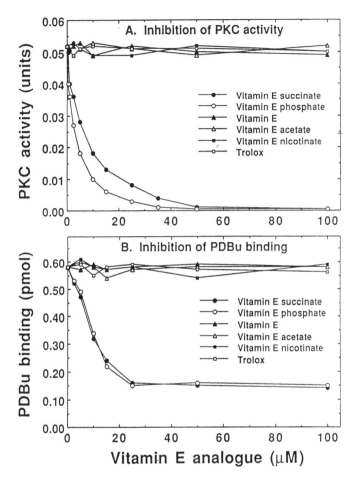

Fig. 2. Effect of various analogues of vitamin E on A) PKC activity and B) phorbol ester binding. The indicated concentrations of various analogues of vitamin E were added to PKC samples first and then the histone phosphotransferase activity was determined by using the multiwell filtration assay as described in the Materials and Methods.

Various analogues of vitamin E, as shown in Fig. 1, were tested for their ability to inhibit kinase activity and PDBu binding of purified PKC from rabbit brain. Vitamin E (alcohol), its acetate or nicotinate esters, and Trolox all did not inhibit PKC activity to any appreciable extent (Fig. 2A). However, vitamin E succinate inhibited PKC activity with an $IC_{50}$ value of 7.5 µM. Vitamin E phosphate, another charged ester which was not previously tested for growth inhibitory activity, also inhibited PKC activity with 2.5-fold higher affinity. Since vitamin E succinate can bind $Ca^{2+}$, to determine whether the inhibition of PKC was due to the chelation of $Ca^{2+}$ present in the reaction mixture, the concentration of $Ca^{2+}$ in the incubation mixture was increased by 10-fold. Nevertheless, a higher concentration of $Ca^{2+}$ did not overcome the vitamin E succinate inhibition. Sodium succinate at this range of concentration did not inhibit PKC. The other analogues, vitamin E (alcohol form) and vitamin E acetate which have no PKC inhibitory activity when tested at high (100 to 250 µM) concentration, did not block the inhibitory effect of succinate or phosphate esters (10 µM) on PKC activity. The lack of inhibition by other charge-free esters such as vitamin E acetate and vitamin E nicotinate suggests that the negative charge associated with succinate or phosphate esters may facilitate high affinity interaction of these vitamin E derivatives with PKC. Furthermore, calpain-derived PKC (M-kinase) possessing only the catalytic domain was also inhibited by vitamin E succinate with an $IC_{50}$ value of 32 µM, a 4-fold lower affinity than that for proenzyme PKC.

The PDBu binding associated with PKC was also inhibited by both vitamin E succinate and phosphate esters, although to a lower extent (Fig. 2B). Unlike the differential rate of inhibition of PKC phosphotransferase activity by succinate and phosphate esters, both these esters were equally effective in inhibiting PDBu binding ($IC_{50}$ value of 12 µM). Other analogues of vitamin E did not show any inhibitory effect on PDBu binding. Conceivably, vitamin E succinate may bind to both catalytic and regulatory domains to influence kinase activity and phorbol ester binding, respectively.

It was also taken into consideration whether vitamin E succinate was behaving as an anionic detergent in this system inducing the inactivation of PKC. Initially an anionic detergent such as sodium dodecylsulfate (SDS) was tested for its effects on PKC activity at concentrations that were comparable to that of vitamin E succinate. Sodium dodecylsulfate had no affect on either PKC activity or PDBu binding up to a 60 µM concentration (data not shown). Nonetheless, it inhibited both kinase activity and PDBu binding at higher concentration (100 µM) which was far below its critical micellar concentration. Therefore, this inhibition was unlikely due to the denaturation of the enzyme. The inhibition of PKC by SDS may be due to phospholipid lamellar-micelle transition and SDS/phosphatidylserine mixed micells are not effective in activation of PKC (20). The SDS-induced inhibition of PKC at a 100 µM concentration was overcome by increasing the phosphatidylserine concentration by two-fold (40 µg/ml). However, the inhibition induced by vitamin E succinate was not overcome by increasing the phosphatidylserine concentration. Conceivably, the inhibition of PKC by low concentrations (1 to 25 µM) of vitamin E succinate is neither due to detergent-like surface effects on the enzyme or due to the phospholipid lamellar-micelle transition.

The possible involvement of $Ca^{2+}$-induced hydrophobic site(s) on PKC in mediating vitamin E succinate-induced inhibition: Similar to other $Ca^{2+}$-binding proteins such as calmodulin, troponin C and S-100 protein, PKC exhibits $Ca^{2+}$-induced hydrophobic sites (21). The functional significance of these $Ca^{2+}$-influenced hydrophobic sites in PKC is not known. Recently we have shown that calphostin C, a specific inhibitor for PKC, binds to these sites to induce site-specific oxidations (22). Therefore, we assessed whether $Ca^{2+}$-induced accessible hydrophobic regions on the PKC surface was involved in mediating the vitamin E succinate-induced inhibition of the enzyme. From a frozen and stored (-20°C for 3 months) preparation of PKC, by using $Ca^{2+}$-dependent hydrophobic chromatography two fractions were separated; one fraction retained the property of exhibiting $Ca^{2+}$-induced hydrophobic binding to phenyl-Sepharose while the other fraction lost this property during storage. Vitamin E succinate inhibited with a three-fold higher affinity ($IC_{50}$ 8 µM) the PKC fraction that $Ca^{2+}$-dependently bound to hydrophobic resin than the PKC fraction that did not exhibit this type of binding. It is possible that vitamin E succinate may bind to these $Ca^{2+}$-induced hydrophobic regions. The negatively charged succinate moiety may interact with the a positively charged residue to complement the hydrophobic interaction between the vitamin E and a hydrophobic site on PKC creating a high affinity stereospecific binding of vitamin E succinate with PKC.

Effect of ionic strength on the inhibition of PKC by vitamin E succinate: The purified preparation of PKC that was used in the above study contained 0.1 M NaCl as it was eluted from the phenyl-

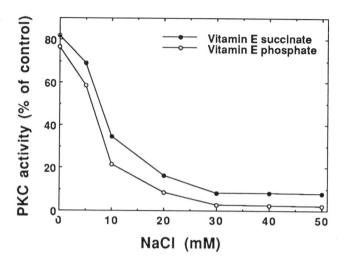

Fig. 3. Effect of ionic strength on vitamin E succinate and phosphate ester mediated inhibition of PKC activity. The indicated final concentrations of NaCl in the reaction were maintained by adding 1 M NaCl to PKC samples. Then vitamin E analogues were added to PKC samples followed by the reaction mixture.

Sepharose hydrophobic chromatography. However, the PKC preparation desalted to remove NaCl was to a less extent inhibited by vitamin E succinate. This prompted us to study the effect of ionic strength on the vitamin E succinate inhibition of PKC. As shown in Fig. 2A, PKC was inhibited only 20% by vitamin E succinate (25 μM) when there was no NaCl in the PKC preparation (Fig. 3). However, by increasing the NaCl in the PKC preparation the extent of PKC inhibition by vitamin E succinate increased. The maximal inhibition was reached at an NaCl final concentration of 30 mM in the reaction mixture. A similar effect of ionic strength in influencing the inhibition of PKC by phosphate ester was observed.

Irreversible nature of inactivation of PKC by vitamin E succinate: Purified preparation of PKC was incubated with vitamin E succinate (20 μM) and then attempts were made to recover PKC activity by removing the excess vitamin E succinate. PKC activity did not recover by subjecting the vitamin E succinate-treated enzyme to extensive dialysis, to hydrophobic chromatography, or to DEAE-

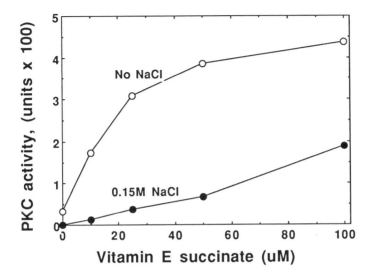

Fig. 4. Vitamin E succinate-induced activation of PKC in a low-ionic-strength buffer. The indicated concentrations of vitamin E succinate were added to reaction mixture and then the reaction was initiated by adding PKC. The assays were done in the presence and absence of 0.15 M NaCl.

cellulose chromatography. Conceivably, the observed decrease in PKC activity was due to the irreversible modification of PKC induced by vitamin E succinate. Similarly, the vitamin E phosphate also induced an irreversible inactivation of the enzyme.

Activation of PKC by vitamin E succinate under nonphysiological conditions: Although an inactivation of PKC occurred when it was incubated with vitamin E succinate in the absence of cofactors, an activation of PKC was observed when the enzyme was added at the end to the reaction mixture containing vitamin E succinate (Fig. 4). Detailed studies revealed that PKC was protected by ATP/Mg$^{2+}$ and substrate protein histone H1 present in the reaction mixture. When the enzyme was protected, vitamin E succinate induced an activation of PKC instead of inhibition. However, this activation occurred only in low-ionic strength buffers with no NaCl. When ionic strength was increased to a physiological level by including 0.15 M NaCl in the

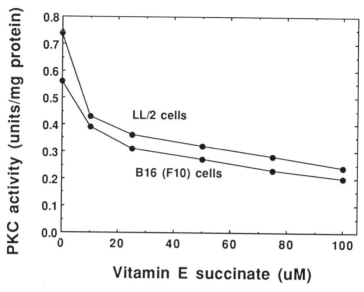

Fig. 5. An irreversible inactivation of PKC in tumor cells treated with vitamin E succinate. Rapidly growing subconfluent LL/2 lung carcinoma and B16 (F10) melanoma cells were treated with vitamin E succinate (25 uM) for 15 h and then total PKC was isolated form the detergent-treated cell extracts by DEAE-cellulose chromatography and the activity was determined.

reaction, there was no appreciable activation of PKC (Fig. 4). Furthermore, under these conditions vitamin E succinate blocked the diolein-sensitized arachidonic acid stimulation of PKC. Thus at the physiological ionic strength the inactivation of PKC by vitamin E succinate is favored, but not the activation.

Effects of vitamin E succinate on PKC in intact cancer cells: Since vitamin E succinate induces either inhibition or activation of PKC in test tube, we determined whether it behaves as an inhibitor or activator of PKC in intact cells. In intact LL/2 lung carcinoma and B16 melanoma cells treated with vitamin E succinate (25 $\mu$M) there was an inactivation of PKC (Fig. 5). However, there was a lag period of 4 to 12 hours depending on the conditions. PKC inactivation was more pronounced in rapidly growing subconfluent cells than confluent cells. To determine the reversible inhibition of PKC activity, the phosphorylation of heat stable 80k protein, a PKC-specific endogenous substrate was measured. Vitamin E succinate (25 μM) treatment resulted in decrease in TPA-stimulated phosphorylation of 80k protein in a short (1 h) period of time prior to the onset of irreversible inactivation of PKC. Due to the presence of ATP, $Mg^{2+}$ and endogenous substrates in the cell, PKC was protected from vitamin E succinate-induced irreversible inactivation. Nonetheless, the physiological ionic strength favored a reversible inhibition of the enzyme. This was followed by a slow irreversible inactivation of the kinase at a later stage. Conceivably, vitamin E succinate is a true antagonist of PKC-mediated cellular events.

Effect of various analogues of vitamin E on the growth of lung carcinoma cells correlating with inhibition of PKC: Exponentially growing LL/2 lung carcinoma cells were used to assess growth inhibitory potential of various vitamin E analogues at a limited

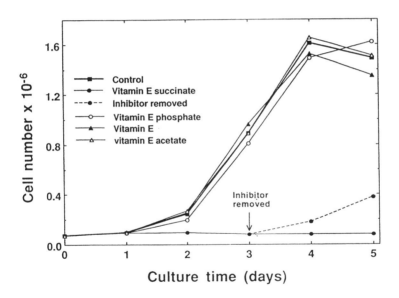

Fig. 6. Growth inhibition of LL/2 lung carcinoma cells by various analogues of vitamin E. LL/2 lung carcinoma cells (74,000) were seeded in 35-mm Petri dishes. The cells were treated with indicated analogues of vitamin E at a 25 μM concentration or solvent control (0.5% ethanol). In one set of cells treated with vitamin E succinate for 48 h, the medium was removed, the cells were washed, and they were then left in a fresh medium without any inhibitor.

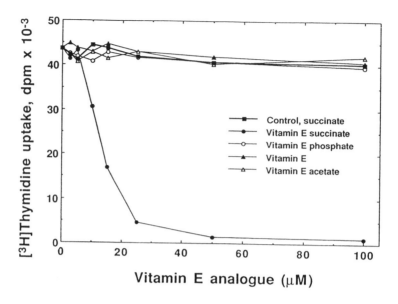

Fig. 7. Effect of various analogues of vitamin E on the [³H]thymidine uptake in lung carcinoma cells. The subconfluent LL/2 lung carcinoma cells were treated with indicated concentrations of vitamin E analogues for a 48-h period. Then the cells were further incubated with [³H]thymidine (0.5 μCi) for 2 h and the thymidine uptake by the cells was determined.

concentration (25 μM). As shown in Fig. 6, only vitamin E succinate significantly inhibited the growth of these cells. The sodium succinate (control), vitamin E or its acetate or nicotinate esters, Trolox all had no effect on the growth rate. Unexpectedly vitamin E phosphate did not show any significant growth inhibition inspite being a potent inhibitor of PKC in the test tube. The ineffective analogues of vitamin E did not prevent the growth inhibitory effect of vitamin E succinate. Furthermore, with pretreatment using these agents only vitamin E succinate decreased [³H]thymidine uptake at 10 to 25 μM concentrations where other analogues had no effect (Fig. 7). However, higher concentrations of vitamin E (250 μM) significantly (20 to 30%) decreased [³H]thymidine uptake (data not shown). The concentrations of vitamin E succinate required to inhibit PKC in the test tube agreed well with the concentrations required to inhibit LL/2 lung carcinoma cell growth. Thus, overall there was a correlation between the ability of vitamin E succinate to inhibit PKC activity and the unique growth inhibitory potential for this vitamin E ester.

## DISCUSSION

Although the unique *in vitro* effects of vitamin E succinate to inhibit growth and transformation or to induce differentiation and cytoprotection were known for several years, the mechanism of its action is not known. There are two views on the possible mechanism to explain growth inhibitory potential for this agent. One assumption is that vitamin E succinate serves as a precursor for vitamin E due to its stability in culture medium and also due to increased cellular uptake. Vitamin E released intracellularly by the hydrolysis of the ester elicits its effects in the cell (7). Such actions of vitamin E may include the well characterized antioxidant function or inhibition of enzymes such as phospholipase $A_2$ and lipoxygenase (23-25). Another view suggests that vitamin E succinate may induce unique effects as an intact molecule (12). This was supported by the fact that in some cell types the rate of hydrolysis of vitamin E succinate was low (3,9). Although the succinate ester was taken up somewhat more readily than free vitamin E, for any equal uptake of both forms of vitamin E, only the succinate derivative could affect growth (3). This difference was attributed to the functionality of the free carboxyl group of the succinate derivative (3,9). Recent studies, using nonhydrolyzable ether analogue of vitamin E succinate in having negative charge, further suggested that the intact molecule of vitamin E succinate may be involved in inducing growth inhibition (26). In another study a binding protein for vitamin E succinate was demonstrated which may play a role in nuclear transcription of growth inhibiting factor similar to transforming growth factor-$\beta$ (2).

Previous studies have shown a synergistic interaction between vitamin E succinate and anticancer drugs such as adriamycin (26,27). PKC activity is high in multidrug resistant cells (28,29) as well as it is known to phosphorylate and regulate membrane P-glycoprotein and thereby increase drug efflux from the cell (30). Therefore, the inhibition and/or inactivation of PKC induced by vitamin E succinate may facilitate increased retention of anticancer drugs in the cell and their therapeutic action. Furthermore, vitamin E succinate unlike parent vitamin E has no significant direct antioxidant action. Therefore, it is unlikely that vitamin E succinate can counteract and prevent any oxidation events that are involved in the anticancer drug action.

In our study we have not seen any appreciable inhibition of PKC by vitamin E or its charge-free analogues up to 250 μM. In another study the inhibition of PKC at supraphysiological amounts ($IC_{50}$ value of 450 μM) was reported (31). Vitamin E succinate was shown to increase the activity of cAMP-dependent protein kinase in B16 melanoma cells (4). In our study the concentration of vitamin E succinate needed to inhibit PKC correlated well with the concentration required to inhibit lung carcinoma cell growth. The negative charge on the vitamin E ester may be required to inhibit both PKC and cell growth. Nevertheless, the negatively charged ester vitamin E phosphate, although it inhibits PKC activity in the test tube, has no growth inhibiting potential. It is possible that the phosphate ester might have rapidly hydrolyzed by various phosphatases present in the cell and thereby it might not have reached PKC or other intracellular targets. This further suggests that increased release of vitamin E inside the cell alone can not induce growth inhibitory affects, but intact charged ester is also required. Although unhydrolyzed vitamin E succinate may have some unique affects on the cell, the hydrolytic product vitamin E, by acting as an antioxidant as well as by other mechanisms, can complement the direct affects induced by the intact ester. Therefore, vitamin E succinate, by having a negative charge and stability in intracellular compartments, induces growth inhibition which may at least in part be due to its inhibition of PKC activity.

Inhibition of carcinogenesis by vitamin E in various experimental models was well documented (32). Nevertheless, there is no consistent relationship between the dietary consumption of vitamin E and the prevention of cancer risk in humans (33). However, many studies have shown that vitamin E succinate is unique and inhibits growth and tumor promotion *in vitro*. Identifying the cellular targets for intact vitamin E succinate is important to elucidate the mechanism of unique chemopreventive effects of these types of agents. Since cell growth is an important process that influences carcinogenesis (34,35), vitamin E succinate has the potential to inhibit carcinogenesis. However, when this ester of vitamin E is orally administered it is hydrolyzed in the intestine and may not reach the target tissues to induce its affects. Nevertheless, when vitamin E succinate is delivered to target tissues without hydrolysis, it may elicit chemopreventive effects. This may be easily achieved in the organs such as skin, oral cavity and eyes where topical administration is possible. Furthermore, both the hydrolysis products of vitamin E succinate, vitamin E and succinate, are nontoxic to the cell. Conceivably, structural modification of the dietary components will lead to the development of new pharmacological agents having greater chemopreventive potential while maintaining low toxicity.

*Acknowledgments*: We thank Mr. Vardkes Karanfilian for his excellent technical assistance. This work was supported in part by a research grant 93B43 from American Institute for Cancer Research, USPHS grant CA62146 from the National Cancer Institute, and by grant RT388 from Tobacco-Related Diseases Research Program, University of California.

## REFERENCES

1. Prasad, K. N., and Edwards-Prasad, J. (1982) Cancer Res. 42, 550-555.
2. Kline, K., and Sanders, B. G. (1990) in Vitamins and Minerals in the Prevention of and Treatment of Cancer (Jacobs M. M. ed.) pp. 189-205. CRC Press, Boca Raton, FL.
3. Slack, R., and Proulx, P. (1989) Nutr. Cancer 12, 75-82.
4. Torelli, S., Masoudi, F., and Prasad, K. N. (1988) Cancer Lett. 39, 129-136.
5. Borek, C., Ong, A., Mason, H., Donahue, L., and Biaglow, J. E. (1986) Proc. Natl. Acad. Sci. USA. 83,1490-1494.
6. Radner, B.S., and Kennedy, A. N. (1986) Cancer Lett. 32, 25-32.
7. Pascoe, G. A., Olafsdottir, K., and Reed, D. J. (1987) Arch. Biochem. Biophys. 256, 150-158.
8. Sugiyama, M., Ando, A., and Ogura, R. (1989) Carcinogenesis 10, 737-741.
9. Fariss, M. W. (1991) Free Rad. Biol. Med. 9, 333-343.
10. Lin, X., Sugiyama, M., and Costa, M. (1991) Mut. Res. 260, 159-164.
11. Nishizuka, Y. (1992) Science 258, 607-613.

12. Gopalakrishna, R., and Anderson, W. B. (1989) Proc. Natl. Acad. Sci. USA. 86, 6758-6762.
13. Gopalakrishna, R., and Anderson, W. B. (1991) Arch. Biochem. Biophys. 285, 382-387.
14. Gopalakrishna, R., Chen, Z. H., and Gundimeda, U. (1992) Biochem. Biophys. Res. Commun. 189, 950-957.
15. Kobayashi, E., Nakano, H., Morimoto, M., and Tamaoki, T. (1989) Biochem. Biophys. Res. Commun. 159, 548-553.
16. O'Brian, C. A., Liskamp, R. M., Solomon, D. H., and Weinstein, I. B. (1985) Cancer Res. 45, 2462-2468.
17. Minana, M. D., Felipo, V., Cortes, F., and Grisolia, S. (1991) FEBS Lett. 284, 60-62.
18. Borek, C., Ong, A., Stevens, V. L., Wang, E., and Merril, A. H., Jr. (1991) Proc. Natl. Acad. Sci. USA. 88, 1953-1957.
19. Gopalakrishna, R.,Chen, Z. H., Gundimeda, U., Wilson, J. C., and Anderson, W. B. (1992) Anal. Biochem. 206, 24-35.
20. Murakami, K., Chan, S. Y., and Routtenberg, A. (1986) J. Biol. Chem. 261, 15424-15429.
21. Anderson, W. B., and Gopalakrishna, R. (1985) in Modulation by covalent modification (Shaltiel, S., and Chock, P. B. eds) Curr. Topics Cell. Reg. vol. 27, 455-469 Academic Press, Orlando.
22. Gopalakrishna, R., Chen, Z. H., and Gundimeda, U. (1992) FEBS Lett. 314, 149-154.
23. Burton, G. W., and Ingold, K. U. (1986) Acc. Chem. Res. 19, 194-201.
24. Pentland, A. P., Morrison, A. R., Jacobs, S. C., Hruza, L. L., Herbert, J. S., and Packer, L. (1992) J. Biol. Chem. 267, 15578-15584.
25. Reddanna, P., Rao, M. K., and and Reddy, C. C. (1985) FEBS Lett. 193, 39-43.
26. Fariss, M. W., Fortuna, M. B., Everett, C. K., Smith, J. D., Trent, D. F., and Djuric, Z. (1994) Cancer Res. 54, 3346-3351.
27. Ripoll, E. A. P., Rama, B. N., and Webber, M. M. (1986) J. Urol. 136, 529-531.
28. Fine, R. L., Patel, J., and Chabner, B. A. (1988) Proc. Natl. Acad. Sci. USA 85, 582-586.
29. Posada, J., Vichi, P., and Tritton, T. R. (1989) Cancer Res. 49, 6634-6639.
30. Chambers, T. C., McAvoy, E. M., Jacobs, J. W., and Elion, G. (1990) J. Biol. Chem. 265, 7679-7686.
31. Mahoney, C. W., and Azzi, A. (1988) Biochem. Biophys. Res. Commun. 154, 694-697.

32. Mergens, W. J., and Bhagavan, H. N. (1989) in Nutrition and Cancer Prevention (Eds. Moon, T. E., Micozzi, M. S.) pp 305-340, Marcell Dekker, New York.
33. Dorgan, J. F., and Schatzkin, A. (1991) Nutr. Cancer 5, 43-68.
34. Preston-Martin, S., Pike, M. C., Ross, R. K., Jones, P. A., and Henderson, B. E. (1990) Cancer Res. 50, 7415- 7421.
35. Kaufmann, W. K., Rice, J. M., MacKenzie, S. A., Smith, G. J., Wenk, M. L., Devor, D., Qaquish, B. F., and Kaufman, D. G. (1991) Carcinogenesis 12, 1587-1593.

# VITAMIN E SUCCINATE: MECHANISMS OF ACTION AS TUMOR CELL GROWTH INHIBITOR[1]

Kimberly Kline[2], Weiping Yu, Bihong Zhao, Karen Israel, April

Charpentier, Marla Simmons-Menchaca and Bob G. Sanders[3]

Division of Nutrition[2] and Department of Zoology[3],

The University of Texas at Austin, Austin, TX 78712

## INTRODUCTION

Vitamin E succinate (VES; RRR-α-tocopheryl succinate; formerly designated d-α-tocopherol acid succinate and d-α-tocopheryl hemisuccinate), a derivative of natural vitamin E, inhibits the proliferation of a number of different types of cells in culture (1, reviewed by 2 ). The antiproliferative properties of VES appear to be unique to this particular tocopherol compound since RRR-α-tocopherol (natural vitamin E, formerly designated d-α-tocopherol), RRR-α-tocopherol acetate (the acetate derivative of natural vitamin E), and all-rac-α-tocopherol (formerly designated dl-α-tocopherol, a synthetic compound that is a mixture of eight different stereoisomers, only one of which is RRR-α-tocopherol) do not exhibit antiproliferative properties in most cell culture systems (1, 2, 3, 4).

VES contains a succinic acid moiety attached to the chroman head structure of RRR-α-tocopherol by an ester linkage (FIGURE 1). This modification eliminates the hydroxyl moiety that

[1]This work was supported by grant number CA59739 from the National Cancer Institute, Bethesda, MD and by The Foundation for Research, Carson City, NV. Its contents are solely the responsibility of the authors and do not necessarily represent the official view of the National Cancer Institute.

RRR-α-tocopherol

| Common names: | d-α-tocopherol, Natural Vitamin E |
|---|---|
| Trivial name: | RRR-α-tocopherol |
| IUPAC name: | 2R,4'R, 8'R-α-tocopherol |
| Chemical name: | 2,5,7,8-tetramethyl-2-(4',8',12'-trimethyltridecyl)-6-chromanol |
| Molecular weight: | 430.69 |
| Empirical formula: | $C_{29}H_{50}O_2$ |

RRR-α-tocopheryl succinate

| Common names: | d-α-tocopheryl succinate, Vitamin E Succinate |
|---|---|
| Trivial name: | RRR-α-tocopheryl succinate |
| Chemical name: | 2,5,7,8-tetramethyl-2-(4',8',12'-trimethyltridecyl)-6-chromanol succinate |
| Molecular weight: | 530.8 |
| Empirical formula: | $C_{33}H_{54}O_5$ |

FIGURE 1. Comparison of RRR-α-tocopherol (natural vitamin E) and RRR-α-tocopheryl succinate (VES). This general information is a compilation of information (5, 6, 7).

mediates RRR-α-tocopherol's classical antioxidant properties. Thus, the intact VES compound does not function as an antioxidant. Only in situations where the esterification is reversed and RRR-α-tocopherol is generated will there be lipid soluble antioxidant activity. Since many cell types have active esterases that can convert VES into RRR-α-tocopherol and succinic acid, it has been unclear whether or not it is the intact VES compound which is the biologically active agent. Recent work by Marc Fariss and co-workers directly establishes the antiproliferative effects of the intact VES compound (4). They prepared vitamin E succinate with a nonhydrolyzable ether linkage and showed it to selectively inhibit leukemia cell proliferation in a manner identical to VES (4).

The mechanisms of action involved in VES-mediated inhibition of tumor cell growth are not known. Several distinct molecular events known to play key roles in the regulation of cell proliferation have been implicated; including alterations of adenylate cyclase and protein kinase C, two compounds known to play key roles in regulation of cell proliferation; and reduced expression of *c-myc* , a ubiquitously expressed nuclear protein that functions as a transcriptional factor controlling cell proliferation, differentiation and apoptosis (reviewed in ref 2). Thus, although VES may well be preventing tumor cell growth by a variety of mechanisms, this paper will focus on recent observations made by this lab documenting VES regulation of the important negative growth control factor, transforming growth factor-beta (TGF-β) as one mechanism whereby VES-induces tumor growth inhibition (1, 3). The ability of VES to induce biologically active TGF-β, places it among a select group of compounds (for example, vitamin D analogs, the antiestrogen: tamoxifen, the synthetic progestin: gestodene, and retinoids) which have been shown to be capable of modulating the endogenous production and activation of TGF-β.

Since the regulated growth of cells is dependent on a dynamic balance between stimulatory and inhibitory signals, escape from autocine or paracrine negative growth control mediated by TGF-β is believed to be a critical event in cancer development in a variety of different cell types, especially cancers of epithelial cell origin (8,9,10). Several possible mechanisms have been described whereby cells may lose responsiveness to the inhibitory effects of TGF-β: (i) cells can no longer produce adequate amounts of TGF-β; (ii) cells can no longer convert the biologically inactive latent TGF-β form which they synthesize and secrete to the biologically active form; (iii) cells no longer express functional cell surface receptor complexes necessary for TGF-β binding and signaling; or (iv) cells have some alteration in the signal transduction pathway for TGF-β mediated growth inhibition (8,10,11). The possibility that certain types of cancer cells cease to produce, activate, or respond to TGF-β and that VES can modulate this pathway of growth control is presently under investigation by our lab.

The TGF-βs are multifunctional polypeptide growth factors that affect a variety of functions in many different cell types (8,9). Five distinct isoforms (subtypes) of TGF-β have been identified, three of which have been shown to be expressed by mammalian tissues, namely TGF-β1, TGF-β2 and TGF-β3. The TGF-β molecules are first synthesized as precursor molecules that are processed to yield a latent molecule consisting of two amino-terminal glycopeptides covalently linked together and non-covalently associated with the mature 25,000 dalton TGF-β

## RESULTS AND DISCUSSION

### VES Causes a Dose-Dependent Inhibition of Proliferation and DNA Synthesis in Various Types of Tumor Cells

VES has been demonstrated to inhibit the proliferation of tumor cells of hematopoietic and epithelial origin, tumor cell types that account for more than 90% of all human malignancies (1,2,3). In our studies, VES has been shown to inhibit tumor cell proliferation in a dose response manner as measured by actual cell numbers or DNA synthesis. The growth inhibitory effects of VES at 5 and 10 µg/ml are evident within 24 hours; whereas, the growth inhibitory effects of VES at 1 µg/ml or lower concentrations require longer periods of time, usually 48-96 hours in order to obtain maximal inhibitory effects (1,3, 22,23).

VES is a hydrophobic molecule that requires solubilization in ethanol. Vehicle controls consisting of equivalent amounts of ethanol and sodium succinate do not induce growth inhibition, implying that growth inhibition is due to VES and not due to ethanol or pH differences. VES's growth inhibitory effects were judged to be cytostatic rather than directly cytotoxic by trypan blue dye exclusion analyses, a measure of cell viability, and the reversibility of VES-mediated growth inhibition since cells can recover proliferative capacity following VES removal (22,23).

It may be of interest to point out that physiologically relevant concentrations of plasma RRR-α-tocopherol (natural vitamin E) are in the 5-16 µg/ml range (24). However, since our studies involve cell cultures in the laboratory and we are using VES, a derivative of vitamin E, which has not been measured in human plasma, it is impossible to comment on the physiologically relevant concentrations of VES at this time.

The growth inhibitory properties of VES on human MCF-7 breast cancer cells are depicted in Figure 2. When the inhibitory effects of VES treatment on MCF-7 breast cancer cell proliferation are measured by tritiated thymidine uptake evidence of decreased DNA synthesis is observed after 1 day of treatment (FIGURE 2A); whereas, when inhibition of proliferation is determined by counting actual cell numbers, a decrease in cell numbers is not evident until after 2 days of treatment (FIGURE 2B).

molecule which consists of two identical 12,500 dalton disulfide-linked monomers (12). To be biologically active the 25,000 dalton TGF-β dimer must be dissociated from the amino-terminal glycopeptides (12). Factors demonstrated to activate TGF-β include pH, heat, and certain enzymes such as plasmin, cathepsin D and glycosidases (12,13).

The TGF-β isoforms elicit a wide spectrum of biological activities and can act as either positive or negative growth factors (reviewed by 8). In general, TGF-βs are stimulatory for cells of mesenchymal origin and inhibitory for cells of lymphoid or epithelial origin. The effects of TGF-β isoforms on a particular target cell are complex and depend on many parameters including the cell type and its stage of differentiation/maturation, state of activation of the cell, and on the presence or absence of other growth factors.

For target cells to be responsive to TGF-β they must have functional cell surface TGF-β receptors. Radiolabeled TGF-β has been shown to bind nine distinct cell membrane proteins (11). Recently, TGF-β receptor type I and type II, glycoproteins of approximate $M_r$ 53,000 and 75,000, respectively, have been shown to function as a heterodimer to signal the diverse effects mediated by TGF-β molecules (11,14,15). TGF-β type III receptors which exhibit high affinity TGF-β binding, do not appear to be associated with TGF-β mediated cell responses. However, the type III receptors may function to sequester biologically active TGF-β and help present it to the receptor type I-type II complex (11).

Less is known about events involved in TGF-β mediated signaling pathways leading to growth inhibition. One major event is suppression of phosphorylation of the retinoblastoma gene product, Rb (16). TGF-β acts to retain Rb in an underphosphorylated state in which Rb remains bound to the transcription factor E2F, preventing E2F from performing its critical role in enhancing the transcription of genes whose products are necessary for entry into the S phase of the cell cycle (17,18,19). More recent evidence indicates that TGF-β-induced cell cycle arrest in G1 are mediated via increased expression of p27 [Kip1], a cyclin-Cdk inhibitor which prevents cyclin-Cdk phosphorylation of Rb (20,21).

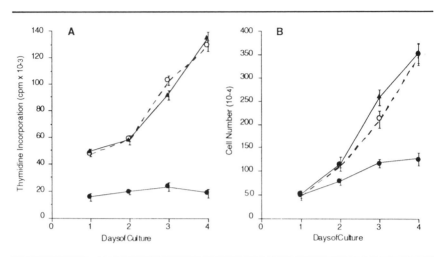

FIGURE 2 A & B.    Inhibition of DNA synthesis and cellular proliferation of human breast cancer cells by VES.  MCF-7 breast cancer cells were monitored for DNA synthesis by tritiated thymidine uptake (Figure 1A) and proliferation by total cell numbers using a hemacytometer (Figure 1B).  A total of 50,000 cells/12-well tissue culture plate was plated in multiple replicas. Freshly prepared media and media with treatments were provided at the beginning of the experiment and at 48 hours after culture initiation.  Cells were harvested and analyzed daily for four days. The data for both figures are presented as the mean ± standard deviation of 5 separate analyses.  closed circles = VES treatment; open circles = vehicle treated; closed triangles = untreated.

## VES does not Function as an Antioxidant

The ability to inhibit the proliferation of tumor cells in culture appears to be a unique property of the succinated form of tocopherol (reviewed by 2;  summarized in TABLE 1).  Studies by this laboratory as well as others show that other forms of vitamin E do not inhibit the proliferation of tumor cells (1,2,3,23). Furthermore, the ability of VES to inhibit the proliferation of tumor cells does not appear to be due to an antioxidant effect since RRR-$\alpha$-tocopherol and other lipid soluble antioxidants have either no detectable effect or a stimulatory rather than inhibitory effect on

TABLE 1.   Comparison of Biological Activities of Vitamin E Compounds

| Name | Structure | Activity Based on Rat Resorption/ Gestation Tests (%) | Anti-oxidant Activity | Inhibition of Proliferation | | |
|------|-----------|----|----|----|----|----|
| | | | | Tumor | Normal Not Act | Normal Act |
| RRR-α-tocopherol | | 100 | 100% | - | - | - |
| RRR-α-tocopheryl-succinate | | 81 | | + | - | + |
| RRR-α-tocopheryloxybutyric acid | | | none | + | - | |
| RRR-α-tocopheryl acetate | | 91 | | - | - | - |
| all-*rac*-α-tocopherol | A mixture of eight stereoisomers | 74 | | - | - | - |
| Trolox | | | 119% | - | - | - |

Compilation of data from  references 3,4, 5,6, 25

tumor cell proliferation (1,2,3,23).   Furthermore, VES in the presence of an inhibitor of cellular esterases,  retains its ability to inhibit tumor cell growth.  Although other lipid soluble antioxidants such as RRR-α-tocopherol, butylated hydroxytoluene and butylated hydroxyanisole do not inhibit proliferation of tumor cells, and VES in the presence of inhibitors of non-specific esterases retains its antiproliferative properties , these type studies are indirect and do not prove that it is the intact VES compound that is responsible for the antiproliferative effects.  As cited in the Introduction, recent research by Marc Fariss and co-workers directly establishes the antiproliferative effects of the intact VES compound (4).  In these studies RRR-α-tocopheryloxybutyric acid (namely,  RRR-α-tocopheryl succinate prepared with a nonhydrolyzable ether linkage), was shown to inhibit murine leukemia cell proliferation in a manner identical to VES while, RRR-α-tocopherol did not exhibit any antiproliferative activity (4).

In addition to inhibiting the proliferation of a wide variety of tumor cells, primarily of epithelial and hematopoietic origin, VES is capable of inhibiting the proliferation of normal T cells that have been activated by mitogen stimulation (25). VES does not inhibit the proliferation of normal, non-activated T cells. The mechanism whereby VES inhibits the proliferation of tumor cells as well as activated normal T cells, but does not inhibit the proliferation of normal non-activated T cells is not understood. The proliferative status of cells appears critical for VES-mediated antiproliferative actions.

## VES causes Tumor Cells to Secrete Biologically Active Antiproliferative Factors

A clue to one possible mechanism of VES's antiproliferative properties came from analyses of the cell culture media obtained from tumor cells cultured in the presence of VES (1,3). Analyses of conditioned media from VES-treated, vehicle control treated or untreated avian, murine and human tumor cells show that cell-conditioned media obtained from the VES-treated cells contain antiproliferative activities that are not detected in the cell-conditioned media from either vehicle control treated cells or from untreated cells. Untreated and vehicle control treated cancer cells either do not secrete antiproliferative factors or secrete low levels of latent (i.e. nonactive) factors.

When cell-conditioned media from VES-treated, vehicle-treated or untreated breast cancer cells are tested for antiproliferative activity, using the TGF-β sensitive Mv1Lu mink lung cell bioassay, no inhibition is seen with either vehicle-treated or untreated samples, while 40-70% inhibition is routinely observed with cell conditioned media from VES-treated cells (FIGURE 3). When the cell-conditioned media are tested back on untreated cells of the same type from which the cell-conditioned media is derived, again inhibition is not seen with cell-conditioned media derived from vehicle or untreated cells while inhibition is seen with cell-conditioned media derived from VES-treated cells, suggesting that the antiproliferative factors can act both in a paracine manner on mink lung bioassay cells as well as in an autocrine manner back on the producer cell type (TABLE 2).

When testing cell conditioned media, the media were concentrated and then either tested directly or heat-activated by boiling for 3 minutes. The best characterized soluble antigrowth factor to date is TGF-β, and it is secreted in a biologically inactive latent form which can be physically activated by either heat or acid treatments (12,26). It is important to note that VES induces increased levels of a biologically active antiproliferative factor that is not destroyed by heating, suggesting that VES is inducing the tumor cells to release biologically active TGF-β from its latent, inactive form (3).

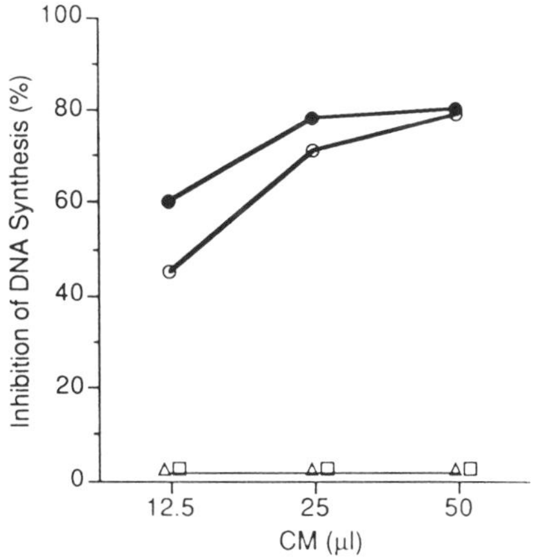

FIGURE 3. Paracrine growth inhibition by antiproliferative factors in conditioned media (CM) from human breast cancer cells treated with VES. Human breast cancer MDA-MB-435 cells were cultured at 1 x $10^5$/ml for 48 hours following the addition of 10 μg/ml of VES, vehicle, or untreated. CM were concentrated/dialyzed 10-fold using Centricon concentrators and aliquots tested for ability to inhibit DNA synthesis of mink lung bioassay cells. CM from VES-treated cells (non-heat-treated and heat activated) inhibited DNA synthesis of the mink lung bioassay cells. CM from vehicle and untreated cells did not inhibit DNA synthesis of the bioassay cells. Percent inhibition of [3]H-TdR uptake of bioassay cells not exposed to CM (i.e. receiving 12.5, 25 or 50 μl of media) is compared to [3]H-TdR uptake of bioassay cells receiving 12.5, 25 or 50 μl aliquots of CM. open circle = CM from VES-treated cells/not-heat-treated; closed circle = CM from VES-treated cells/heat activated; open square = CM from vehicle treated cells/heat activated; open triangle = CM from untreated cells/heat activated.

TABLE 2. Autocrine Growth Inhibition of Human Breast Cancer
Cells by Antiproliferative Factors in Conditioned Media from VES-
Treated Cells

| Conditioned Media | DNA Synthesis (cpm) | Inhibition (%) |
|---|---|---|
| Vehicle | | |
| 20 μl | 118,464 ± 13,180 | |
| 40 μl | 141,090 ± 2,159 | |
| VES | | |
| 20 μl | 53,342 ± 5,717 | 49 |
| 40 μl | 48,180 ± 1,857 | 65 |

The addition of 20 μl or 40 μl of 10X concentrated, dialyzed CM
from MDA-MB-435 cells treated for 24 hours with VES or vehicle
to untreated MDA-MB-435 cells produced 49% and 65%
inhibition, respectively, after a 24 hour incubation period. DNA
synthesis was determine by $^3$H-TdR uptake.

## VES Induction of Biologically Active TGF-β as a Mechanism of Tumor Cell Growth Inhibition

The ability of the antiproliferative activity in conditioned
media from VES-treated tumor cells to withstand both heat and
acid treatments, two characteristics of the well characterized TGF-β
family of antiproliferative factors, suggested that VES could be
causing the secretion of biologically active TGF-β. Several lines of
evidence support this possibility: i) growth inhibition of TGF-β-
responsive Mv1Lu mink lung and murine CTLL-2 cell lines; ii)
combination of physical characteristics including heat stability,
acid stability, and Bio-Gel P60 column chromatography elution
profile; iii) neutralization of the antiproliferative activity of a Mr
14,000 factor isolated from CM from VES-treated cells fractionated
on a Bio-Gel-P60 filtration column by antibodies specific for TGF-
βs and (iv) immunoprecipitation of metabolically-labeled proteins
from CM from VES-treated cells with antibodies specific for TGF-βs
(3, and unpublished data).

The mechanisms whereby VES causes tumor cells to
increase secretion of latent TGF-β and free the biologically active
mature dimer from the pro-peptide is not known at this time.
Activation of purified, recombinant latent TGF-β in vitro can be
accomplished by plasmin digestion, acid or heat-treatments
(12,26). Possible in vivo cellular mechanisms of activation of

latent TGF-β are thought to involve disruption of latent TGF-β by enzymes such as plasmin or cathepsins (13) or removal of carbohydrate structures in latent TGF-β by glycosidases such as endoglycosidase F or sialidase (27,28).

We know, from metabolic labeling studies, that VES-treated cells are producing and secreting newly made biologically active TGF-β. We also know, from Northern blot analyses, that VES is not acting at the transcriptional level since VES does not increase levels of the constitutively produced TGF-β 1, 2 or 3 messenger RNA. The specific TGF-β isoforms induced by VES as well as the mechanism for production and secretion of active TGF-β remain to be elucidated.

Another line of evidence that supports a TGF-β mediated mechanism for VES-induced growth inhibition comes from cell cycle analyses of VES-treated tumor cells. Like TGF-βs which have been demonstrated to cause late G1 cell cycle arrest in cells of different lineages from different species (9,29), VES inhibits tumor cell proliferation by arresting cells in the $G_0/G_1$ cell cycle phase (22; TABLE 3).

TABLE 3. Cell Cycle Analyses of MDA-MB-435 Cells

| Treatments | G0/G1 | S | G2/M |
|---|---|---|---|
| Untreated | 62 | 28 | 10 |
| Vehicle | 58 | 29 | 13 |
| VES | 72 | 18 | 10 |
| TGF-β1 | 70 | 24 | 6 |
| TGF-β2 | 77 | 15 | 8 |

Data are presented as percentage of cells per cell cycle phase.

Progression through the cell cycle is regulated by cyclin-dependent protein kinases (30). Studies suggest that the phosphorylation and dephosphorylation events carried out by cell cycle dependent kinases and phosphatases are critical events in cell cycle progression (16-19). These studies suggest that cyclin E-Cdk2 activity phosphorylates the retinoblastoma gene product, Rb, during the mid to late G1 cell cycle, promoting progression from late G1 into the S cell cycle phase (31); while underphosphorylated Rb is associated with growth-suppression (16,18,31,32). Thus, it is relevant to the VES story that TGF-β treatments have been shown to block cells in the G1 cell cycle and to retain Rb in a hypophosphorylated state (31,32). While the mechanism of growth ihhibition by TGF-β is not fully known, the hypophosphorylation of Rb is considered to be a critical event (16,35). Thus it is of interest that in VES-treated cells like TGF-β-treated cells Rb remains in a hypophosphorylated condition.

## Evidence that VES is Modulating TGF-β Receptor Expression

Evidence that VES is up-regulating TGF-β receptors/binding proteins comes from two experiments. First, combinations of suboptimal levels of VES with a suboptimal dose of TGF-β1 greatly increases the antiproliferative activity when compared to treatment with VES or TGF-β alone. Second, $^{125}$I-TGF-β binding experiments show that VES treatment of tumor cells increases their ability to bind radiolabeled TGF-β. Although one interpretation of these studies is that VES is up-regulating TGF-β receptor/binding proteins, northern blot analyses of messenger RNA levels for TGF-β receptor type III or western immunoblotting analyses of protein levels of TGF-β receptor type II do not support the hypothesis that VES is up-regulating these two receptors.

## Evidence that VES is Inhibiting the Proliferation of Tumor Cells via a Mechanism Independent of TGF-β

VES induction of biologically active TGF-β and its subsequent signaling via the TGF-β receptor complex to block tumor cells in the G1 cell cycle phase does not appear to be the only way that VES can inhibit the proliferation of tumor cells. The antiproliferative actions of VES appear to be more complex and involve inhibition of proliferation by mechanisms yet to be fully understood. Support for the hypothesis that VES can inhibit tumor cell proliferation via a mechanism independent from TGF-β comes from several lines of evidence.

First, not all of the antiproliferative activity in CM from VES-treated tumor cells can be neutralized by anti-TGF-β reagents. Neutralizing antibodies added to VES-treated cells in culture have been shown to reduce but not totally block growth inhibition. Furthermore, antibody neutralization studies performed on partially purified antiproliferative factors isolated from the CM of VES treated tumor cells fails to neutralize all of the antiproliferative activity. These studies suggest that VES is inducing soluble antiproliferative factors that cannot be neutralized by anti-TGF-β reagents.

Second, VES is a more potent inhibitor of cell proliferation than TGF-β. Our studies show that VES inhibits the proliferation of tumor cells within 24 hours; whereas, inhibition of tumor cell proliferation by purified TGF-βs is not detectable until after 48-72 hours of culture. This suggests that VES is affecting cell proliferation by some mechanism in addition to TGF-β.

Third, and most important, VES is capable of inhibiting the proliferation of tumor cells with defective TGF-β receptors (TABLE 4). Two tumor cell lines, chemically mutated Dra-27 mink lung cells with a defective TGF-β type II receptor and LnCAP human prostate cancer cells that are non-responsive to treatments with purified TGF-βs; however, both cell lines are growth inhibited by VES. Growth inhibition of these two cell lines by VES occurs in a similar time course and level as control cells of the same cell lineages that possess responsive TGF-β receptors.

Fourth, VES has the ability to inhibit the proliferation of tumor cells in which both Rb alleles are mutated (TABLE 4). Human prostate Du-145 tumor cells, in which both Rb alleles are mutated and nonfunctional, are non-responsive to TGF-βs; yet, VES inhibits the proliferation of these cells.

Also of importance, these studies show VES can inhibit the proliferation of tumor cells in which both alleles of the tumor suppressor gene, p53, is defective (TABLE 4). This observation maybe important since in vivo studies by Schwartz and co-workers show that VES administered orally by pipette in the hamster buccal pouch squamous cell carcinoma tumor model significantly inhibited tumor development and found that there was

TABLE 4. Ability of Vitamin E Succinate to Inhibit Growth of Tumor Cell Lines With Various Alterations in Growth Regulator Pathways

|  | Prostate Cancer Cell Lines | | | Mink Lung Cell Lines | |
|  | PC-3 | LnCap | Du-145 | DRa27 | Mv1Lu |
|---|---|---|---|---|---|
| **Trait** | | | | | |
| TGF-β Receptor | + | - | + | - | + |
| pRb | + | + | - | + | + |
| p53 | - | + | - | + | + |
| **Growth Inhibition** | | | | | |
| TGF-β | + | - | - | - | + |
| VES | + | + | + | + | + |

increased expression of "wild type" p53 and decreased levels of "mutant" p53 (36).    Our studies show that PC-3 human prostate cells that have both p53 alleles mutated can be inhibited from proliferating by VES.    Thus, it appears that even though VES can directly affect p53, growth inhibition can be induced by VES independent of the mutated state of p53 (TABLE 4). The inhibition of growth of tumor cells with defective p53 alleles may be of significance since many tumors have sustained p53 mutations (37).

    Taken together, these studies point to VES as having anti-proliferative properties independent of TGF-β.    The fact that VES can induce biologically active TGF-β ; can inhibit tumor cell proliferation, independently of TGF-β, in tumor cell lines with either defective TGF-β receptors or defective pRb; and can inhibit the proliferation of tumor cells with mutated p53 alleles suggest a potentially important therapeutic role for the succinated form of vitamin E.

## Summary of VES Actions in Tumor Growth Inhibition

    Studies to date suggest that VES's antiproliferative effects are unique to this form of vitamin E,  and appear to not involve antioxidant effects.    VES blocks tumor cells of epithelial and hematopoietic-lymphoid lineage in the $G_0/G_1$ cell cycle phase and induces the secretion of biologically active TGF-βs. In addition, VES appears to be capable of up-regulating the cell surface expression of TGF-β binding proteins.    Whether or not VES may also directly influence some critical event(s) in the multistep intracellular signaling pathway whereby TGF-βs mediate their antiproliferative actions is under investigation.        Evidence supporting the possibility that VES's antiproliferative effects are mediated by activation of the potent TGF-β growth-inhibitory signaling system is summarized in the top section of TABLE 5. Studies showing that TGF-β is not the only mechanism for VES antiproliferative actions are summarized in the second part of TABLE 5.

TABLE 5.  Summary of VES Inhibition of Tumor Growth

*VES Inhibits Tumor Growth Via Activation of the TGF-$\beta$ Growth-Inhibitory Pathway*

o    Presence of biologically active TGF-$\beta$ in CM from VES-treated tumor cells

o    Cell cycle blockage in $G_1$

o    Increased binding of $^{125}$I-TGF-$\beta$ by VES-treated tumor cells

o    Reduction of VES-mediated growth inhibition by TGF-$\beta$ neutralizing antibody

*VES Inhibits Tumor Growth Via Actions other than TGF-$\beta$*

o    Presence of unique antiproliferative factors in conditioned media from VES-treated tumor cells

o    VES inhibits growth of TGF-$\beta$ receptor negative/TGF-$\beta$ nonresponsive cells

o    VES inhibits growth of Rb negative (Rb$^-$/Rb$^-$) tumor cells

## Future Directions

On-going studies in the lab are outlined in TABLE 6.  We are interested in determining how VES is functioning as an antiproliferative factor and as a biological response modifier of cells involved in mediating immune responses.  Studies designed to determine how VES is functioning as an antiproliferative factor are focused on VES-induced soluble antiproliferative factors that act as inhibitors of cell proliferation.  Studies in the lab show VES to have multiple effects on important cellular growth regulatory components, including retention of Rb in a hypophosphorylated state, reduction of *c-myc* messenger RNA expression, interference with transcription factor binding to DNA, and induction of apoptosis.  Although not the  subject of this review, studies in the lab are also designed to investigate  how  VES modulates immune responses, ameliorates retrovirus-induced immune suppressed states, enhances T cell cytokine production and secretion, and induces fibronectin secretion and expression of a novel fibronectin receptor.

TABLE 6.
### FUTURE DIRECTIONS

*Inhibition of Cell Proliferation*
  enhancer of secretion/activation of autocrine/paracrine
      acting antiproliferative factors
  inducer of cell cycle blockage
  modulator of growth inhibitory signaling pathways
  inducer of apoptosis

*Modulator of Immune Response System*
  enhancer of anti-tumor immunity
  regulator of cytokine expression
  enhancer of cell adhesion factors and receptors
  modifier of eicosanoid biosynthesis

*Vitamin E Succinate-Gene Interactions*
  role of VES binding proteins
  modifier of NF-$\kappa$B/Rel transcriptional factor regulatory
      system

## REFERENCES

1.     Kline, K & BG Sanders. 1991. "Anti-tumor proliferation properties of vitamin E." In:  Vitamins and Minerals in the Prevention and Treatment of Cancer. MM Jacobs, ed. CRC Press, Boca Raton, FL. pp 189-205.
2.     Prasad, KN & J Edwards-Prasad. 1992. J. Am. Coll. Nutr. 11: 487-500.
3.     Charpentier, A, S Groves, M Simmons-Menchaca, J Turley, B Zhao, BG Sanders & K Kline. 1993. Nutr. Cancer 19:225-239.
4.     Fariss, MW, MB Fortuna, CK Everett, JD Smith, DF Trent & Z Djuric. 1994. Cancer Res. 54:3346-3351.
5.     Machlin, LJ. 1991. "Chapter 3 Vitamin E." In:  Handbook of Vitamins. LJ Machlin (ed). Marcel Dekker, Inc. NY.  pp 99-144.
6.     Horwitt, MK. 1992. "The Forms of Vitamin E" In:  1992 Vitamin E Abstracts.  Vitamin E Research & Information Service, LaGrange, IL. pp vii-xiv.
7.     The Merck Index-Tenth Edition.  1983.  M Windholz (ed). Merck & Co., Inc. Rahway, NJ.

8.     Roberts, AB & MB Sporn. 1990. "The transforming growth factor-βs." In: Peptide Growth Factors and Their Receptors I. MB Sporn & A B Roberts (eds). Springer-Verlag, NY, pp 419-472.
9.     Massague, J. 1990. Annu. Rev. Cell Biol. 6:597-641.
10.    Wakefield, L M, AA Colletta, BK McCune & MB Sporn. 1991. "Roles for transforming growth factors-β in the genesis, prevention, and treatment of breast cancer." In: Genes, Oncogenes, and Hormones: Advances in Cellular and Molecular Biology of Breast Cancer. RB Dickson & ME Lippman (eds). Kluwer Academic Publishers, Boston, MA, pp 97-136.
11.    Massague, J, J Andres, L Attisano, S Cheifetz, F Lopez-Casillas, M Ohtsuki & JL Wrana. 1992. Mol. Reprod. Develop. 32:99-104.
12.    Lyons, RM, LE Gentry, AF Purchio & HL Moses. 1990. J. Cell Biology 110: 1361-1367.
13.    Lyons, RM, J Keski-Oja & HL Moses. 1988. J. Cell Biol. 106:1659-1665.
14.    Massague, J. 1992. Cell 69:1067-1070.
15.    Wrana, J L, L Attisano, J Carcamo, A Zentella, J Doody, M Laiho, X-F Wang & J Massague. 1992. Cell 71:1003-1014.
16.    Laiho, M, JA DeCaprio, JW Ludlow, DM Livingston & J Massague. 1990. Cell 62:175-185.
17.    Cooper, J.A. and P. Whyte. 1989. Cell. 58:1009-1011.
18.    DeCaprio, J.A , JW Ludlow, D Lynch, Y Furukawa, J Griffin, H Piwnica-Worms, C-M Huang & D M Livingston. 1989. Cell 58: 1085-1095.
19.    Furukawa, Y, JA DeCaprio, A Freedman, Y Kanakura, M Nakamura, TJ Ernst, D M Livingston & JD Griffin. 1990. Proc. Natl. Acad. Sci. USA 87:2770-2774.
20.    Polyak, K, MH Lee, H Erdjument-Bromage, A Koff, J M Roberts, P Tempst & J Massague. 1994. Cell 78:59-66.
21.    Polyak, K, J Kato, M J Solomon, C J Sherr, J Massague, J M Roberts & A Koff. 1994. Genes & Develop. 8:9-22.
22.    Kline, K, GS Cochran & BG Sanders. 1990. Nutr. Cancer 14:27-41.
23.    Turley, JM, B G Sanders & K Kline. 1992. Nutr. Cancer 18:201-213.
24.    Carpenter, D 1985. Sem. Neurol. 5:283-287.
25.    Kline, K & BG Sanders.1993. Nutr. Cancer 19:241-252.
26.    Brown, PD, LM Wakefield, A D Levinson & MB Sporn. 1990. Growth Factors 3:35-43.
27.    Miyazono, K & C-H Heldin. 1989. Nature 338:158-160.

28.    Miyazono, K & C-H Heldin. 1991. Latent forms of TGF-β: molecular structure and mechanisms of activation. In: Clinical applications of TGF-β. GR Bock & J Marsh (eds). (Ciba Foundation Symposium). John Wiley & Sons, Chichester. 157: 81-92.

29.    Sporn, MB & A B Roberts. 1990. Cell Regulation 1:875-882.

30.    Cross, F, J Roberts & H Weintraub. 1989. Annual Rev. Cell Biol. 5: 341-395.

31.    Koff, A, M Ohtsuki, K Polyak, JM Roberts & J Massague. 1993. Science 260:536-539.

32.    Ahuja, SS, F Paliogianni, H Yamada, JE Balow & DT Boumpas. 1993. J. Immunol. 150:3109-2118.

33.    Ludlow, JW, JA DeCaprio, CM Huang, WH Lee, E Paucha & DM Livingston. 1989. Cell 56:57-65.

34.    Ludlow, JW, J Shon, JM Pipas, DM Livingston & JA DeCaprio. 1990. Cell 60: 387-396.

35.    Chen, R, R Ebner & R Derynck.1993.Science 260:1335-1338.

36.    Schwartz, J, G Shklar & D Trickler. 1993. Oral. Oncol. Eur. J. Cancer 29B:313-318.

37.    Allred, DC, GM Clark & R Elledge. 1993. J. National Cancer Instit. 85:200-206.

# Vitamin D, Gene Expression, and Cancer

Hector F. DeLuca

Department of Biochemistry, University of Wisconsin-Madison, 420 Henry Mall, Madison, WI 53706 U.S.A.

## I    Introduction

Classically, vitamin D was discovered because in its absence the disease rickets, osteomalacia, and hypocalcemic tetany resulted (1, 2). Clearly, vitamin D functions in the regulation of plasma calcium and plasma phosphorus, which in turn results in normal mineralization of the skeleton and the normal functioning of the neuromuscular junction. Vitamin D carries out these functions following its metabolism, as described below, to its active or hormonal form, i.e. 1,25-dihydroxyvitamin $D_3$ (1,25-$(OH)_2D_3$). This hormone directly stimulates intestinal calcium transport and independently intestinal phosphate transport by mechanisms not yet fully understood (1, 2). In addition, 1,25-$(OH)_2D_3$ acts on the osteoblasts together with parathyroid hormone (PTH) to facilitate the mobilization of calcium from bone into the plasma compartment when required. More recently it has been demonstrated that 1,25-$(OH)_2D_3$ facilitates the reabsorption of calcium in the distal renal tubule in a mechanism also dependent upon the presence of the PTH (1-3). These actions result in an elevation of plasma calcium and phosphorus, resulting in normal mineralization of the skeleton and neuromuscular function (Figure 1).

Since the mid-1970s with the realization that this steroid hormone, 1,25-$(OH)_2D_3$, functions through a nuclear receptor, it has become known that vitamin D functions beyond regulating calcium and phosphorus homeostasis (4). Certainly one of the more exciting developments was the discovery that it suppresses growth and stimulates differentiation of stem cells (4, 5). Thus, vitamin D must also be considered a developmental hormone as well. In addition, this vitamin functions in the immune system, the female reproduction system, the islet cells of the pancreas; it carries out many different functions on the osteoblast, and suppresses the preproparathyroid gene, illustrating that vitamin D has profound and diverse actions (1-5). One of these diverse actions, namely the suppression of growth and the stimulation of differentiation has interesting applications in the treatment of various forms of cancer.

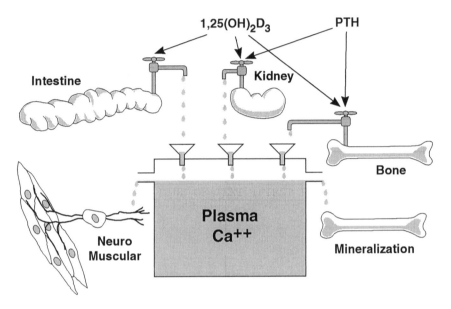

Figure 1. Diagrammatic representation of the sites of action of 1,25-$(OH)_2D_3$ and PTH in calcium homeostasis.

## I.    Metabolism

Vitamin D must be metabolized first in the liver to 25-hydroxyvitamin D (25-OH-D) by two enzymes, one of which has been cloned (6), and subsequently it must be 1-hydroxylated in the kidney by the 25-OH-D-1α-hydroxylase that has yet to be cloned or isolated (1-4). Although it has been reported in culture that 1α-hydroxylation can take place in cells other than the proximal convoluted tubule cells of the kidney, *in vivo* experiments fail to support the relevance of these determinations (7, 8). However, certainly under conditions of sarcoidosis or certain lymphomas, ectopic production of 1,25-$(OH)_2D_3$ does occur and contributes to the disease process (9, 10).

The vitamin D system is tightly regulated at the renal $1\alpha$-hydroxylation step (1, 2). When calcium is needed, the parathyroid glands secrete PTH that, in turn, stimulates the $1\alpha$-hydroxylase resulting in the production of $1,25\text{-}(OH)_2D_3$. When calcium is not needed, the $1\alpha$-hydroxylase is shut off presumably because of low levels of PTH and instead another enzyme, the $1,25\text{-}(OH)_2D_3\text{-}24$-hydroxylase is stimulated. This enzyme is believed to carry out the initial step in the degradation of the vitamin D hormone to its excretion product, calcitroic acid, that appears primarily in the bile (11). $1,25\text{-}(OH)_2D_3$ itself stimulates the 24-hydroxylase and thus programs its own destruction. $1,25\text{-}(OH)_2D_3$ also suppresses the $1\alpha$-hydroxylase. This exquisitely regulated endocrine system located in the proximal convoluted tubule cells is probably the major component of the calcium regulating system (1-4, 12).

## II. Molecular Mechanism of Action of $1,25\text{-}(OH)_2D_3$

Using high specific activity radiolabeled $1,25\text{-}(OH)_2D_3$, it was shown that this compound localizes specifically in the nuclei of target tissues of the intestinal enterocyte, the osteoblasts of bone, and the distal renal tubule cells (13). In addition, it localized in other cells not previously appreciated to be targets of vitamin D action (14). Since $1,25\text{-}(OH)_2D_3$ is a steroid and it localizes in the nuclei of target tissues, a steroid hormone-type mechanism was anticipated. Thus, a receptor was sought and found (14). The receptor is likely nuclear, although there have been reports of cytoplasmic occurrences of the receptor (15). This receptor is in extremely low abundance and was cloned through the route of generation of monoclonal antibodies which were then used to screen $\lambda$ gt11 expression libraries (16, 17). As a result, the full length coding sequence of the rat receptor was identified and the full coding sequence of the human receptor was identified (18, 19). This receptor is a protein of molecular weight 55,000, and has in it the usual domains attributed to a steroid hormone receptor (18, 19). Especially notable is that it contains a DNA binding domain (C domain) and a ligand binding domain (E domain) separated by a hinge region (D domain). In addition, there are domains at the N-terminus called the AB domain and at the carboxy terminus called the F domain. Although deletion analysis has been carried out on this receptor, little is known concerning its actual 3-dimensional structure (14). The receptor has been successfully expressed in mammalian cells, baculovirus infected insect cells, yeast, and bacteria (20). By far, the most promising appears the baculovirus-infected insect cells where large amounts of native receptor can be produced and attempts at 3-dimensional structural analysis is currently underway (21). The receptor can also be quickly purified to homogeneity by affinity chromatography using anti-receptor antibodies (21).

The essentiality of the receptor to the vitamin D system is illustrated by the autosomal recessive disorder, vitamin D dependency rickets Type II. Several kindreds have been described, all representing mutations in the vitamin D receptor (VDR) (22, 23). Single-base mutations have been described for virtually all of the known kindreds, most resulting in nonsense codons causing termination of translation. In any case, affected children fail to respond to 1,25-(OH)$_2$D$_3$, illustrating that the major if not sole mechanism of action of the vitamin D hormone is through its receptor (24). Many reports have appeared regarding possible non-genomic actions of 1,25-(OH)$_2$D$_3$. These are largely *in vitro* experiments using high and unphysiologic concentrations of the hormone and have yet to be shown to have *in vivo* relevance. The remainder of this presentation will deal with the molecular mechanism of the vitamin D hormone utilizing the receptor.

As might be expected, like other steroid hormones, binding sites for the VDR have been located in the promoter region of target genes (20). This is done largely by two techniques: one involving the binding of the receptor in a specific manner to segments of DNA called gel shift experiments, and the other technique is the splicing of such regions proximal to the promoter of a reporter gene in an expression plasmid and by transfection experiments determine hormonal stimulation of a reporter gene. Using this functional assay and the gel shift experiments, specific VDR binding and functional sites have been described for approximately 6 genes shown in Table 1 (20, 25). The vitamin D system, unlike the other steroid hormones, generally utilizes direct repeat sequences of six nucleotides for each sequence separated by 3 nonspecific bases as described by Umesono et al. (26). By far the most interesting and most powerful vitamin D response system has been located in the 24-hydroxylase gene as illustrated in Figure 2. This responsive system is silent in the presence of receptor and is stimulated as much as 15-30-fold by addition of the hormone (27, 28).

Binding of the VDR to these responsive elements requires the presence of a nuclear accessory factor (NAF). This NAF can be replaced by another family of steroid hormone receptors known as the RXR proteins that bind 9-*cis*-retinoic acid (29-32) We recently have completed isolation of the nuclear accessory factor from a vitamin D target organ, namely porcine intestine. This protein reacts with an anti-RXR receptor antibody and furthermore the highly purified protein binds 9-cis-retinoic acid. This illustrates that from a target organ, the functional NAF is either an RXR or a closely related protein. Of special interest is that the binding of the VDR to its response element in the presence of the nuclear accessory protein does not require the presence of the vitamin D hormone (33).

Table 1. The 1,25-(OH)$_2$D Response Elements

| Gene | Position | Sequence |
|------|----------|----------|
| **Activation** | | |
| Rat Osteocalcin | -456 to -442 | GGGTGA ATG AGGACA |
| Human Osteocalcin | -511 to -486 | GGGTGA ACT GGGGCA |
| Mouse Osteopontin | -757 to -743 | GGTTCA CGA GGTTCA |
| Rat Calbindin 9k | -488 to -474 | GGGTGT CGG AAGCCC |
| Rat 24-OHase I | -459 to -245 | CGCACC CGC TGAACC |
| Rat 24-OHase II | -151 to -137 | GCGGGA GTG AGTGGA ... CTGAG |
| | | 3 spaces / required    3 spaces / required |
| **Suppression** | | |
| Human PTH | -100 to -106 | NNNNN TGAACC |

Another important event is phosphorylation of the receptor. In an organ culture system that is responsive to the vitamin D hormone by increasing intestinal calcium transport, Brown and DeLuca were able to show that within 15 minutes to 1 hour following addition of the hormone to the organ culture system, the receptor becomes phosphorylated (34). Thus, the phosphorylation is ligand dependent in that it does not take place unless ligand is added, and secondly it occurs very quickly which indicates it is an early event in the mechanism of 1,25-(OH)$_2$D$_3$ action in the intestine. Several sites of phosphorylation of the VDR have been reported from *in vitro* experiments (35-38) but they do not correspond to the site of phosphorylation occurring in this functional organ culture system. This phosphorylation is on a serine and in the ligand binding domain but has not been characterized further (39). Stimulation of protein kinase A by 8-bromo-cAMP or it inhibition by H9 or other inhibitors of that kinase suggest that the phosphorylation is an essential step in the molecular events resulting in gene expression in response to 1,25-(OH)$_2$D$_3$ (40). Thus, in a reporter gene experiment, stimulation of protein kinase A by 8-bromo-cAMP markedly stimulates reporter gene response in a VDR-dependent manner. H9 inhibits 1,25-(OH)$_2$D$_3$ induced response (40). These results argue that this specific phosphorylation occurring in the ligand binding domain is an essential step in the molecular mechanism of action of vitamin D. Figure 3 illustrates the current thinking of the molecular mechanism of action of the vitamin D hormone.

Thus, the receptor binds with the nuclear accessory factor probably an RXR to the response element in a ligand-independent process. The next step is the binding of ligand that increases the affinity of the binding to the response element and which then converts this complex to an appropriate substrate for phosphorylation. Phosphorylation then results in activation of this transcriptively active protein. What other factors are involved remain unknown, although it is speculated that some of the factors illustrated by analogy probably operate. Whether the ligand remains bound to the phosphorylated receptor or not has yet to be determined.

**25-OH-VITAMIN D$_3$-24-HYDROXYLASE GENE STRUCTURE**

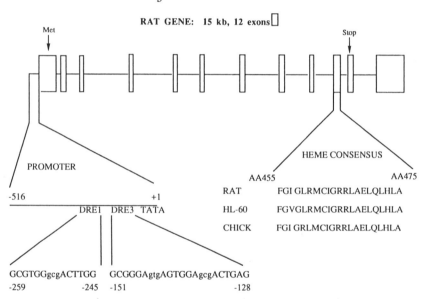

## IV.  Role of the Vitamin D Hormone in Differentiation and Suppression of Growth

Abe and Suda (41) discovered that M1 promyelocyte cells when incubated with 1,25-(OH)$_2$D$_3$ undergo differentiation to monocytes and their growth is suppressed. A similar observations was made in the case of the HL-60 human promyelocyte line (42) and now several similar systems are well known. This important discovery illustrates that the vitamin D hormone is an important differentiating agent and plays a role in the generation of the monocyte which is the precursor of the giant osteoclast, the bone resorbing cell.

Suda and colleagues, Teitelbaum, and others have provided strong evidence that the vitamin D hormone functions at 2 additional sites in the generation of an active osteoclast (43). Most important, however, from a cancer point of view, is that the vitamin D hormone can suppress growth of cancer cells lines while causing their differentiation (44). This has excited many scientists with the idea that the vitamin D hormone or a derivative might be useful in the treatment of malignancies. However, because of the extremely high calcium activity of 1,25-$(OH)_2D_3$, the concentrations needed to suppress cancer growth would result in lethal hypercalcemia. This has led investigators to attempt to synthesize analogs of the vitamin D hormone that no longer stimulate calcium absorption or mobilization of calcium from bone while retaining their ability to cause differentiation. Thus, the group at Wisconsin developed three classes of such compounds; Hoffmann-La Roche, two classes; Chugai, one class; and Leo Pharmaceuticals, a number of such compounds (45).

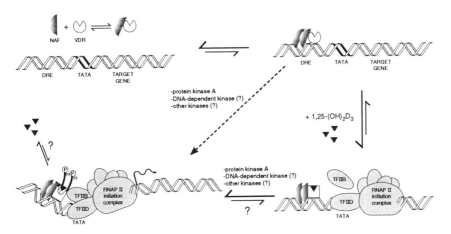

Figure 3. Diagrammatic representation of the molecular events occurring in the 1,25-$(OH)_2D_3$ stimulation of target gene expression.

Of particular interest is that the keratinocyte is a site of vitamin D action where it is induced to differentiate and its growth is suppressed (46). This has led to the topical application of the vitamin D hormone or its analogs to the disease psoriasis with excellent results (47). However, the treatment of malignancies remains a major question. Virtually every cell line examined has high levels of the VDR (48). Certainly fresh breast tissue explants show much higher levels of VDR than adjacent tissue (49). Colon, lung, and other types of carcinomas also show high levels of the VDR (50). Of particular importance is the study of Eisman and his colleagues that show that transplantable cancers

*DeLuca*

having receptor can be suppressed by 1,25-$(OH)_2D_3$ (51). Eisman and colleagues were able to carry out this experiment by restricting calcium in the diet. These results show that tumor growth can be suppressed by the vitamin D hormone if hypercalcemia is not a problem. We have attempted to study N-nitroso-N-methylurea-induced breast cancers. Using 19-nor-1,25-$(OH)_2D_3$ given three times a week, the incidence of breast tumors as a result of N-nitroso-N-methylurea is markedly suppressed without inducing hypercalcemia (Table 2). On the other hand in the same experiments, extreme vitamin D deficiency has little or no influence on the induction of tumors by N-nitroso-N-methylurea. These results and those of Eisman as well as some recent results on 16-ene-1,25-$(OH)_2D_3$ from Uskokovic and colleagues (52) demonstrate that possible utility of vitamin D compounds in the treatment of induced cancers.

---

Table 2. Reduction of Tumor Incidence in N.M.U.-Treated Female Rats by $\Delta^{22}$-22,23-Dehydro-19-Nor-1,25-Dihydroxyvitamin $D_3$[*]

| Treatment | Avg. Size | Tumor Bearing Rats/ Rats per Group | % |
|---|---|---|---|
| Vehicle | 4 cm$^2$ | 9/11 | 82 |
| $\Delta^{22}$-22,23-Dehydro-19-Nor 1,25-$(OH)_2D_3$ | 3 cm$^3$ | 2/15 | 13 |

[*]Given at 200 ng/dose I.P. three times week for two months.

## V.    Summary

Much has been learned on the mechanism of action of the vitamin D hormone. It acts as a steroid hormone, interacting with a nuclear receptor of 55,000 molecular weight. This receptor binds to response elements in the promoter region of target genes. This binding requires the presence of an RXR type protein followed by interaction with the ligand resulting in phosphorylation. This converts the VDR to a transcriptively active agent, stimulating gene expression or suppression in the case of the preproparathyroid gene. The vitamin D hormone has actions far beyond stimulating calcium transport and serum calcium in that it certainly causes the differentiation of a variety of precursor cells and suppresses growth. The presence of VDR in high concentrations in cancer tissue and the suppression of growth of cancer cells in culture by the hormone suggest it or an analog's use in the treatment of cancer. Preliminary results are promising that the vitamin D hormonal analogs may be of therapeutic value in the treatment of malignant tissue that expresses the 1,25-(OH)$_2$D$_3$ receptor.

## VI.    Acknowledgments

This work was supported in part by a program project grant no. DK14881 from the National Institutes of Health, a fund from the National Foundation for Cancer Research, and a fund from the Wisconsin Alumni Research Foundation.

## VII.    References

1.      DeLuca, H. F. The transformation of a vitamin into a hormone: The vitamin D story. The Harvey Lectures, Series 75, pp. 333-379. New York:Academic Press, 1981.

2       DeLuca, H. F. The vitamin D-calcium axis--1983. In: R.P. Rubin, G. B. Weiss, and J.W. Putney, Jr. (eds.), Calcium in Biological System, pp. 491-511. New York: Plenum , 1985.

3.      Yamamoto, M., Kawanobe, Y., Takahashi, H., Shimazawa, E., Kimura, S., and Ogata, E, Vitamin D deficiency and renal calcium transport in the rat. J. Clin. Invest., 74: 507-513, 1984.

4.      DeLuca, H. F. New concepts of vitamin D functions. In: H.E. Sauberlich and K.J. Machlin (eds.), Beyond Deficiency. New Views on the Function and Health Effects of Vitamins, vol. 669, pp. 59-69. The New York Academy of Sciences, New York, 1992.

5.      Suda, T. The role of 1$\alpha$,25-dihydroxyvitamin D$_3$ in the myeloid cell differentiation. Proc. Soc. Exp. Biol. Med., 191: 214-220, 1989.

6.      Usui, E., Noshiro, M., and Okuda, K. Molecular cloning of cDNA for vitamin D$_3$ 25-hydroxylase from rat liver mitochondria. FEBS Lett., 262: 135-138, 1990.

7.      Reeve, L., Tanaka, Y., and DeLuca, H. F. Studies on the site of 1,25-dihydroxyvitamin D$_3$ synthesis in vivo. J. Biol. Chem., 258: 3615-3617, 1983.

8.      Shultz, T. D., Fox, J., Heath, H. III, and Kumar, R. Do tissues other than the kidney produce 1,25-dihydroxyvitamin D3 in vivo? A reexamination. Proc. Natl. Acad. Sci. USA, 80: 1746-1750, 1983.

9.      Barbour, G. L., Coburn, J. W., Slatopolsky, E., Norman, A. W., and Horst, R. L. Hypercalcemia in an anephric patient with sarcoidosis; Evidence

for extrarenal generation of 1,25-dihydroxyvitamin D. New Engl. J. Med., 305: 440-443, 1981.

10.   Adams, J. S., Gacad, M. A., Singer, F. R., and Sharma, O. P. Production of 1,25-dihydroxyvitamin D3 by pulmonary alveolar macrophages from patients with sarcoidosis. In: C.J. Johns (ed.), Tenth International Conference on Sarcoidosis and Other Granulomatous Disorders, vol. 465, pp. 587-. New York:New York Academy of Sciences, 1986.

11.   Lohnes, D., and Jones, G. Side chain metabolism of vitamin D3 in osteosarcoma cell line UMR-106. Characterization of products. J. Biol. Chem., 262: 14394-14401, 1987.

12.   DeLuca, H. F. The vitamin D story: A collaborative effort of basic science and clinical medicine. FASEB J., 2: 224-236, 1988.

13.   Stumpf, W.E., Sar, M., Reid, F.A., Tanaka, Y., and DeLuca, H. F. Target cells for 1,25-dihydroxyvitamin D3 in intestinal tract, stomach, kidney, skin, pituitary and parathyroid. Science, 206: 1188-1190, 1979.

14.   Link, R., and DeLuca, H. F. The vitamin D receptor. In: P.M. Conn (ed.), The Receptors, vol. II, pp. 1-35. New York: Academic Press, 1985.

15.   Barsony, J., Pike, J. W., DeLuca, H. F., and Marx, S. J. Immunocytology with microwave-fixed fibroblasts shows $1\alpha$,25-dihydroxyvitamin D3-dependent rapid and estrogen-dependent slow reorganization of vitamin D receptors. J. Cell Biol., 111: 2385-2395, 1990.

16.   Dame, M. C., Pierce, E. A., Prahl, J. M., Hayes, C. E., and DeLuca, H. F. Monoclonal antibodies to the porcine intestinal receptor for 1,25-dihydroxyvitamin D3: Interaction with distinct receptor domains. Biochemistry, 25: 4523-4534, 1986.

17.   Pike, J. W., Marion, S. L., Donaldson, C. A., and Haussler, M. R. Serum and monoclonal antibodies against the chick intestinal receptor for 1,25-dihydroxyvitamin D3. J. Biol. Chem., 258: 1289-1296, 1983.

18.   Burmester, J. K., Wiese, R. J., Maeda, N., and DeLuca, H. F. Structure and regulation of the rat 1,25-dihydroxyvitamin D3 receptor. Proc. Natl. Acad. Sci. USA, 85: 9499-9502, 1988.

19.   Baker, A. R., McDonnell, D. P., Hughes, M., Crisp, T. M., Mangelsdorf, D. J., Haussler, M. R., Pike, J. W., Shine, J., and O'Malley, B. W. Cloning and expression of full-length cDNA encoding human vitamin D receptor. Proc. Natl. Acad. Sci. USA, 85: 3294-3298, 1988.

20.   Darwish, H., and DeLuca, H. F. Vitamin D-regulated gene expression. In: G.S. Stein, J.L. Stein, and J.B. Lian (eds.), Critical Reviews in Eukaryotic Gene Expression, vol. 3(2), pp. 89-116. Boca Raton, FL: CRC Press, 1993.

21.   Li, Z., Prahl, J. M., Hellwig, W., and DeLuca, H. F. Immunoaffinity purification of active rat recombinant 1,25-dihydroxyvitamin D3 receptor. Arch. Biochem. Biophys., 310: 347-351, 1994.

22. Wiese, R. J., Goto, H., Prahl, J. M., Marx, S. J., Thomas, M., Al-Aqeel, A., and DeLuca, H. F. Vitamin D-dependency rickets type II: Truncated vitamin D receptor in three kindreds. Mol. Cell. Endocrinol., 90: 197-201, 1993.

23. Malloy, P. J., Hochberg, Z., Tiosano, D., Pike, J. W., Hughes, M. R., and Feldman, D. The molecular basis of hereditary 1,25-dihydroxyvitamin $D_3$ resistant rickets in seven related families. J. Clin. Invest., 86: 2071-2079, 1990.

24. Brooks, M. H., Bell, N. H., Love, L., Stern, P. H., Orfei, E., Queener, S. F., Hamstra, A. J., and DeLuca, H. F. Vitamin D-dependent rickets type II. Resistance of target organs to 1,25-dihydroxyvitamin D. New Engl. J. Med., 298: 996-999, 1978.

25. Ross, T. K., Darwish, H. M., and DeLuca, H. F. Molecular biology of vitamin D action. In: G. Litwack (ed.), Vitamins and Hormones, vol. 49, pp. 281-326. New York:Academic Press, 1994.

26. Umesono, K., Murakami, K. K., Thompson, C. C., and Evans, R. M. Direct repeats as selective response elements for the thyroid hormone, retinoic acid, and vitamin $D_3$ receptors. Cell, 65: 1255-1266, 1991.

27. Zierold, C., Darwish, H. M., and DeLuca, H. F. Identification of a vitamin D-response element in the rat calcidiol (25-hydroxyvitamin $D_3$) 24-hydroxylase gene. Proc. Natl. Acad. Sci. USA, 91: 900-902, 1994.

28. Ohyama, Y., Zono, K., Uchida, M., Shinki, T., Kato, S., Suda, T., Yamamoto, O., Noshiro, M., and Kato, Y. Identification of a vitamin D-responsive element in the 5'-flanking region of the rat 25-hydroxyvitamin $D_3$ 24-hydroxylase gene. J. Biol. Chem., 269: 10545-10550, 1994.

29. Ross, T. K., Moss, V. E., Prahl, J. M., and DeLuca, H. F. A nuclear protein essential for binding of rat 1,25-dihydroxyvitamin $D_3$ receptor to its response elements. Proc. Natl. Acad. Sci. USA, 89: 256-260, 1992.

30. Sone, T., Ozono, K., and Pike, J. W. A 55-kilodalton accessory factor facilitates vitamin D receptor DNA binding. Mol. Endocrinol., 5: 1578-1586, 1991.

31. Kliewer, S. A., Umesono, K., Mangelsdorf, D. J., and Evans, R. M. Retinoid X receptor interacts with nuclear receptors in retinoic acid, thyroid hormone and vitamin $D_3$ signaling. Nature, 355: 446-449, 1992.

32. Zhang, S. K., Hoffmann, B., Tran, P. B. V., Gaupner, G., and Pfahl, M. Retinoid X receptor is an auxiliary protein for thyroid hormone and retinoic acid receptors. Nature, 355: 441-446, 1992.

33. Ross, T. K., Darwish, H. M., Moss, V. E., and DeLuca, H. F. Vitamin D-influenced gene expression via a ligand-independent, receptor-DNA complex intermediate. Proc. Natl. Acad. Sci. USA, 90: 9257-9260, 1993.

34. Brown, T. A., and DeLuca, H. F. Phosphorylation of the 1,25-dihydroxyvitamin $D_3$ receptor: A primary event in 1,25-dihydroxyvitamin $D_3$ action. J. Biol. Chem., 265: 10025-10029, 1990.

35.    Jurutka, P. W., Terpening, C. M., and Haussler, M. R. The 1,25-dihydroxy-vitamin D3 receptor is phosphorylated in response to 1,25-dihydroxyvitamin D3 and 22-oxacalcitriol in rat osteoblasts, and by casein kinase II, in vitro. Biochemistry, 32: 8184-8192, 1993.

36.    Jurutka, P. W., Hsieh, J-C., MacDonald, P. N., Terpening, C. M., Haussler, C. A., Haussler, M. R., and Whitfield, G. K. Phosphorylation of serine 208 in the human vitamin D receptor. The predominant amino acid phosphorylated by casein kinase II, *in vitro*, and identification as a significant phosphorylation site in intact cells. J. Biol. Chem., 268: 6791-6799, 1993.

37.    Hsieh, J-C., Jurutka, P. W., Galligan, M. A., Terpening, C. M., Haussler, C. A., Samuels, D. W., Himizu, Y., Shimizu, N., and Haussler, M. R. Human vitamin D receptor is selectively phosphorylated by protein kinase C on serine 51, a residue crucial to its trans-activation function. Proc. Natl. Acad. Sci. USA, 88: 9315-9319, 1991.

38.    Hsieh, J-C., Jurutka, P. W., Nakajima, S., Galligan, M. A., Haussler, C. A., Shimizu, Y., Himizu, N., Whitfield, G. K., and Haussler, M. R. Phosphorylation of the human vitamin D receptor by protein kinase C. Biochemical and functional evaluation of the serine 51 recognition site. J. Biol. Chem., 268: 15118-15126, 1993.

39.    Brown, T. A., and DeLuca, H. F. Sites of phosphorylation and photoaffinity labeling of the 1,25-dihydroxyvitamin D3 receptor. Arch. Biochem. Biophys., 286: 466-472, 1991.

40.    Darwish, H. M., Burmester, J. K., Moss, V. E., and DeLuca, H. F. Phosphorylation is involved in transcriptional activation by the 1,25-dihydroxyvitamin D3 receptor. Biochim. Biophys. Acta, 1167: 29-36, 1993.

41.    Abe, E., Miyaura, C., Sakagami, H., Takeda, M., Konno, K., Yamazaki, T., Yoshiki, S., and Suda, T. Differentiation of mouse myeloid leukemia cells induced by $1\alpha$,25-dihydroxyvitamin D3. Proc. Natl. Acad. Sci. USA, 78, 4990-4994, 1981.

42.    Tanaka, H., Abe, E., Miyaura, C., Kuribayashi, T., Konno, K., Nishii, Y., and Suda, T. $1\alpha$,25-Dihydroxycholecalciferol and a human myeloid leukaemia cell line (HL-60). The presence of a cytosol receptor and induction of differentiation. Biochem. J., 204: 713-719, 1982.

43.    Suda, T., Takahashi, N., and Martin, T. J. Modulation of osteoclast differentiation. Endocrine Rev., 13: 66-80, 1992.

44.    Eisman, J. A., Koga, M., Sutherland, R. L., Barkla, D. H., and Tutton, P. J. M. 1,25-Dihydroxyvitamin D3 and the regulation of human cancer cell replication. Proc. Soc. Exp. Biol. Med., 191: 221-226, 1989.

45.    DeLuca, H. F. Application of new vitamin D compounds to disease. Drug News and Perspectives, 5: 87-92, 1992.

46. Smith, E. L., Walworth, N. C., and Holick, M. F. Effect of $1\alpha,25$-dihydroxyvitamin $D_3$ on the morphologic and biochemical differentiation of cultured human epidermal keratinocytes grown in serum-free conditions. J. Invest. Dermatol., 86: 709-714, 1986.

47. Holick, M. F. 1,25-Dihydroxyvitamin $D_3$ and the skin: A unique application for the treatment of psoriasis. Proc. Soc. Exp. Biol. Med., 191: 246-257, 1989.

48. Frampton, R. J., Suva, L. J., Eisman, J. A., Findlay, D. M., Moore, G. E., Moseley, J. M., and Martin, T. J. Presence of 1,25-dihydroxyvitamin D3 receptors in established human cancer cell lines in culture. Cancer Res., 42: 1116-1119, 1982.

49. Sandgren, M., Danforth, L., Plasse, T. F., and DeLuca, H. F. 1,25-Dihydroxyvitamin $D_3$ receptors in human carcinomas: A pilot study. Cancer Res., 51, 2021-2024, 1991.

50. Eisman, J. A. 1,25-Dihydroxyvitamin $D_3$ receptor and role of 1,25-$(OH)_2D_3$ in human cancer cells. In: R. Kumar (ed.), Vitamin D, Chapter 14, pp. 365-382. Boston: Martinus Nijhoff, 1984.

51. Eisman, J. A., Barkla, D. H., and Tutton, P. J. M. Suppression of in vivo growth of human cancer solid tumor xenografs by 1,25-dihydroxyvitamin $D_3$. Cancer Res., 47, 21-26, 1987.

52. Anzano, M. A., Smith, J. M., Uskokovic, M. R., Peer, C. W., Mullen, L. T., Letterio, J. J., Welsh, M. C., Shrader, M. W., Logsdon, D. L., Drive, C. L., et al. $1\alpha,25$-Dihydroxy-16-ene-23-yne-26,27-hexafluorocholecalciferol (Ro24-5531), a new deltanoid (vitamin D analogue) for prevention of breast cancer in the rat. Cancer Res., 54(7): 1653-1656, 1994.

# MECHANISMS OF CANCER PREVENTION: EFFECTS OF PROTEASE INHIBITORS ON PROTEASES AND GENE EXPRESSION

Ann R. Kennedy

Dept. of Radiation Oncology, University of
Pennsylvania School of Medicine
Philadelphia, PA 19104

## Abstract

Our studies utilizing different types of protease inhibitors as anticarcinogenic agents in in vivo and in vitro systems have recently been reviewed (1). These studies suggest that the protease inhibitors which prevent carcinogenesis are affecting processes in the early stages of carcinogenesis, although they can be effective at long time periods after carcinogen exposure in both in vitro and in vivo systems. While there is strong evidence that these protease inhibitors can affect both the initiation and promotion stages of carcinogenesis, they have no effect on cells which are already transformed. Our results have suggested that the first event in carcinogenesis is a high frequency epigenetic event and that a later event, presumably genetic, leads to the malignant state. Protease inhibitors appear to be capable of reversing the initiating event, presumably by stopping an ongoing cellular process begun by carcinogen exposure. The major lines of investigation on the mechanism of the protease inhibitor suppression of carcinogenesis relate to the ability of anticarcinogenic protease inhibitors to affect: 1) the expression of certain oncogenes, and 2) the levels of certain types of proteolytic activities. The anticarcinogenic protease inhibitors have no observable effects on normal cells, but have the ability to reverse carcinogen-induced cellular changes for several different

71

endpoints studied.

The most direct method of determining the mechanism of action of the anticarcinogenic protease inhibitors is to identify and characterize the proteases with which they interact. In the cells of the in vivo and in vitro systems in which we've observed that protease inhibitors can prevent carcinogenesis, only a few proteases have been observed to interact with the anticarcinogenic protease inhibitors. Proteases have been identified by both substrate hydrolysis and affinity chromatography. Utilizing substrate hydrolysis, we have examined the ability of cell homogenates to cleave specific substrates and have then determined the ability of various protease inhibitors to affect that hydrolyzing activity. Utilizing affinity chromatography, specific proteases directly interacting with the anticarcinogenic protease inhibitors can be identified. The Boc-Val-Pro-Arg-MCA hydrolyzing activity was identified by substrate hydrolysis and a 43 kDa protease has been identified by affinity chromatography. There is evidence that both of these different proteolytic activities are playing a role in the prevention of carcinogenesis by protease inhibitors.

Our studies on anticarcinogenic protease inhibitors have suggested that the Bowman-Birk Inhibitor (BBI), derived from soybeans, is a particularly effective anti-carcinogenic protease inhibitor. BBI has been studied both as a pure protease inhibitor, purified BBI (PBBI), and as an extract of soybeans enriched in BBI, termed BBI concentrate (BBIC). PBBI and/or BBIC have been shown to suppress carcinogenesis: 1) in three different species (mice, rats and hamsters), 2) in several organ systems/tissue types (colon, liver, lung, esophagus and cheek pouch [oral epithelium]), 3) in cells of both epithelial and connective tissue origin, 4) when given to animals by several different routes of administration (including the diet), 5) leading to different types of cancer (e.g., squamous cell carcinomas, adenocarcinomas, angiosarcomas, etc.), and 6) induced by a wide variety of chemical and physical carcinogens (1). We originally identified BBI as an anticarcinogenic agent in an in vitro transformation assay system. BBI, as BBIC, has recently risen to the human trial stage. In human trials, elevated levels of proteolytic activities known to be affected by BBI are serving as intermediate marker endpoints human trials, elevated levels of proteolytic activities known to be affected by BBI are serving as intermediate marker endpoints (IME) in the cells of tissues at higher than normal risks of cancer development. In previous animal studies, we have observed that BBI is capable of bringing such elevated levels of proteolytic activity back to normal levels in normal appearing tissues. We have recently observed that BBI treatment can increase the levels of proteolytic activities in pre-malignant tissues. We hypothesize that the increased levels of proteolytic activities in pre-malignant cells and tissues are associated with a cell killing effect, leading to a degradation of the pre-malignant lesions. Although the mechanism for the anticarcinogenic effect(s) of BBI is unclear, BBI is a highly promising human cancer chemopreventive agent.

Introduction
Many vegetables contain protease inhibitors which could be useful as cancer chemopreventive agents, as has been reviewed (1). Soybeans are unusually rich in protease inhibitor activity; protease inhibitors comprise as much as 6% of the total soybean protein. Several protease inhibitors are present in soybeans. The best characterized of these inhibitors are soybean trypsin inhibitor (SBTI) (2) and BBI (3). SBTI has a molecular weight of about 21,000 and has primarily trypsin inhibitory activity; BBI has a molecular weight of about 8000 and inhibits chymotrypsin and trypsin (3). The other soybean protease inhibitors have not been as fully characterized as BBI and SBTI, but are known to inhibit trypsin (4). BBI is the only known protease inhibitor in soybeans with the ability to inhibit chymotrypsin. BBI serves as the best characterized protease inhibitor of the Bowman-Birk family of protease inhibitors, present primarily in legumes. Other members of the Bowman-Birk family of molecules, such as the chick pea inhibitor, are equally as effective as BBI in chymotrypsin inhibitor activity (3) and the ability to suppress transformation in vitro (5).

It is believed that the ability to inhibit chymotrypsin is the anticarcinogenic activity of the BBI family of molecules (5). The BBI family of protease inhibitors have extraordinary properties. BBI has 7 disulfide bonds which make it an exceptionally stable molecule. The ability to inhibit trypsin and chymotrypsin is maintained in BBI-type molecules during the like molecules survive the digestive process. After the ingestion of BBI by animals, BBI reaches the intestines in an intact form and is taken up into the bloodstream (presumably via paracellular transport). BBI excreted into the urine has the same molecular weight and the same ability to inhibit proteases as native BBI (7, 8). It is believed that BBI will have the ability to prevent cancer in many different organ systems in the body, as has been reviewed (1). BBI has recently risen to the human trial stage as a cancer chemopreventive agent as an extract of soybeans enriched in BBI, called Bowman Birk Inhibitor Concentrate (BBIC). Although it would be preferable to study BBI as purified BBI (PBBI) in human cancer prevention trials, this would be prohibitive in cost at present. BBIC works as well as PBBI in various in vivo and in vitro carcinogenesis assay systems, as has been reviewed elsewhere (1, 9, 10).

BBIC is far better than soybeans themselves as a human cancer chemopreventive agent for the following reasons.
1) There are several agents in soybeans, in soybean flour, and in various commercial preparations of soybeans that have the ability to promote transformation in vitro, and presumably, the ability to enhance carcinogenesis in vivo (as discussed to some extent in refs. 5 and 10). The assay system in which BBI was originally identified as an anticarcinogenic agent (7) was used to develop the methods of production of BBIC so that its cancer preventive ability would be maintained during the manufacturing process (while soybean constituents which enhance transformation are removed) (6).
2) Compounds are removed from BBIC which are known to mask the anticarcinogenic activity of BBI, as has been discussed (5, 10). These low molecular weight compounds are removed from BBIC by dialysis or ultrafiltration.
3) Other activities are removed from BBIC which are likely to be harmful, including much of the trypsin inhibitor activity. There is far more trypsin inhibitor activity in soybeans than chymotrypsin inhibitory activity. As discussed above, our publications have shown that it is the chymotrypsin inhibitory activity of BBI that is responsible for the anticarcinogenic effect (e.g., 5). There are 2 protease inhibitor sites in BBI; the chymotrypsin inhibitory site is distant and separable from the trypsin inhibitory site (3). The

many other soybean protease inhibitors are known to inhibit trypsin but, presumably, do not inhibit chymotrypsin. Thus, normal soybean-derived preparations are known to have far more trypsin inhibitory activity than chymotrypsin inhibitory activity. Trypsin inhibitory activity is the activity associated with pancreatic pathology in rats, while the chymotrypsin inhibitory activity of the soybean protease inhibitors is not associated with rat pancreatic pathology (3). In BBIC, the trypsin inhibitory activity of the soybean preparation has been greatly reduced such that it is only a small fraction of the protease inhibitory activity present in BBIC. (The strength of BBIC as a cancer preventive agent is measured in Chymotrypsin Inhibitor [C.I.] units [10].) No pancreatic pathology or other pathology attributable to BBIC has been observed in three species of animals in studies performed in our laboratory (1, 10-20) or in the two species of animals (dogs and rats) studied over a period of months at the Southern Research Institute (SRI). The SRI dog and rat studies were performed with doses of BBIC which were orders of magnitude above those proposed for use in human populations, as has been reviewed (10-12).

Our mechanistic studies on the protease inhibitor suppression of carcinogenesis have primarily focused on the ability of the anticarcinogenic protease inhibitors to affect the levels of expression of certain proto-oncogenes (21-27) and proteolytic activities (16, 28-37), as has been recently reviewed (1, 10-12, 38-41). The findings that protease inhibitors suppress the levels of expression of novel proteases and proto-oncogenes have now been confirmed by many other investigators (e.g. 42-46). Our mechanistic studies have led directly to the development of appropriate intermediate marker endpoints (IME) being utilized in human trials using BBIC as the cancer preventive agent. An example of our use of levels of proteolytic activities as IME for BBIC clinical trials is given in ref. 47. At this point in our research program, the results on IME in people (and animals) are driving the major mechanistic studies which are currently being performed, so these studies will be briefly described here.

Our studies of levels of proteolytic activities in people with a pre-malignant oral lesion (leukoplakia) have led to some surprising

results (47). One of the expectations in these studies was that
tissues with a higher than normal cancer risk, such as leukoplakia,
would have elevated levels of proteolytic activity compared to
normal tissue--and this would be an indication that they
represented an "initiated" cell population. This was clearly the
case for many patients with leukoplakia (47). Another
expectation was that cancer preventive agents such as BBI and β-
carotene would be able to reduce the elevated levels of proteolytic
activities to normal levels in parallel with reducing the risk of
cancer development, as BBI is clearly able to reduce the
carcinogen-elevated levels of proteolytic activity (in normal-
appearing areas of buccal mucosa) in parallel with the
suppression of carcinogenesis (16, 17). β-carotene and BBI have
similar suppressive effects on hamster oral carcinogenesis (16, 17,
48) and β-carotene is known to cause the regression of
leukoplakia in some patients (as reviewed in ref. 49). The
surprising finding in our IME studies was that some patients
treated with β-carotene had extremely high levels of proteolytic
activities, which were far higher than expected for the elevated
levels occurring in patients with leukoplakia (47). We have
hypothesized that it is the induction of extremely high levels of
proteolytic activities by β-carotene that causes the tissue
destruction necessary for the regression of leukoplakia (47).

We have now performed many studies in several different cell
culture systems representative of pre-malignant tissue in vivo and
observed that BBI increases the levels of the marker proteolytic
activities which have been described (47). These results suggest a
new hypothesis for cancer prevention by BBI--i.e., that BBI
induces proteases involved in the destruction of pre-malignant
tissue. This effect could explain the mechanism by which
BBI/BBIC prevents cancer and reduces the levels of many
different types of pre-malignant lesions even when applied to
tissue many months after carcinogen treatment and at a time
when it is known that such pre-malignant tissue is present in
tissues (e.g. 17). The reason that the BBI induction of proteolytic
activity was not observed in our previous studies is that we have
focused on carcinogen-treated normal tissues for our studies of
levels of proteolytic activity in vivo (e.g. 16). It is now clear that

BBI/BBIC has opposite effects in normal tissue exposed to carcinogens and pre-malignant lesions in the same tissue. It reduces the levels of proteolytic activity in carcinogen-treated normal appearing tissue (which has elevated levels of activity in response to carcinogen exposure (e.g. 16) and it increases these same activities in pre-malignant tissues.

Our new finding that BBI can either increase or decrease the levels of proteolytic activities in cells suggests that the relationship between BBI and the levels of proteolytic activities in cells is more complicated than a simple enzyme inhibition by the protease inhibitor. There may well be more than one mechanism by which BBI serves as an anticarcinogenic agent. It is also conceivable that more than one type of proteolytic activity is measured by the proteolytic activities serving as IME in our studies. From our present perspective, BBI appears to be affecting the levels of proteolytic activities serving as IME in our studies by affecting the levels of expression of the genes coding for these proteolytic activities in cells, and thus, could be expected to either increase or decrease the expression levels of such genes. As clearly observed and described above, BBI treatment results in both increases or decreases in the levels of proteolytic activities serving as IME. For these IME, it is known from various in vivo and in vitro studies that BBI does not affect the endogenous levels of these proteolytic activities, but has the ability to result in either increased or decreased levels of these activities depending on the status of the cells/tissues being studied (i.e., whether the cells are normal or pre-malignant in nature). It has been observed that the BBI produced changes in levels of the IME never go below the endogenous levels of the proteolytic activities routinely observed in normal cells or tissues of the types being studied, again suggesting that it is not simply the effect of a protease/protease inhibitor interaction that we have been studying, but instead the ability of BBI to regulate the expression of genes coding for certain types of proteolytic activities.

Our current hypothesis is that BBI is affecting the levels of proteolytic activities serving as IME in our studies by its effects on gene expression. Whatever the mechanism or mechanisms, BBI is clearly a highly effective cancer preventive agent in the carcinogenesis model systems studied in our laboratory.

Acknowledgments. The research investigations discussed here have been supported by NIH Grants CA-22704 and CA-46496.

1.  Kennedy, A.R.: Overview: Anticarcinogenic activity of protease inhibitors. In: Protease Inhibitors as Cancer Chemopreventive Agents, edited by Walter Troll and Ann R. Kennedy, Plenum Publishing Corporation, pp. 9-64, 1993.
2.  Kunitz, M.: Crystalline soybean trypsin inhibitor. J. Gen. Physiol. 30:291-310, 1947.
3.  Birk, Y.: Proteinase inhibitors from plant sources. In: Methods in Enzymology, Vol. 45:695-751, 1975.
4.  Hwang, D.L.R., Davis-Lin, K.T., Yang, W.K. and Foard, D.T.: Purification, partial characterization and immunological relationships of multiple low molecular weight proteinase inhibitors of soybean. Biochem. Biophy. Acta. 495:369-382, 1977.
5.  Yavelow, J., Collins, M., Birk, Y., Troll, W. and Kennedy, A.R.: Nanomolar concentrations of Bowman-Birk soybean protease inhibitor suppress X-ray induced transformation in vitro. Proc. Natl. Acad. Sci. USA 82: 5395-5399, 1985.
6.  Yavelow, J., Gidlund, M., and Troll, W.: Protease inhibitors from processed legumes effectively inhibit superoxide generation in response to TPA. Carcinogenesis 3: 135-138, 1982.
7.  Yavelow, J., Finlay, T.H., Kennedy, A.R. and Troll, W.: Bowman-Birk soybean protease inhibitor as an anticarcinogen. Cancer Res. 43: 2454-2459, 1983.
8.  Billings, P.C., St. Clair, W.H., Maki, P.A. and Kennedy, A.R.: Distribution of the Bowman Birk protease inhibitor in mice following oral administration. Cancer Letters 62: 191-197, 1992.
9.  Kennedy, A.R.: In vitro studies of anticarcinogenic protease inhibitors. In: Protease Inhibitors as Cancer Chemopreventive Agents, edited by Walter Troll and Ann R. Kennedy, Plenum Publishing Corporation, pp. 65-91, 1993.
10. Kennedy, A.R., Szuhaj, B.F., Newberne, P.M. and Billings, P.C.: Preparation and production of a cancer chemopreventive agent, Bowman-Birk Inhibitor

Concentrate. Nutr. Cancer 19: 281-302, 1993.

11. Kennedy, A.R.: Prevention of carcinogenesis by protease inhibitors. Cancer Res. (suppl.). 54:1999s-2005s, 1994.

12. Kennedy, A.R.: Cancer prevention by protease inhibitors. Preventive Medicine 22: 796-811, 1993.

13. Weed, H., McGandy, R.B. and Kennedy, A.R.: Protection against dimethylhydrazine induced adenomatous tumors of the mouse prostate by the dietary addition of an extract of soybeans containing the Bowman-Birk protease inhibitor. Carcinogenesis 6: 1239-1241, 1985.

14. St. Clair, W., Billings, P., Carew, J., Keller-McGandy, C., Newberne, P. and Kennedy, A.R.: Suppression of DMH-induced carcinogenesis in mice by dietary addition of the Bowman-Birk protease inhibitor. Cancer Res. 50: 580-586, 1990.

15. Billings, P.C., Newberne, P. and Kennedy, A.R.: Protease inhibitor suppression of prostate and anal gland carcinogenesis induced by dimethylhydrazine. Carcinogenesis 11: 1083-1086, 1990.

16. Messadi, P.V., Billings, P., Shklar, G. and Kennedy, A.R.: Inhibition of oral carcinogenesis by a protease inhibitor. J. Natl. Cancer Inst. 76: 447-452, 1986.

17. Kennedy, A.R., Billings, P.C., Maki, P.A. and Newberne, P.: Effects of various protease inhibitor preparations on oral carcinogenesis in hamsters induced by 7,12-dimethylbenz(a)anthracene. Nutr. Cancer 19: 191-200, 1993.

18. Witschi, H. and Kennedy, A.R.: Modulation of lung tumor development in mice with the soybean-derived Bowman-Birk protease inhibitor. Carcinogenesis 10: 2275-2277, 1989.

19. von Hofe, E., Newberne, P.M. and Kennedy, A.R.: Inhibition of N-nitrosomethylbenzylamine induced esophageal neoplasms by the Bowman-Birk protease inhibitor. Carcinogenesis 12: 2147-2150, 1991.

20. Evans, S.M., Szuhaj, B.F., Van Winkle, T., Michel, K. and Kennedy, A.R.: Protection against metastasis of radiation induced thymic lymphosarcoma and weight loss in C57Bl/6NCr1BR mice by an autoclave resistant factor present in soybeans. Radiation Res. 132: 259-262, 1992.

21. Chang, J.D., Billings, P. and Kennedy, A.R.: C-myc expression is reduced in antipain-treated proliferating C3H10T1/2 cells. Biochem. Biophys. Res. Comm. 133: 830-835, 1985.

22. Chang, J.D. and Kennedy, A.R.: Cell cycle progression of C3H10T1/2 and 3T3 cells in the absence of a transient increase in c-myc RNA levels. Carcinogenesis 9: 17-20, 1988.

23. Caggana, M. and Kennedy, A.R.: C-fos mRNA levels are reduced in the presence of antipain and the Bowman-Birk inhibitor. Carcinogenesis 10: 2145-2148, 1989.

24. Chang, J.D., Li, J.-H., Billings, P.C. and Kennedy, A.R.: Effects of protease inhibitors on c-myc expression in normal and transformed C3H10T1/2 cells. Molec. Carc. 3: 226-232, 1990.

25. St. Clair, W.H., Billings, P.C. and Kennedy, A.R.: The effects of the Bowman-Birk protease inhibitor on c-myc expression and cell proliferation in the unirradiated and irradiated mouse colon. Cancer Letters 52: 145-152, 1990.

26. Li, J.-H., Billings, P.C. and Kennedy, A.R.: Induction of oncogene expression by sodium arsenite in C3H/10T1/2 cells; inhibition of c-myc expression by protease inhibitors. The Cancer Journal 5: 354-358, 1992.

27. Chang, J.D. and Kennedy, A.R.: Suppression of c-myc by anticarcinogenic protease inhibitors. In: Protease Inhibitors as Cancer Chemopreventive Agents, edited by Walter Troll and Ann R. Kennedy, Plenum Publishing Corporation, pp. 265-280, 1993.

28. Long, S., Quigley, J., Troll, W. and Kennedy, A.R.: Protease inhibitor antipain suppresses TPA induction of plasminogen activator in transformable mouse embryo fibroblasts. Carcinogenesis 2: 933-936, 1981.

29. Billings, P.C., Carew, J.A., Keller-McGandy, C.E., Goldberg, A. and Kennedy, A.R.: A serine protease activity in C3H/10T1/2 cells that is inhibited by anticarcinogenic protease inhibitors. Proc. Natl. Acad. Sci. 84: 4801-4805, 1987.

30. Billings, P.C., St. Clair, W., Owen, A.J. and Kennedy, A.R.: Potential intracellular target proteins of the anticarcinogenic Bowman-Birk protease inhibitor identified by affinity chromatography. Cancer Res. 48: 1798-1802, 1988.

31. Billings, P.C., Morrow, A.R., Ryan, C.A. and Kennedy, A.R.: Inhibition of radiation-induced transformation of C3H/10T1/2 cells by carboxypeptidase Inhibitor I and Inhibitor II from potatoes. Carcinogenesis 10: 687-691, 1989.

32. Carew, J.A. and Kennedy, A.R.: Identification of a proteolytic activity which responds to anticarcinogenic protease inhibitors in C3H10T1/2 cells. Cancer Letters 49: 153-163, 1990.

33. Billings, P.C., Habres, J.M. and Kennedy, A.R.: Inhibition of radiation-induced transformation of C3H10T1/2 cells by specific protease substrates. Carcinogenesis 11: 329-332, 1990.

33. Oreffo, V.I.C., Billings, P.C., Kennedy, A.R. and Witschi, H.: Acute effects of the Bowman-Birk protease inhibitor in mice. Toxicology 69: 165-176, 1991.

34. Billings, P.C., Habres, J.M., Liao, D.C. and Tuttle, S.W.: A protease activity in human fibroblasts which is inhibited by the anticarcinogenic Bowman-Birk protease inhibitor. Cancer Res. 51: 5539-5543, 1991.

35. Billings, P.C. and Habres, J.M.: A growth regulated protease activity which is inhibited by the anticarcinogenic Bowman-Birk protease inhibitor. Proc. Nat. Acad. Sci. USA 89: 3120-3124, 1992.

36. Billings, P.C.: Approaches to studying the target enzymes of anticarcinogenic protease inhibitors. In: Protease Inhibitors as Cancer Chemopreventive Agents, edited by Walter Troll and Ann R. Kennedy, Plenum Publishing Corporation, 1993.

37. Habres, J.M. and Billings, P.C.: Intestinal epithelial cells contain a high molecular weight protease subject to inhibition by anticarcinogenic protease inhibitors. Cancer Letters 135-142, 1992.

38. Kennedy, A.R. and Billings, P.C.: Anticarcinogenic actions of protease inhibitors. In: Anticarcinogenesis and Radiation Protection, edited by P. A. Cerutti, O.F. Nygaard, and M.G. Simic, Plenum Press, New York, pp. 285-295, 1987.

39. Kennedy, A.R.: Promotion and other interactions between agents in the induction of transformation in vitro in fibroblasts. In: Mechanisms of Tumor Promotion, Vol. III, "Tumor Promotion and Carcinogenesis In Vitro" edited by T.J. Slaga, CRC Press, Inc., Chapter 2, pp. 13-55, 1984.

40. Kennedy, A.R.: Is there a critical target gene for the first step in carcinogenesis? Environ. Health Perspectives 93: 199-203, 1991.

41.  Kennedy, A.R.: Potential mechanisms of antitumorigenesis by protease inhibitors. In: <u>Antimutagenesis and Anticarcinogenesis Mechanisms: III</u>, edited by G. Bronzetti, A. Hayatsu, S. DeFlora, M.D. Waters, D.M. Shankel, pp. 301-308. Plenum Publishing Corporation, 1993.

42.  Yavelow, J., Caggana, M. and Beck, K.A.: Proteases occurring in the cell membrane: a possible receptor for the Bowman Birk type of protease inhibitors. Cancer Res. 47:1598-1601, 1987.

43.  Yavelow, J., Schepis, L.T., Nichols, J., Jr. and Ritchie, G.: Cell membrane enzymes containing chymotrypsin-like activity. In: <u>Protease Inhibitors as Cancer Chemopreventive Agents</u>, edited by Walter Troll and Ann R. Kennedy, Plenum Publishing Corporation, pp. 217-226, 1993.

44.  Garte, S.J., Currie, D.C. and Troll, W.: Inhibition of H-ras oncogene transformation of NIH3T3 cells by protease inhibitors. Cancer Res. 47: 3159-3162, 1987.

45.  Garte, S.J. and Troll, W.: Protease inhibitor suppression of <u>ras</u> oncogene transformation. In: <u>Protease Inhibitors as Cancer Chemopreventive Agents</u>, edited by Walter Troll and Ann R. Kennedy, Plenum Publishing Corporation, pp. 251-264, 1993.

46.  St. Clair, W.H. and St. Clair, D.K.: Effect of the Bowman-Birk protease inhibitor on the expression of oncogenes in the irradiated rat prostate. Cancer Res. 51: 4539-4543, 1991.

47.  Manzone, H., Billings, P.C., Cummings, W.N., Feldman, R., Odell, C.S., Horan, A., Atiba, J.O., Meyskens, F.L., Jr., and Kennedy, A.R.: Levels of proteolytic activities as intermediate marker endpoints in oral carcinogenesis. Cancer Epidemiology Biomarkers & Prevention (in press).

48.  Suda, D., Schwartz, J. and Shklar, G.: Inhibition of experimental oral carcinogenesis by topical β-carotene. Carcinogenesis 7: 711-715, 1986.

49.  Garewal, H.S. and Meyskens, F., Jr.: Retinoids and carotenoids in the prevention of oral cancer: a critical appraisal. Cancer Epidem. Biomarkers Prevention 1: 155-159, 1992.

# ANTIOXIDANTS AND CANCER PREVENTION

## *IN VIVO* AND *IN VITRO*

Andrija Kornhauser, Lark A. Lambert, Wayne G. Warner,
Rong Rong Wei, Sukadev Lavu and William C. Timmer

Center for Food Safety and Applied Nutrition, U.S. Food and Drug
Administration, Washington, D.C. 20204.

## INTRODUCTION

The role of dietary factors in modulating cancer continues to be vigorously investigated. In particular there has been increased interest in various potential anticancer agents, including biological antioxidants such as carotenoids, retinoids, ascorbic acid, and $\alpha$-tocopherol.

Possible mechanisms for the induction of cancer include the effects of free radicals and activated oxygen species, which can damage cells and tissues. These highly reactive molecules can be produced as a result of cellular metabolism or from environmental factors such as pollution and certain dietary components. Biological defenses against free radicals and reactive oxygen species include endogenous enzymes such as superoxide dismutase, catalase, and glutathione peroxidase. In addition, other factors that may play a role in disease prevention are micronutrients such as ß-carotene, selenium, zinc, and vitamins A, C, and E.

ß-Carotene, a micronutrient known for its ability to quench singlet oxygen and scavenge free radicals, is found in foods such as carrots, broccoli, spinach, kale, and sweet potatoes. Although ß-carotene is an important precursor for vitamin A, an increasing number of studies have indicated that protection against cancer may be due to the ß-carotene molecule itself and not its provitamin A function (1). Epidemiological studies involving ß-carotene have shown a strong protective association most consistently against lung cancer (1). ß-Carotene has been associated with the delay or reduction of tumors in other cancers, including those of

*83*

the breast (2), cervix (3), stomach, and esophagus (4). Experimental evidence for protective effects of ß-carotene against various cancers in animals includes delayed or reduced tumors of the colon (5), skin (6,7), and buccal pouch (8). Research has also indicated ß-carotene's ability to enhance the immune defense system (9).

Vitamin E, which is found in foods such as vegetable oils, nuts, seeds, green leafy vegetables, and wheat germ, is important for scavenging free radicals. Vitamin E intercalates into the lipid bilayers of cell membranes, where it terminates free radical chain reactions and confines membrane damage. Epidemiological studies have shown protective associations of vitamin E against cancers of the breast (10), lung (11), female reproductive organs (12), and other organs (13). Animal studies have shown protective effects of vitamin E in reducing chemically induced colon tumors in mice (14), oral tumors in hamsters (15), and UV-induced skin cancer in mice (16).

In this report we describe our *in vivo* and *in vitro* research results for ß-carotene and vitamin E. Our *in vivo* study involved the investigation of the individual effects of these antioxidants as well as the possible synergistic effects of the combination of ß-carotene and vitamin E. Our *in vitro* work involved the examination of uptake, metabolism, and distribution of ß-carotene in mouse fibroblasts and preliminary studies of psoralen + ultraviolet A light (PUVA)-induced biomarkers.

## *IN VIVO* STUDY

Protective but Nonsynergistic Effect of ß-Carotene and Vitamin E on Skin Tumorigenesis in SKH Mice.

Materials and Methods. Forty-five, female Skh-1 hairless mice, 80 days old, were placed in each of four diet groups. The control group received standard mouse chow (pellets). The three other groups received mouse chow fortified with one of the following: (*1*) ß-carotene (0.5%, wt/wt, type 1, all *trans*, synthetic, crystalline, Sigma Chemical Co., St. Louis, MO), (*2*) vitamin E (d-α-tocopheryl acid succinate, 0.12%, wt/wt, Henkel Corp., Kankakee, IL), or (*3*) ß-carotene (0.5%) + vitamin E (0.12%). Each batch of fortified diet was analyzed for $\beta$-carotene and/or α-tocopheryl succinate. Details for this study can be found in Lambert *et al.* (17).

Mouse skin tumors were generated by a two-stage, initiation-promotion treatment regimen. After receiving the diets for 11 weeks, mice were treated topically on the dorsal skin with the carcinogen (initiator), 7,12-dimethylbenz[*a*]anthracene (DMBA), followed 1 week later by the promotion regimen with phorbol 12-myristate 13-acetate (PMA).

After treatment with the carcinogen, the tumors on each animal were counted once per week for 27 weeks. Tumors were first counted when they reached approximately 1 mm in height. The approximate location of each growth was plotted on a diagram of each mouse. The total number of tumors observed on each mouse during its lifetime, regardless of whether the tumors later regressed, was defined as "cumulative tumors."

Results. The week of appearance of tumors 1-8 in the ß-carotene + vitamin E diet group was significantly delayed (Kruskal-Wallis Test, $p <$ 0.05) compared with the weeks in which the first 10 tumors appeared in the standard diet group. Also, the week of appearance of the first tumor in the ß-carotene diet group was delayed. The cumulative numbers of tumors found each week in the supplemented diet- and standard diet-fed mice are shown in Figure 1.Cumulative tumor totals at week 27 were 733 for the standard diet group, 579 for the ß-carotene + vitamin E diet group (21% less than the number for the control), 551 for the vitamin E diet group

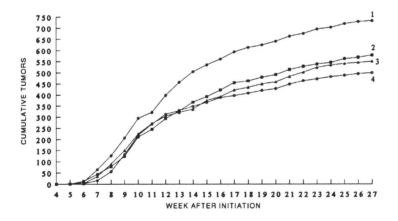

Figure 1. Tumors resulted from a DMBA–initiated (150 μg/mouse), PMA–promoted (5 μg/mouse, multiple applications), two–stage tumorigenesis treatment regimen. Mice were fed one of four diets 10 weeks before chemical initiation and for the remainder of the study: (**1**) standard (Ralston Purina Rodent Chow), (**2**) 0.5% β– carotene (all *trans*, crystalline) + 0.12% vitaimn E succinate, (**3**) 0.12% vitamin E succinate, and (**4**) 0.5% β–carotene. Supplements were mixed with standard chow. After DMBA treatment, mice were examined for tumors once per week for 27 weeks.

(25% less than the number for the control), and 500 for the ß-carotene diet group (32% less than the number for the control). The results of statistical analyses, which compared the cumulative tumor data for the standard-diet group with the data for the three supplemented-diet groups, yielded $p =$ 0.03, 0.06, and 0.04 for the ß-carotene, vitamin E, and ß-carotene + vitamin E diet groups, respectively.

Mice in the various groups were weighed 17 times during the study. Statistical analyses showed that the rate of growth was not significantly different between dietary groups. An analysis of covariance showed that body weight did not affect the cumulative tumor data.

Levels of accumulated ß-carotene and/or α-tocopherol were determined in serum, skin, and livers of noncarcinogen-treated mice. Higher levels of α-tocopherol were found in both serum and skin, compared with levels for the standard-diet group. The two groups that received β-carotene showed higher skin levels of β-carotene in all determinations. In contrast, levels of β-carotene in the serum of animals receiving β-carotene remained near the detection limit of the analysis (16 ng/ml) until the end of the study. α-Tocopherol levels in both skin and serum of mice that received only ß-carotene supplementation were lower than those for the standard-diet controls. Supplementation with 0.12% α-tocopheryl succinate did not result in consistently greater storage of α-tocopherol in the liver. However, dietary supplementation with β-carotene resulted in significantly more liver β-carotene for both the ß-carotene and ß-carotene + vitamin E diet groups. Dietary supplementation with β-carotene resulted in lower levels of α-tocopherorol in the liver.

Discussion. Although animal experiments (5-8,14-16) and epidemiological studies (1-4,10-13) have demonstrated the protective effects of ß-carotene and vitamin E for a variety of cancers, few studies have investigated possible synergistic effects of the combination of these nutrients.

Shklar and co-workers (18) showed that a combination of β-carotene and vitamin E was more effective in regressing epidermoid carcinomas than the separate administration of these micronutrients. Our laboratory was interested in determining if a synergistic protective effect against skin tumorigenesis could be observed in a system in which the individually fed supplements were also effective in reducing the number of tumors. Our previous work (7) demonstrated a 39% reduction in skin tumors in Skh mice by a 3% dietary supplement of ß-carotene. In the present study, the ß-carotene concentration fed to the mice was reduced to 0.5%. The 32% decrease in the number of skin tumors confirms our previous findings of the tumor inhibitory properties of ß-carotene, even at this lower level of supplementation. A 0.12% supplement of vitamin E also had a similar effect. The number of skin tumors decreased 25% compared with that for animals fed the standard diet. The group fed the dietary combination of ß-carotene + vitamin E, although showing a statistically significant reduction in tumors compared with the number for the standard-diet group, showed no synergistic effect. The degree of protection against tumorigenesis in the ß-carotene + vitamin E group was not greater than that for either the ß-carotene or vitamin E diet group.

An explanation for the lack of a synergistic effect against tumorigenesis may be obtained from our previous study (7) in which a six-times greater amount of crystalline ß-carotene was fed to the mice. As previously mentioned, the degree of tumor inhibition was similar for both ß-carotene groups in the two studies. This finding indicates that either an upper limit for protection was reached or the biological system was saturated with antioxidant. Therefore, no further protective effect was possible by the addition of the antioxidant vitamin E to a diet already fortified with ß-carotene. In addition, because differences in the number of tumors between any of the diet-supplemented groups were not statistically significant, we reasoned that the protection resulted from nonspecific antioxidant effects rather than the actions of ß-carotene or vitamin E through different mechanisms.

Studies by other investigators have shown that restricted caloric intake provides protective effects against carcinogenesis (19). Therefore, we were concerned that supplementation of the diet might affect the amount or utilization of food eaten by the animals. Mice were weighed 17 times throughout our study to determine if the various diets affected body weights. The growth rates of the mice in the four diet groups were statistically analyzed for 3 weeks before and for weeks 2-10 of the dietary regimen, before chemical initiation. During these weeks the effects of chemical treatments and the added weight of tumors would not be factors in body weight change. Results of the analyses showed that differences in the growth rates of the animals between any of the four dietary groups were not statistically significant.

As an indication of absorption and distribution of vitamin E and ß-carotene in the animals, levels of these supplements were determined in liver, serum, and skin. Liver levels of both ß-carotene and vitamin E were higher with the ß-carotene + vitamin E diet supplementation. The ß-carotene diet resulted in higher ß-carotene levels but lower $\alpha$-tocopherol levels in the liver. Supplementation with vitamin E resulted in little difference in α-tocopherol or ß-carotene liver levels compared with those for animals fed the standard diet. Skin levels of ß-carotene and α-tocopherol were greater for animals that received these supplements than for animals fed the standard diet. Only animals fed the vitamin E diets had consistently higher serum levels. The small increases in ß-carotene serum levels, which were observed only at week 43, emphasize the difficulty in obtaining elevated serum titers in rodents for the level of this micronutrient fed in our study. Supplementation with ß-carotene resulted in lower α-tocopherol levels in skin and serum.

The chemical two-stage, DMBA-PMA treatment regimen used in our experiment involves complex mechanisms with numerous molecular events for the induction of tumors. The carcinogen DMBA, used for initiation, is thought to act by inducing somatic cell mutation. The promoter, PMA, completes the process of tumorigenesis. Mechanisms for this process include the induction of reactive oxygen species and free radicals, especially as a result of the inflammatory response (20). ß-Carotene or vitamin E has been found to eliminate or modify some of the products, effects, or events involved in the tumorigenesis process in various systems. Both ß-carotene and vitamin E are considered important chain-breaking antioxidants for lipid peroxidation (21,22), thus stabilizing membrane structures and functions. Vitamin E inhibits PMA-stimulated protein kinase C activity, the main phorbol ester receptor, in mouse skin (23), inhibits PMA-induced ornithine decarboxylase, a key regulatory enzyme in the growth process, *in vivo* and *in vitro* (24), and shows limited enhancement of gap junctional communication (25), which can be inhibited by tumor promoters. ß-Carotene effects include increasing the expression of a gene that encodes a major gap junction protein in mouse cells (26), inhibiting PMA-induced arachidonic acid, which can be metabolized to produce free radicals, in chick embryo fibroblasts (27), inhibiting DMBA-induced transformation of mouse mammary cells *in vitro* (28), and providing anticlastogenic effects against direct-acting mutagens in hamsters (29).

## *IN VITRO* STUDIES

### β-Carotene Uptake, Metabolism, and Distribution in BALB/c 3T3 Cells

The need to clarify the role of β-carotene in protection against carcinogenesis has given rise to an increasing interest in more controllable animal and *in vitro* studies. *In vitro* studies of β-carotene have increasingly proven valuable for evaluating the role and mechanism of β-carotene protection. In a general sense, similar problems are encountered in the development of both animal and *in vitro* studies of β-carotene protection. Since β-carotene is a highly lipophilic compound, poorly absorbed by most animals (30) and cells in culture (31), uptake of β-carotene and distribution to the target site are, therefore, of primary importance in developing experimental models. In addition, a central question with regard to mechanism is the importance of provitamin A activity in the protective function of β-carotene. The present investigation was designed to address these questions in pursuit of an *in vitro* system appropriate for studying how β-carotene functions as a protective agent at the cellular level.

We have examined several critical features in designing an *in vitro* system for studying the protective action of β-carotene. These include (*1*) the form of β-carotene used for cellular uptake, (*2*) the cellular metabolism of β-carotene, and (*3*) the subcellular distribution of β-carotene. It was determined that β-carotene in a water-dispersible formulation is readily taken up by BALB/c 3T3 cells. In contrast, the uptake of β-carotene added to media in an organic solvent is greatly reduced. This dependence of cellular uptake on the form of β-carotene should be considered when dose-response relationships derived from *in vitro* studies are evaluated. A significant increase in intracellular retinol was observed following a 3-day exposure of BALB/c 3T3 cells. This result suggests that the ability to metabolize β-carotene to retinoids is not limited to cells of intestinal or hepatic origin.

Materials and Methods. Crystalline β-carotene (synthetic, all *trans*, type I, Sigma Chemical Co.) was dissolved in acetone (46 $\mu$g/ml, 86 $\mu$M) or ethanol (7.6 $\mu$g/ml, 14.2 $\mu$M). Sufficient β-carotene in acetone or ethanol was added to culture media to yield a final β-carotene concentration of 0.3 $\mu$M or 0.16 $\mu$g/ml. The medium was then incubated for 30 min at 37°C, and passed through a 0.45 $\mu$m filter. The concentration of β-carotene in media was measured by HPLC analysis after extraction of media.

β-Carotene and canthaxanthin, formulated as water-dispersible beadlets, were kindly provided by Hoffmann-LaRoche, Nutley, NJ. A beadlet formulation, containing all components except the carotenoids, was used as the control. Stock solutions of these formulations were prepared and analyzed as described earlier (32).

BALB/c 3T3 clone A31-1-1 cells were cultured in Eagle's minimum essential medium (Gibco, Grand Island, NY) supplemented with 7.5% fetal bovine serum (Microbiological Associates Inc., Rockville, MD), antibiotics (100 U/ml penicillin, 100 µg/ml streptomycin), and 2 mM L-glutamine. Cells were used between passages 5 and 12. As required for uptake and metabolism studies, confluent monolayers of cells were treated with media containing the appropriate preparation of β-carotene, canthaxanthin, or control. At selected times after initial treatment, an aliquot of the medium was removed for β-carotene and retinol determinations. Extraction and quantitation of β-carotene, canthaxanthin, and retinol as well as cell fractionation procedures were performed as previously described (32).

Results and Discussion. The method of β-carotene media supplementation greatly affected cellular uptake. Crystalline β-carotene added in an organic solvent was accumulated much less readily than when added in a water-dispersible beadlet formulation.

Cellular accumulation of β-carotene increased rapidly during the first 48 hr of treatment and then appeared to plateau thereafter. However, we found that upon replenishing media at Day 5 with freshly supplemented media, continued accumulation was observed. No β-carotene was found in cells cultured in media containing control beadlets. In addition, none of the described treatments resulted in significant cytotoxicity as measured by cell numbers. β-Carotene was also quantitated in media incubated with cells, as well as without cells, for up to 5 days. A rapid loss of β-carotene was noted in media without cells, while the presence of cells appeared to retard the disappearance of β-carotene.

The effect of media supplementation with β-carotene (3 $\mu$M) or control beadlets on cellular retinol levels is shown in Figure 2. After an apparent lag phase, retinol levels were significantly higher in β-carotene-exposed cells than in control cells. Retinol levels in cells exposed to β-carotene for 5 days were approximately threefold higher than those in cells treated with control beadlets. Addition of β-carotene at Day 5 resulted in an initial decrease in cellular retinol levels, consistent with the well-established rapid exchange of retinol between cells and media (33).

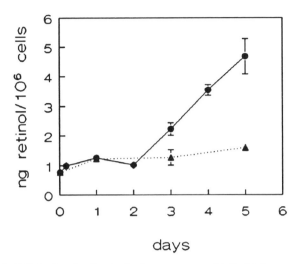

Figure 2. Cellular levels of retinol after treatment with 3 $\mu$M β-carotene (solid line) or control (broken line) beadlets. Data are averages of 3 determinations.

Elevated cellular levels of retinol were maintained for 14 days of continued culture of cells with β-carotene, with media changes every 5 days. Treatment of cells with canthaxanthin (the 4,4'-dioxo analogue of β-carotene, which lacks provitamin A activity (*in vivo*), failed to yield similarly elevated retinol levels, even though cellular uptakes of these two carotenoids were similar (data not shown).

The need to examine the extent and mechanisms of the anticarcinogenic activity of β-carotene has resulted in an increasing number of *in vitro* studies. Both the level and method of media supplementation with β-carotene vary widely in published studies appearing to date. We chose a level of β-carotene supplementation that is similar to those reported for the sera of human subjects receiving β-carotene dietary supplementation and comparable to sera levels of total carotenoids derived from dietary sources (34). The uptake of β-carotene by cells that were incubated in media containing a physiologically relevant level of β-carotene was strongly dependent on the type of β-carotene used. Levels of β-carotene were approximately 15-fold higher in cells incubated with media containing a water-dispersible beadlet formulation of β-carotene than in cells incubated with media containing β-carotene in an organic solvent.

Measurement of cellular uptake of β-carotene can provide valuable information for designing and evaluating both short-duration (e.g. metabolism, antiproliferation, moderation of cytotoxicity) and long-duration (e.g. antimutagenesis) *in vitro* studies. Because of the extremely low water solubility of β-carotene, its decomposition during cell culture, and the effect on cellular uptake of the method of its addition to media, measurement of cellular β-carotene levels is the most direct and reliable indicator of β-carotene exposure *in vitro*. In addition, knowledge of β-carotene cellular levels greatly facilitates comparison of *in vitro* studies with *in vivo* studies, which are beginning to report cellular β-carotene levels (35, 36).

In all *in vitro* studies of the mechanism of β-carotene protective effects, the role of β-carotene's provitamin A activity must be evaluated. Both *in vitro* and *in vivo* studies have demonstated that retinoids are extremely potent modulators of cell toxicity, differentiation, and proliferation. For this reason, even a low level of β-carotene conversion to retinoids may play an important role in the mechanism of β-carotene protective effects. Our results demonstrate that continued culture of BALB/c 3T3 fibroblasts in media containing 3 μM β-carotene results in significant increases in retinol levels both in culture media and in cells, indicating net production of retinol. Because the elevation in levels of retinol in media is dependent on the presence of cells, abiotic decomposition of β-carotene is not responsible for the retinol formation observed.

In conclusion, both animal and epidemiological studies indicate that the biological activity of β-carotene may involve multiple, complex mechanisms. *In vitro* studies of β-carotene are rapidly becoming valuable for elucidating these mechanisms. Carefully designing future *in vitro* studies to incorporate measurements of the cellular uptake, metabolism, and distribution of β-carotene can significantly increase their value.

## Biomarkers and Antioxidants

In this section we describe our preliminary work on the application of molecular probes or biomarkers as endpoints to measure cellular stress. We have chosen to investigate one biochemical and three genetic markers: the DNA product 8-hydroxy-2'-deoxyguanosine (8-OHdG), and three stress response genes: *gadd*45, *gadd*153 (*gadd* = growth arrest and DNA damage), and a heat-shock protein (70 kD gene). Expression of these markers has been shown to be elevated in response to oxidative stress and/or DNA damage. Because of our previous experience in photobiology, we have chosen the PUVA protocol as a model for investigating these biomarkers. In brief, we irradiated cell cultures of human skin fibroblasts (Hs27) with various fluences of ultraviolet A light in the presence of 8-methoxypsoralen (8-MOP). This procedure was used because of indications that PUVA induces oxidative stress. Interestingly, we found that the described PUVA treatment did not increase the 8-OHdG level, compared with that of the control. This result indicated that in this system PUVA treatment did not result in substantial oxidative damage. The 8-OHdG was measured by HPLC with electrochemical detection (37).

The genetic biomarkers were studied by conventional gene expression (Northern analysis) techniques. Typically, RNA was isolated from fibroblasts at various times post-PUVA treatment. The RNA was size-fractionated by gel electrophoresis, capillary blotted to a nitrocellulose filter, hybridized to a $^{32}$P-labeled probe (biomarker), washed at high stringency, and exposed to autoradiographic film. Three probes for stress response genes were used in this preliminary investigation: *gadd*45, *gadd*153, and *hsp*70.

The *gadd* genes were obtained from a library of DNA damage-inducible genes (38). Both of these genes are induced by ultraviolet light radiation as well as agents that alkylate DNA (39). Interestingly, *gadd*153 was not induced in Hs27 fibroblasts up to 5 hours post-PUVA treatment, while *gadd*45 was very weakly induced 1 hour post-PUVA treatment. As a positive control we used methane methanesulfonate (MMS), which is known to produce an increase in expression of the described genetic markers.

Present studies are in progress to examine the effects of selected antioxidants on the described biomarkers. They may yield useful information regarding mechanisms of protection by antioxidants at the molecular level.

## EPILOGUE

The dramatic progress in the understanding of basic biologic and genetic knowledge of normal and transformed cellular growth, which evolved in the last decade, has still not resulted in significant breakthroughs in cancer prevention or therapy. This fact was highlighted in the controversial article by Bailar and Smith (40), which stated that we are losing the war on cancer.  The authors suggested that research on the treatment of cancer be shifted to emphasize prevention if substantial progress against cancer is to be achieved.  Certainly, the war on cancer should be continued on both fronts:  research on therapy as well as prevention.  The use of preventative measures is also supported by the hypothesis that the human diet, as well as lifestyle factors, contributes to up to 70% of cancer deaths, which at least in theory could be prevented (41). It is understandable, therefore, that the concept of chemoprevention has come of age.  Chemoprevention of cancer may be defined as the prevention of various forms of cancers by the use of chemical-pharmaceutical agents that inhibit, delay, or reverse the process of carcinogenesis.  ß-Carotene together with antioxidant vitamins such as α-tocopherol and ascorbic acid is among the agents that have been the focus of an increased number of studies for their possible chemopreventive properties.

Evidence is increasing that free radical reactions are implicated in the development of various degenerative diseases, including cancer.  Along with α-tocopherol, ß-carotene is one of the most efficient free radical scavengers (21).  Although the relevance of animal studies to human experience remains uncertain, *in vivo* studies in our laboratory involving dietary ß-carotene and vitamin E have shown protective effects of these micronutrients against two-stage skin carcinogenesis in mice (7,17).

Important evidence for the role of antioxidant micronutrients in various human chronic diseases is derived from epidemiologic studies which have shown an inverse relationship between human cancer incidence and the intake of food high in carotenoids and antioxidant vitamins.  In the past several years there appears to be a great increase in the number of epidemiological studies reported in the literature, assessing a variety of diseases.  Why are so many studies of this kind being conducted?  One of the reasons is that the major diseases now affecting humans are chronic, degenerative diseases that probably result from several contributing causes, many of which are lifestyle related such as dietary habits, smoking, and exercise.  We must also understand that today's clinical trials involving dietary supplementation generally test agents that may offer only modest improvements to an already healthy diet and, therefore, may give minimal or inconsistent results.

While this manuscript was in preparation, two clinical studies on the effects of antioxidants on human health were published.  One of them described the role of ß-carotene and vitamin E in a large cohort of smokers in Finland, and found that supplementation with ß-carotene resulted in a higher incidence of lung cancer than did supplementation with the placebo

(42). A second study, involving a much smaller population, reported that antioxidants had no effect in preventing cancer of the colon (43), although earlier studies had found a protective antioxidant effect (44,45).

Although the results of these trials do not disprove the possible benefits of antioxidants, they do suggest caution and the need for further studies. The Finish study in particular was the subject of extensive media coverage in the United States, probably because its results were contrary to previously reported findings. This increased media exposure contributed to the confusion of the public, who had previously been informed as to possible beneficial relationships between antioxidants and chronic diseases. As with all scientific evaluations, it is important that we make decisions concerning antioxidants based on the totality of information from all research. In particular, we should not change our diets or habits on the basis of the conclusions of a small number of studies.

It must be remembered that although protective effects of diet-supplemented antioxidants have been observed in many rodent studies and clinical trials, the reduction in cancer risk indicated in many epidemiological studies continues to be strongly related to diets containing high amounts of fruits and vegetables.

In summary, it is hoped that continued intensive research through the combined efforts of epidemiologists, biochemists, toxicologists, and other scientists in related basic disciplines will provide more definitive conclusions regarding the effects of antioxidant vitamins and micronutrients on reducing risk for cancer and other human degenerative diseases. Based on the totality of evidence from epidemiologic, animal, and *in vitro* studies, a relationship is indicated between reduced risk of some diseases, including various cancers, and increased levels of carotenoids along with other antioxidants. In most human studies, however, this relationship is strongest for diets containing high amounts of fruits and vegetables, indicating a possible multiplicity of dietary factors, including those of the antioxidants.

## REFERENCES

1.   Zeigler, RG, Subar, AF, Craft, NE, Ursin, G, Patterson, BH, and Graubard, BI:  "Does ß-Carotene Explain Why Reduced Cancer Risk Is Associated with Vegetable and Fruit Intake?" *Cancer Res* (suppl) **52**, 2060s-2066s, 1992.

2.  Potischman, N, McCulloch, CE, Byers, T, Nemoto, T, Stubbe, N, Milch, R, Parker, R, Rasmussen, KM, Root, M, Graham, S, and Campbell, TC: "Breast Cancer and Dietary and Plasma Concentrations of Carotenoids and Vitamin A." *Am J Clin Nutr* **52**, 909-915, 1990.

3.  Palan, PR, Mikhail, MS, Basu, J, and Romney, SL: "Plasma Levels of Antioxidant ß-Carotene and α-Tocopherol in Uterine Cervix Dysplasias and Cancer." *Nutr Cancer* **15**, 13-20, 1991.

4.  Gaby, SK, and Singh, VN: "ß-Carotene." In *Vitamin Intake and Health, A Scientific Review*, SK Gaby, A Bendich, VN Singh and L Machlin (eds). New York: Marcel Dekker, Inc., 1991, pp 29-57.

5.  Temple, NJ, and Basu, TK: "Protective Effect of ß-Carotene Against Colon Tumors in Mice." *J Natl Cancer Inst* **78**, 1211-1214, 1987.

6.  Mathews-Roth, MM: "Antitumor Activity of ß-Carotene, Canthaxanthin and Phytoene." *Oncology* **39**, 33-37, 1982.

7.  Lambert, LA, Koch, WH, Wamer, WG, and Kornhauser, A: "Antitumor Activity in Skin of Skh and Sencar Mice by Two Dietary ß-Carotene Formulations." *Nutr Cancer* **13**, 213-221, 1990.

8.  Suda, D, Schwartz, J, and Shklar, G: "Inhibition of Experimental Oral Carcinogenesis by Topical ß-Carotene." *Carcinogenesis* **7**, 711-715, 1986.

9.  Bendich, A: "Carotenoids and the Immune Response." *J Nutr* **119**, 112-115, 1989.

10. Wald, NJ, Boreham, J, Hayward, JL, and Bulbrook, RD: "Plasma Retinol, ß-Carotene and Vitamin E Levels in Relation to the Future Risk of Breast Cancer." *Br J Cancer* **49**, 321-324, 1984.

11. Menkes, MS, Comstock, GW, Vuilleumier, JP, Helsing, KJ, Rider, AA, and Brookmeyer, R: "Serum ß-Carotene, Vitamins A and E, Selenium, and the Risk of Lung Cancer." *N Engl J Med* **315**, 1250-1254, 1986.

12. Verreault, R, Chu, J, Mandelson, M, and Shy, K: "A Case-Control Study of Diet and Invasive Cervical Cancer." *Int J Cancer* **43**, 1050-1054, 1989.

13. Gaby, SK, and Machlin, LJ: "Vitamin E." In *Vitamin Intake and Health, A Scientific Review*, SK Gaby, A Bendich, VN Singh and L Machlin (eds). New York: Marcel Dekker, Inc., 1991, pp 71-101.

14. Cook, MG, and McNamara, P: "Effect of Dietary Vitamin E on Dimethylhydrazine-Induced Colonic Tumors in Mice." *Cancer Res* **40**, 1329-1331, 1980.

15. Shklar, G, Schwartz, JL, Trickler, D, and Reid, S: "Prevention of Experimental Cancer and Immunostimulation by Vitamin E (Immunosurveillance)." *J Oral Pathol Med* **19**, 60-64, 1990.

16. Gensler, HL, and Magdaleno, M: "Topical Vitamin E Inhibition of Immunosuppression and Tumorigenesis Induced by Ultraviolet Irradiation." *Nutr Cancer* **15**, 97-106, 1991.

17. Lambert, LA, Warner, WG, Wei, RR, Lavu, S, Chirtel, SJ, and Kornhauser, A: "The Protective but Nonsynergistic Effect of Dietary ß-Carotene and Vitamin E on Skin Tumorigenesis in Skh Mice." *Nutr Cancer* **21**, 1-12, 1994.

18. Shklar, G, Schwartz, J, Trickler, D, and Reid, S: "Regression of Experimental Cancer by Oral Administration of Combined α-Tocopherol and ß-Carotene." *Nutr Cancer* **12**, 321-325, 1989.

19. Kritchevsky, D: "Influence of Caloric Restriction and Exercise on Tumorigenesis in Rats." *Proc Soc Exp Biol Med* **193**, 35-38, 1990.

20. Ward, PA, Warren, JS, and Johnson, KJ: "Oxygen Radicals, Inflammation, and Tissue Injury." *Free Rad Biol Med* **5**, 403-408, 1988.

21. Burton, GW: "Antioxidant Action of Carotenoids." *J Nutr* **119**, 109-111, 1989.

22. Machlin, LJ: "Vitamin E." In *Handbook of Vitamins*, 2nd Ed., LJ Machlin (ed). New York: Marcel Dekker, Inc., 1991, pp 99-144.

23. Ham, Y-K, Choe, M, and Kim, S-W: "Effects of Vitamin A and E on the Protein Kinase Activity and Antioxidative Parameters During Carcinogenesis Induced by DMBA and TPA." *Korean Biochem J* **23**, 486-491, 1990.

24. Perchellet, J-P, Owen, MD, Posey, TD, Orten, DK, and Schneider, BA: "Inhibitory Effects of Glutathione Level-Raising Agents and d-α-Tocopherol on Ornithine Decarboxylase Induction and Mouse Skin Tumor Promotion by 12-O-Tetradecanoylphorbol-13-Acetate." *Carcinogenesis* **6**, 567-573, 1985.

25. Zhang, L-X, Cooney, RV, and Bertram, JS: "Carotenoids Enhance Gap Junctional Communication and Inhibit Lipid Peroxidation in C3H/10T½ Cells: Relationship to Their Cancer Chemopreventive Action." *Carcinogenesis* **12**, 2109-2114, 1991.

26. Zhang, L-X, Cooney, RV, and Bertram, JS: "Carotenoids Up-Regulate *Connexin43* Gene Expression Independent of Their Provitamin A or Antioxidant Properties." *Cancer Res* **52**, 5707-5712, 1992.

27. Mufson, RA, DeFeo, D, and Weinstein, IB: "Effects of Phorbol Ester Tumor Promoters on Arachidonic Acid Metabolism in Chick Embryo Fibroblasts." *Mol Pharmacol* **16**, 569-578, 1979.

28. Som, S, Chatterjee, M, and Banerjee, MR: "ß-Carotene Inhibition of 7,12-Dimethylbenz[*a*]anthracene-Induced Transformation of Murine Mammary Cells *In Vitro*." *Carcinogenesis* **5**, 937-940, 1984.

29. Renner, HW: "Anticlastogenic Effect of ß-Carotene in Chinese Hamsters. Time and Dose Response Studies with Different Mutagens." *Mutat Res* **144**, 251-256, 1985.

30. Warner, W, Giles, A, and Kornhauser, A: "Accumulation of Dietary β-Carotene in the Rat." *Nutr Rep Int* **32**, 295-301, 1985.

31.  Renner, HW: "Anticlastogenic Effect of β-Carotene in Chinese Hamsters: Time and Dose Response Studies with Different Mutagens." *Mutat Res* **144**, 251-256, 1985.

32.  Warner, WG, Wei, RR, Matusik, JE, Kornhauser, A, and Dunkel, VC: "β-Carotene Uptake, Metabolism, and Distribution in BALB/c 3T3 Cells." *Nutr Cancer* **19**, 31-42, 1993.

33.  Rundhaug, J, Gubler, ML, Sherman, MI, Blaner, WS, and Bertram, JS: "Differential Uptake, Binding, and Metabolism of Retinol and Retinoic Acid by 10T1/2 Cells." *Cancer Res* **47**, 5637-5643, 1987.

34.  Willett, WC, Stampfer, MJ, Underwood, BA, Speizer, FE, Rosner, B, and Hennekens, CH: "Validation of a Dietary Questionnaire with Plasma Carotenoid and α-Tocopherol Levels." *Am J Clin Nutr* **38**, 631-639, 1983.

35.  Mathews-Roth, MM: "Carotenoids in the Leukocytes of Carotenemic and Non-Carotenemic Individuals." *Clin Chem* **24**, 700-701, 1978.

36.  Stich, HF, Hornby, AP, and Dunn, BP: "Beta-Carotene Levels in Exfoliates of Human Mucosal Cells of Population Groups at Low and Elevated Risk for Oral Cancer." *Int J Cancer* **37**, 389-393, 1986.

37.  Floyd, RA, Watson, JJ, Wong, PK, Altmiller, DH, and Rickard, RC: "Hydroxyl Free Radical Adduct of Deoxyguanosine: Sensitive Detection and Mechanism of Formation," *Free Rad Res Commun* **1**, 163-172, 1986.

38.  Fornace, AJ, Alamo, I, and Hollander, MC: "DNA Damage Inducible Transcripts in Mammalian Cells," *Proc Natl Acad Sci, USA* **85**, 8800-8804, 1988.

39.  Holbrook, NJ, and Fornace, AJ: "Response to Adversity: Molecular Control of Gene Activation Following Genotoxic Stress," *The New Biologist* **3**, 825-833, 1991.

40.   Bailar, JC, III, and Smith, EM: "Progress Against Cancer?" *N Engl J Med* **314**, 1226-1232, 1986.

41.   Peto, R, Doll, R, Buckley, JD, and Sporn, MB: "Can Dietary Beta-Carotene Materially Reduce Human Cancer Rates?" Nature **290**, 201-208, 1981.

42.   Heinonen, OP, *et al.*: "The Effect of Vitamin E and Beta Carotene on the Incidence of Lung Cancer and Other Cancers in Male Smokers." *N Engl J Med* **330**, 1029-1035, 1994.

43.   Greenberg, RE, *et al.*: "A Clinical Trial of Antioxidant Vitamins to Prevent Colorectal Adenoma." *N Engl J Med* **331**, 141-147, 1994.

44.   Bostick, RM, *et al.*: "Reduced Risk of Colon Cancer with High Intake of Vitamin E: The Iowa Women's Health Study." *Cancer Res* **53**, 4230-4237, 1993.

45.   Roncucci, L: "Antioxidant Vitamins or Lactulose for the Prevention of the Recurrence of Colorectal Adenomas." *Dis Colon Rectum* **36**, 227-234, 1993.

# ASCORBIC ACID AND GASTROINTESTINAL CANCER

Marvin Cohen and Hemmi N. Bhagavan

Hoffmann-La Roche Inc.

Nutley, NJ 07110

## ABSTRACT

A literature review was made to critically evaluate the ability of ascorbic acid to modulate the incidence of gastrointestinal cancer. A comparison of preclinical, clinical, and epidemiological studies indicated that evidence for ascorbic acid as an inhibitor of carcinogenesis is stronger with regard to gastric cancer and weaker with regard to esophageal and colon/rectal cancer. Insufficient evidence currently exists regarding the oral cavity and the use of ascorbic acid in precancerous conditions such as polyposis.

## INTRODUCTION

A large body of literature exists on the role of ascorbic acid as a modulator of tumor development. While many of these studies suggest a preventive or therapeutic effect of ascorbic acid under certain conditions, much inconclusive or contradictory data have been reported. In a effort to critically examine one aspect of this area of research, a literature review was conducted for studies relating to ascorbic acid and gastrointestinal cancer.

*101*

## METHODS

An extensive MEDLINE search was conducted for all preclinical and clinical studies relating to effects of ascorbic acid on gastrointestinal cancer; the reference sections of all reprints received were also checked to detect any relevant research missed on-line. The topic of gastrointestinal cancer was subdivided into tumors of the oral cavity, pharynx, esophagus, stomach, and colon/rectum. Epidemiological studies were included only if some estimate of ascorbic acid intake had been reported. Studies on selected precancerous lesions (atrophic gastritis, polyposis) were also included. Literature on the inhibitory effects of ascorbic acid on nitrosamine formation was included because of its possible relevance to ascorbic acid effects on gastric cancer.

## RESULTS

### Oral/Pharyngeal Cancer

Two case-control epidemiological studies found an inverse correlation between ascorbic acid intake and cancer risk (McLaughlin et al 1988, Rossing et al (1989).

### Esophageal Cancer

Three case-control epidemiological studies found an inverse correlation between ascorbic acid intake and cancer risk (Ziegler et al 1981, Mettlin et al 1981, Brown et al 1988). Another epidemiological survey found a significant inverse correlation between plasma vitamin C levels and esophageal cancer mortality (Guo et al 1990). Four epidemiological/ nutritional surveys concluded that inhabitants of "high-risk" esophageal cancer areas had below normal intakes of ascorbic acid (Greenwald et al 1981, Hormozdiari et al 1975, Van Rensberg 1981, Yang et al 1982). However, a study of subjects with or without a family history of esophageal cancer found a similar incidence of vitamin C deficiency (Yang et al 1984). One intervention study found no change in the incidence of esophageal dysplasia or cancer when 120 mg/day ascorbic acid was administered for 5.25 yr (Taylor et al 1994, Wang et al 1994).

Gastric Cancer

Preclinical Studies. In 8/10 animal studies, ascorbic acid had no, equivocal, or stimulatory effects on chemically induced gastric tumors (Fukushima et al 1987, Imaida et al 1984, Kawasaki et al 1982, Mirvish et al 1983, Shibata et al 1992a, Shirai et al 1985a, Werner et al 1981, Yoshida et al 1994). In one mouse and one rat study, ascorbic acid significantly decreased tumor incidence (Wang et al 1984, Balansky et al 1986).

Human Studies. In 7/8 case-control epidemiological studies, a significant inverse correlation was found between ascorbic acid intake and cancer risk (Bjelke 1974, Buiatti et al 1990, Correa et al 1985, Fontham et al 1986, Kono et al 1988, LaVecchia et al 1987, You et al 1988); an equivocal relationship was reported in one study (Risch et al 1985). In 8/9 epidemiological surveys that were not of the case-control type, a similar relationship was found when ascorbic acid intake or plasma ascorbic acid levels were compared to cancer risk or cancer incidence (Bjelke 1974, Burr et al 1987, Dungal & Sigurjonssen 1967, Eichholzer-Helbling & Stahelin 1991, Gey et al 1987, Kolonel et al 1981, 1983, Stahelin 1989, Stahelin et al 1984, 1986, 1987, 1991); in one study, no correlation was found between ascorbic acid intake and cancer risk (Correa et al 1983).

Other studies have found decreased plasma or gastric ascorbic acid levels in cancer patients (Krasner & Dymock 1974, O'Connor et al 1989, Shi et al 1991) and in precancerous conditions such as chronic gastritis, hypochlorhydria, or intestinal metaplasia (Rathbone et al 1989, Schorah et al 1991, Sobala et al 1989, 1991, UK Subgroup 1992, Zhang et al 1994, Jaskiewicz et al 1990). One study found no correlation between plasma ascorbic acid levels and gastric pathology (Haenszel et al 1985).

Three intervention studies were reported. In one, administration of 1000 mg/day ascorbic acid for 4 weeks to patients with hypochlorhydria or partial gastrectomy significantly reduced gastric N-nitroso compound concentrations (Reed et al 1983). Administration of 1000 mg/day ascorbic acid for 28 days to patients with asymptomatic benign peptic ulcer disease significantly decreased DNA damage in 28 of 43 subjects (Dyke et al 1994). However, there was no correlation between intragastric ascorbic acid levels and DNA adducts. Administration of 120 mg/day ascorbic acid for 5.25 years in a study involving 29,584 adults did not change the incidence of gastric dysplasia or cancer as determined by 391 biopsies (Taylor et al 1994).

Recent studies have implicated Helicobacter pylori as a factor in gastric cancer through its effect on gastric ascorbic acid levels. Ruiz et al (1994a) and Banerjee et al (1994) found that patients positive for H. pylori had significantly lower gastric ascorbic acid levels than H. pylori-negative subjects. When the bacteria were cleared by appropriate therapy, gastric ascorbic acid levels rose to levels equivalent to those found in the control group. An epidemiological study by Ruiz et al (1994b) found a higher prevalence of H. pylori infection and lower gastric ascorbic acid levels in black subjects than in white subjects. The authors suggested that this pattern could be related to the higher incidence of gastric carcinoma in blacks.

### Colorectal Cancer

    Preclinical Studies. Two in vitro studies concluded that rat colonic mucosa contained a reductase that regenerated ascorbic acid from dehydroascorbic acid (Choi & Rose 1989, Rose 1990). In two mouse studies, ascorbic acid had no effect on transplanted colon carcinoma cells (Silverman et al 1983) or 1,2-dimethylhydrazine induced colonic tumors (Jones et al 1981). In one rat study, ascorbic acid produced a significant decrease in the number of chemically produced tumors (Colacchio & Memoli, 1986); in a second study, ascorbic acid inhibited tumor formation after single but not multiple doses of carcinogens (Reddy et al 1982). In a third study, ascorbic acid enhanced the carcinogenic activity of 1,2-dimethylhydrazine (Shirai et al 1985b).

    Human Studies. In 7 of 12 case-control epidemiological studies, an inverse correlation was found between ascorbic acid intake and cancer risk (Benito et al 1991, Freudenheim et al 1990, Heilburn et al 1989, Jain et al 1980, Kune et al 1987, LaVecchia et al 1988, Lee et al 1989, Macquardt-Moulin et al 1986, Potter & McMichael 1986, Tuyns 1986). In three case-control epidemiological studies, no significant difference was found for ascorbic acid intake in cancer patients and controls (Howe et al 1982, Bristol et al 1985, West et al 1989). In 1 of 3 epidemiological surveys not of the case-control type, a significant decrease in cancer risk was found with increase in ascorbic acid intake (Gey et al 1987, Shibata et al 1992, Stahelin et al 1986). In one study that compared leukocyte ascorbic acid levels, 46 of 50 cancer patients (8 with colorectal cancer) had levels below the lower limit of normal (Krasner & Dymock 1974).

In two intervention studies, ascorbic acid did not affect the time to disease progression or survival in advanced cancer patients who had not received any chemotherapy (Moertel et al 1985) and did not affect the incidence of colorectal adenomas over a 4 year period (Greenberg et al 1994). One intervention study reported that ascorbic acid administered to colorectal cancer patients improved functional activity of lymphocytes (Sergeev 1983); another study indicated that administration of 400 mg/day ascorbic acid for 2 weeks significantly reduced fecal mutagenicity (Dion et al 1982).

### Ascorbic Acid and Nitrosamine Formation

Animal and in Vitro Studies. Nine in vitro studies consistently showed that ascorbic acid inhibited nitrosation reactions (Archer et al 1975, Dikun et al 1991, Leach et al 1991, Mackerness et al 1989, Marquardt et al 1977, Weisburger & Raineri 1975, Raineri & Weisburger 1975, Ziebarth & Teichman 1980). One rat study and two dog studies indicated that ascorbic acid could inhibit the nitrosation of amines such as aminopyrine, proline and dimethylamine (Kamm et al 1975, Licht et al 1988, Lintas et al 1982).

Human Studies. In 3 of 4 studies, ascorbic acid reduced the urinary excretion of nitrosoproline; ascorbic acid dosage did not appear to be a factor in the results of positive and negative studies (Oshima & Bartsch 1981, Stich et al 1984, Wu et al 1993, Wagner et al 1985). Administration of ascorbic acid reduced the mutagenic activity of gastric fluid (O'Connor et al 1985) and significantly reduced gastric concentrations of N-nitroso compounds (Reed et al 1983, 1991).

Treatment of Polyposis

In two open studies and one double-blind study, ascorbic acid appeared to inhibit polyp formation (Bussey et al 1992, DeCosse et al 1975, Watne et al 1977). Equivocal results were obtained in two placebo-controlled studies (DeCosse et al 1989, McKeowyn-Eyssen et al 1988). In one placebo-controlled study, ascorbic acid was reported to significantly reduce cell proliferation in patients up to 6 months after complete polypectomy (Paganelli et al 1992).

CONCLUSIONS

The available epidemiological evidence suggests that ascorbic acid deficiency is a predisposing factor in the development of gastrointestinal cancer. It is strongest for gastric cancer, and the limited data on esophageal and oral/pharyngeal cancer are consistent with this interpretation. The evidence with respect to colorectal cancer is less convincing and additional studies are needed. There is also evidence that ascorbic acid may inhibit the progression of precancerous gastrointestinal conditions to tumors. One example is gastric dysplasias especially as they relate to H. pylori infection and nitrosamine production.

There are certain important factors affecting the outcome of such intervention trials. One appears to be the rather short duration chosen in some of the trials, and this window may have been too narrow considering that it takes 25 to 30 years to develop cancer. Another variable is the dose of ascorbic acid used. It is possible that while doses in the RDA range may not be effective, pharmacologic doses would exert a beneficial effect.

Animal studies have many yielded mixed results. One confounding factor is that of the models used are capable of ascorbic acid synthesis. Future research directed towards precancerous lesions in human subjects and employing well-defined intermediate biomarkers should yield definitive data.

REFERENCES

Archer MC, Tannenbaum SR, Fan TY, Weisman M: Reaction of nitrite with ascorbate and its relation to nitrosamine formation. J Natl Cancer Inst 54:1203-1205, 1975.

Balansky RM, Blagoeua PM, Mircheva ZI, Stoitchev I, Chernozemski I: The effect of antioxidants on MNNG-induced stomach carcinogenesis in rats. J Cancer Res Clin Oncol 112:272-275, 1986.

Benito E, Stiggelbout A, Bosch FX, Obrador A, Kaldor J, Mulet M, Munoz, N: Nutritional factors in colorectal cancer risk: A case-control study in Majorca. Int J Cancer 49:161-167, 1991.

Bjelke E: Epidemiologic studies of cancer of the stomach, colon, and rectum, with special emphasis on the role of diet. Scand J Gastroenterol 31 (Suppl):1-235, 1974.

Bristol JB, Emmett PM, Heaton KW, Williamson RCN: Sugar, fat, and the risk of colorectal cancer. Br Med J 291:1467-1471, 1985.

Brown LM, Blot WJ, Schuman SH, Smith VM, Ershow AG, Marks RD, Fraumeni JF, Jr: Environmental factors and high risk of esophageal cancer among men in coastal South Carolina. J Natl Cancer Inst 80(20):1620-1625, 1988.

Buiatti E, Palli D, Decarli A, Amadori D, Avellini C, Bianchi S, Bonaguri C, Cipriani F, Cocco P, Giacosa A: A case-control study of gastric cancer and diet in Italy: II. Association with nutrients. Int J Cancer 45:896-901, 1990.

Burr ML, Samloff IM, Bates CJ, Holliday RM: Atrophic gastritis and vitamin C status in two towns with different stomach cancer death-rates. Br J Cancer 56:163-167, 1987.

Bussey HJR, DeCosse JJ, Deschna EE, Eyers AA, Lesser ML, Morson BC, Ritchie SM, Thomson JPS, Wadsworth J: A randomized trial of ascorbic acid in polyposis coli. Cancer 50:1434-1439, 1982.

Choi JL, Rose RC: Regeneration of ascorbic acid by rat colon. Proc Soc Exp Biol Med 190:369-374, 1989.

Colacchio TA, Memoli VA: Chemoprevention of colorectal neoplasms. Ascorbic acid and beta-carotene. Arch Surg 121:1421-1424, 1986.

Correa P, Cuello C, Fajardo LF, Haenszel W, Bolanos O, de Ramirez B: Diet and gastric cancer:nutrition survey in a high-risk area. J Natl Cancer Inst 70:673-678, 1983.

Correa P, Fontham E, Pickle LW, Chen V, Lin YP, Haenszel W: Dietary determinants of gastric cancer in south Louisiana inhabitants. J Natl Cancer Inst 75:645-654, 1985.

DeCosse JJ, Adams MB, Kuzma JF, LoGerfo P, Condon RE: Effect of ascorbic acid on rectal polyps of patients with familial polyposis. Surgery 78:608-612, 1975.

DeCosse JJ, Miller HH, Lesser ML: Effect of wheat fiber and vitamins C and E on rectal polyps in patients with familial adenomatous polyposis. J Nat Cancer Inst 81:1290-1297, 1989.

Dikun PP, Ermilov VB, Shendrikova IA: Some approaches to prevention of endogenous formation of N-nitrosamines in humans. In: IK O'Neill et al (Eds), Relevance to human cancer of N-nitroso compounds, tobacco smoke, and mycotoxins, IARC, Lyon, p. 552-557, 1991.

Dion PW, Bright-See, EB, Smith CC, Bruce WR: The effect of dietary ascorbic acid and alpha-tocopherol on fecal mutagenicity. Mutat Res 102:27-37, 1982.

Dungal N, Sigurjonsson J: Gastric cancer and diet. A pilot study on dietary habits in two districts differing markedly in respect of mortality from gastric cancer. Br J Cancer 21:270-276, 1967.

Dyke GW, Craven JL, Hall R, Garner RC: Effect of vitamin C supplementation on gastric mucosal damage. Carcinogenesis 15:291-295, 1994.

Eichholzer-Helbling M, Stahelin HB: Plasma antioxidant vitamins and cancer risk: 12 year followup of the Basle Prospective Study. Int J Vit Nutr Res 61:271, 1991.

Fontham E, Zavala D, Correa P, Rodriguez E, Hunter F, Haenszel W, Tannenbaum SR: Diet and chronic atrophic gastritis: a case-control study. J Natl Cancer Inst 76:621-627, 1986.

Freudenheim JL, Graham S, Marshall JR, Haughey BP, Wilkinson G: A case-control study of diet and rectal cancer in western New York. Am J Epidemiol 131:612-624, 1990.

Fukushima S, Sakata T, Tagawa Y, Shibata MA, Hirose M, Ito N: Different modifying response of butylated hydroxyanisole, butylated hydroxytoluene, and other antioxidants in N,N-dibutylnitrosamine esophagus and forestomach carcinogenesis of rats. Cancer Res 47:2113-2116, 1987.

Gey KF, Brubacher GB, Stahelin HB: Plasma levels of antioxidant vitamins in relation to ischemic heart disease and cancer. Am J Clin Nutr 45:1368-1377, 1987.

Graham S, Marshall J, Haughey B, Mittelman A, Swanson M, Zielezny M, Byers T, Wilkinson G, West D: Dietary epidemiology of cancer of the colon in Western New York. Am J Epidemiol 128:490-503, 1988.

Greenberg ER: A clinical trial of antioxidant vitamins to prevent colorectal adenoma. N Eng J Med 331:141-147, 1994.

Groenewald G, Langenhoven ML, Beyers MJC, DuPlessis JP, Ferreira JJ, VanRensburg J: Nutrient intakes among rural Transkeians at risk for oesophageal cancer. S Afr Med J 60:964-967, 1981.

Guo W, Li J-Y, Blot WJ, Hsing AW, Chen J, Fraumeni JF, Jr: Correlations of dietary intake and blood nutrient levels with esophageal cancer mortality in China. Nutr Cancer 13:121-127, 1990.

Haenszel W, Correa P, Lopez A, Cuello C, Zarama G, Zavala D, Fontham E: Serum micronutrient levels in relation to gastric pathology. Int J Cancer 36:43-48, 1985.

Heilbrun LK, Nomura A, Hankin JH, Stemmermann GW: Diet and colorectal cancer with special reference to fiber intake. Int J Cancer 44:1-6, 1989.

Hormozdiari H, Day NE, Aramesh B, Mahboubi E: Dietary factors and esophageal cancer in the Caspian Littoral of Iran. Cancer Res 35:3493-3498, 1975.

Howe GR, Miller AB, Jain M, Cook G: Dietary factors in relation to the etiology of colorectal cancer. Cancer Detect Prevent 5:331-334, 1982.

Imaida K, Fukushima S, Shirai T, Masui T, Ogiso T, Ito N: Promoting activities of butylated hydroxyanisole, butylated hydroxytoluene and sodium L-ascorbate on forestomach and urinary bladder carcinogenesis initiated with methylnitrosourea in F344 male rats. Gann 75:769-775, 1984.

Jain M, Cook GM, Davis FG, Grace MG, Howe GR, Miller AB: A case-control study of diet and colorectal cancer. Int J Cancer 26:757-768, 1980.

Jaskiewicz K, Van Helden PD, Wiid IJF, SteenKamp HJ, VanWyk MJ: Chronic atropic gastritis, gastric pH, nitrites and micronutrient levels in a population at risk for gastric carcinoma. Anticancer Res 10:833-836, 1990.

Jones FE, Komorowski RA, Condon RE: Chemoprevention of 1,2-dimethylhydrazine-induced large bowel neoplasms. Surg Forum 31:435-437, 1981.

Jones FE, Komorowski RA, Condon RE: The effects of ascorbic acid and butylated hydroxyanisole in the chemoprevention of 1,2-dimethylhydrazine-induced large bowel neoplasms. J Surg Oncol 25:54-60, 1984.

Kamm JJ, Dashman T, Conney AH, Burns JJ: Effect of ascorbic acid on amine-nitrite toxicity. Ann NY Acad Sci 258:169-174, 1975.

Kawasaki H, Morishige F, Tananka H, Kimoto E: Influence of oral supplementation of ascorbate upon the induction of N-methyl-N'-nitro-N-nitrosoguanidine. Cancer Lett 16:57-63, 1982.

Kolonel LN, Nomura AM, Hirohata T, Hankin JH, Hinds MW: Association of diet and place of birth with stomach cancer incidence in Hawaii Japanese and Caucasians. Am J Clin Nutr 34:2478-2485, 1981.

Kolonel LN, Nomura AMY, Hinds MW, Hirohata T, Hankin JH, Lee J: Role of diet in cancer incidence in Hawaii. Cancer Res 43(Suppl):2397S-2402S, 1983.

Kono S, Ikeda M, Tokudome S, Kuratsune M: A case-control study of gastric cancer and diet in Northern Kyushu, Japan. Jpn J Cancer Res 79:1067-1074, 1988.

Krasner N, Dymock IW: Ascorbic acid deficiency in malignant diseases: a clinical and biochemical study. Br J Cancer 30:142-145, 1974.

Kune S, Kune GA, Watson LF: Case-control study of dietary etiological factors: the Melbourne Colorectal Cancer Study. Nutr Cancer 9:21-42, 1987.

La Vecchia C, Negri E, Decarli A, D'Avanzo B, Franceschi S: A case-control study of diet and gastric cancer in northern Italy. Int J Cancer 40:484-489, 1987.

La Vecchia C, Negri E, Decarli A, D'Avanzo B, Gallotti L, Gentile A, Franceschi S: A case-control study of diet and colo-rectal cancer in northern Italy. Int J Cancer 41:492-498, 1988.

Leach SA, Mackerness CW, Hill MJ, Thompson MH: Inhibition of bacterially mediated N-nitrosation by ascorbate: therapeutic and mechanistic considerations. In: IK O'Neill et al (Eds), Relevance to human cancer of N-nitroso compounds, tobacco smoke and mycotoxins, IARC, Lyon, p. 571-578, 1991.

Lee HP, Gourley L, Duffy SW, Esteve J, Lee J, Day NE: Colorectal cancer and diet in an Asian population--A case-control study among Singapore Chinese. Int J Cancer 43:1007-1016, 1989.

Licht WR, Fox JG, Deen WM: Effects of ascorbic acid and thiocyanate on nitrosation of proline in the dog stomach. Carcinogenesis 9:373-377, 1988.

Lintas CL, Clark A, Fox J, Tannenbaum SR, Newberne PM: In vivo stability of nitrite and nitrosamine formation in the stomach: effect of nitrite and amine concentration and of ascorbic acid. Carcinogenesis 3:161-165, 1982.

Mackerness CW, Leach SA, Thompson MH, Hill MJ: The inhibition of bacterially mediated N-nitrosation by vitamin C: relevance to the inhibition of endogenous N-nitrosation in the achlorhydric stomach. Carcinogenesis 10:397-399, 1989.

Macquart-Moulin G, Riboli E, Cornee J, Charnay B, Berthezene P, Day N: Case-control study on colorectal cancer and diet in Marseilles. Int J Cancer 38:183-191, 1986.

Marquardt H, Rufino F, Weisburger JH: Mutagenic activity of nitrite-treated foods: human stomach cancer may be related to dietary factors. Science 196:1000-1001, 1977.

McKeown-Eyssen G, Holloway C, Jazmaji V, Bright-See E, Dion P, Bruce WR: A randomized trial of vitamins C and E in the prevention of recurrence of colorectal polyps. Cancer Res 48:4701-4705, 1988.

McLaughlin JK, Gridley G, Block G, Winn DM, Preston-Martin S, Schoenberg JB, Greenberg RS, Stemhagen A, Austin DF, Ershow AG: Dietary factors in oral and pharyngeal cancer. J Natl Cancer Inst 80:1237-1243, 1988.

Mettlin C, Graham S, Priore R, Marshall J, Swanson M: Diet and cancer of the esophagus. Nutr Cancer 2:143-147, 1981.

Mirvish SS, Wallcave L, Eagen M, Shubik P: Ascorbate-nitrite reaction: possible means of blocking the formation of carcinogenic N-nitroso compounds. Science 177: 65-68, 1972.

Mirvish SS, Pelfrene AF, Garcia H, Shubik P: Effect of sodium ascorbate on tumor induction in rats treated wtih morpholine and sodium nitrite, and with nitrosomorpholine. Cancer Lett 2:101-108, 1976.

Mirvish SS, Salmasi S, Cohen SM, Patil K, Mahboubi E: Liver and forestomach tumors and other forestomach lesions in rats treated with morpholine and sodium nitrite, with and without sodium ascorbate. J Nat Cancer Inst 71:81-85, 1983.

Moertel CG, Fleming TR, Creagan ET, Rubin J, O'Connell MJ, Ames MM: High-dose vitamin C versus placebo in the treatment of patients with advanced cancer who have had no prior chemotherapy. N Eng J Med 312:137-141, 1985.

O'Connor HJ, Habibzedah N, Schorah CJ, Axon AT, Riley SE, Garner RC: Effect of increased intake of vitamin C on the mutagenic activity of gastric juice and intragastric concentrations of ascorbic acid. Carcinogenesis 6:1675-1676, 1985.

O'Connor HJ, Schorah CJ, Habibzedah N, Axon ATR, Cockel RL: Vitamin C in the human stomach: relation to gastric pH, gastroduodenal disease, and possible sources. Gut 30:436-442, 1989.

Ohshima H, Bartsch H: Quantitative estimation of endogenous nitrosation in humans by monitoring N-nitrosoproline excreted in the urine. Cancer Res 41:3658-3662, 1981.

Paganelli GM, Biasco G, Brandi G, Santucci R, Gizzi G, Villani V, Cianci M, Miglioli M, Barbara L: Effect of vitamin A, E, and E supplementation on rectal cell proliferation in patients with colorectal adenomas. J Natl Cancer Inst. 84:47-51, 1992.

Potter JD, McMichael AJ: Diet and cancer of the colon and rectum: a case-control study. J Natl Cancer Inst 76:557-569, 1986.

Raineri R, Weisburger JH: Reduction of gastric carcinogens with ascorbic acid. Ann NY Acad Sci 258:181-189, 1975.

Rathbone BJ, Johnson AW, Wyatt JI, Kelleher J, Heatley RV, Losowsky MS: Ascorbic acid: a factor concentrated in human gastric juice. Clin Sci 76:237-241, 1989.

Reddy BS, Hirota N, Katayama S: Effect of dietary sodium ascorbate on 1,2-dimethylhydrazine- or methylnitrosourea-induced colon carcinogenesis in rats. Carcinogenesis 3:1097-1099, 1982.

Reed PI, Summers K, Smith PLR: Effect of ascorbic acid treatment of gastric juice, nitrite, and N-nitroso compound concentrations in achlorhydric subjects. Gut 24:492-493, 1983.

Reed PI, Summers K, Smith PLR, Walters CL, Bartholomew BA, Hill MJ, Venitt S, House FR, Hornig DH, Bonjour JP: Effect of gastric surgery for benign peptic ulcer and ascorbic acid therapy on concentrations of nitrite and N-nitroso compounds in gastric juice. IARC 57:975-979, 1984.

Reed PI, Johnston BJ, Walters CL, Hill MJ: Effect of ascorbic acid on the intragastric environment in patients at increased risk of developing gastric cancer. In: O'Neill IK et al (Eds), Relevance to human cancer of N-nitroso compounds, tobacco smoke and mycotoxins, IARC, p. 139-142, 1991.

Risch HA, Jain M, Choi NW, Fodor JG, Pfeiffer CJ, Howe GR, Harrison LW, Craib KJ, Miller AB: Dietary factors and the incidence of cancer of the stomach. Am J Epidemiol 122:947-959, 1985.

Rose RC: Ascorbic acid metabolism in protection against free radicals: a radiation model. Biochem Biophys Res Commun 169:430-436, 1990.

Rossing MA, Vaughan TL, McKnight B: Diet and pharyngeal cancer. Int J Cancer 44:593-597, 1989.

Schorah CJ, Sobala GM, Sanderson M, Collis N, Primrose JN: Gastric juice ascorbic acid: effects of disease and implications for gastric carcinogenesis. Am J Clin Nutr 53(Suppl):287S-293S, 1991.

Sergeev AV: Correction of the biochemical and immunological indices in colonic cancer using optimal doses of retinyl acetate and ascorbic acid. Biull Eksp Biol Med 96:90-92, 1983.

Shi KX, Mao DJ, Cheng WF, Ji YS, Xu LE: An approach to establishing N-nitroso compounds as the cause of gastric cancer. In: Relevance to human cancer of N-nitroso compounds, tobacco smoke and mycotoxins, O'Neill IK et al (eds), IARC, Lyon, p. 143-145, 1991.

Shibata MA, Fukushima S, Asakawa E, Hirose M, Ito N: The modifying effects of indomethacin or ascorbic acid on cell proliferation induced by different types of bladder tumor promoters in rat urinary bladder and forestomach mucosal epithelium. Jpn J Cancer Res 83:31-39, 1992a.

Shibata A, Paganini-Hill A, Ross RK, Hendersen BE:Intake of vegetables, fruits, beta-carotene, vitamin C and vitamin supplements and cancer incidence among the elderly: a prospective study. Br J Cancer 66:673-679, 1992b.

Shirai T, Masuda A, Fukushima S, Hosoda K, Ito N: Effects of sodium L-ascorbate and related compounds on rat stomach carcinogenesis initiated by N-methyl-N'-nitro-N-nitrosoguanidine. Cancer Lett 29:283-288, 1985a.

Shirai T, Ikawa E, Hirose, Thamavit W, Ito N: Modification by five antioxidants on 1,2-dimethylhydrazine-initiated colon carcinogenesis in F344 rats. Carcinogenesis 6:637-639, 1985b.

Silverman J, Rivenson A, Reddy B: Effect of sodium ascorbate on transplantable murine tumors. Nutr Cancer 4:192-197, 1983.

Sobala GM, Schorah CJ, Sanderson M, Dixon MF, Tompkins DS, Godwin P, Axon AT: Ascorbic acid in the human stomach. Gastroenterology 97:357-363, 1989.

Sobala GM, Pignatelli B, Schorah CJ, Bartsch H, Sanderson M, Dixon MF, Shires S, King RF, Axon AT: Levels of nitrite, nitrate, N-nitroso compounds, ascorbic acid, and total bile acids in gastric juice of patients with and without precancerous conditions of the stomach. Carcinogenesis 12:193-198, 1991.

Stahelin HB: Vitamins and cancer:results of the Basel Study. Soz Praeventivmed 34:75-77, 1989.

Stahelin HB, Rosel F, Buess E, Brubacher G: Cancer, vitamins, and plasma lipids: prospective Basel study. J Natl Cancer Inst 73:1463-1468, 1984.

Stahelin HB, Rosel F, Buess E, Brubacker G: Dietary risk factors for cancer in the Basel study. Biblthca Nutr Dieta No. 37., 144-153, 1986.

Stahelin HB, Gey KF, Brubacher G: Plasma vitamin C and cancer death: the prospective Basel Study. Ann NY Acad Sci 498:124-131, 1987.

Stahelin HB, Gey KF, Eichholzer M, Ludin E, Bernasconi F, Thurneysen J, Brubacher G: Plasma antioxidant vitamins and subsequent cancer mortality in the 12 year follow-up of the prospective Basel Study. Am J Epidemiol 133:766-775, 1991.

Stich HF, Hornby AP, Dunn BP: The effect of dietary factors on nitrosoproline levels in human urine. Int J Cancer 33:625-628, 1984.

Tannenbaum SR, Mergens W: Reaction of nitrite with vitamins C and E. Ann NY Acad Sci 355: 267-279, 1980.

Taylor PR, Li B, Dawsey SM, Li JY, Yang CS, Guo W, Blot WJ: Prevention of esophageal cancer; the nutrition intervention trials in Linxian, China. Cancer Res 54(Suppl):2029S-2031S, 1994.

Tuyns AJ: A case-control study on colorectal cancer in Belgium. Preliminary results. Soz Praventivmed 31:81-82, 1986.

UK Sub-Group of ECP-EURONUT-IM Study Group: Plasma vitamin concentrations in patients with intestinal metaplasia and in controls. Europ J Cancer Prev 1:177-186, 1992.

van Rensberg SJ: Epidemiologic and dietary evidence for a specific nutritional predisposition to esophageal cancer. J Natl Cancer Inst 67:243-251, 1981.

Wagner DA, Shuker DE, Bilmazes C, Obiedzinski M, Baker I, Young VR, Tannenbaum SR: Effect of vitamins C and E on endogenous synthesis of N-nitrosamino acids in humans:precursor-product studies with [15N]nitrate. Cancer Res 45:6519-6522, 1985.

Wang XH, Zhang XY, Chen XT: Ascorbic acid inhibition of 3-methylcholanthrene induced carcinoma of glandular stomach in mice. Chin Med J 97:215-222, 1984.

Wang GQ, Dawsey SM, Li JY, Taylor PR, Li B, Blot WJ, Weinstein WM, Liu FS, Lewin KJ, Wang H: Effects of vitamin/mineral supplementation on the prevalence of histological dysplasia and early cancer of the esophagus and stomach: results from the General Population Trial in Linxian, China. Cancer Epidemiol Biomarker Prev 3:161-166, 1994.

Watne AL, Lai HY, Carrier J, Coppula W: The diagnosis and surgical treatment of patients with Gardner's syndrome. Surgery 82:327-333, 1977.

Weisburger JH, Raineri R: Dietary factors and the etiology of gastric cancer. Cancer Res 35:3469-3474, 1975.

Werner B, Denzer U, Mitschke H, Brassow F: Ascorbic acid and cancer of the duodenum: an experimental study. Langenbeck's Arch Chir 354:101-109, 1981.

West DW, Slattery ML, Robison LM, Schuman KL, Ford MH, Mahoney AW, Lyon JL, Sorensen AW: Dietary intake and colon cancer; sex- and anatomic site-specific associations. Am J Epidemiol 130:883-894, 1989.

Wu Y, Chen J, Ohshima H, Pignatelli B, Boreham J, Li J, Campbell TC, Peto R, Bartsch H: Geographic associations between urinary excretion of N-nitroso compounds and oesophageal cancer mortality in China. Int J Cancer 54:713-719, 1993.

Yang CS, Miao J, Yang W, Huang M, Wang T, Xue H, You S, Lu J, Wu J: Diet and vitamin nutrition of the high esophageal cancer risk population in Linxian, China. Nutr Cancer 4:154-164, 1982.

Yang CS, Sun Y, Yang QU, Miller KW, Li GY, Zheng SF, Ershow AG, Blot WJ, Li JY: Vitamin A and other deficiencies in Linxian, a high esophageal cancer incidence area in northern China. J Natl Cancer Inst 73:1449-1453, 1984.

Yoshida Y, Hirose M, Takaba K, Kimura J, Ito N: Induction and promotion of forestomach tumors by sodium nitrite in combination with ascorbic acid or sodium ascorbate in rats with or without N-methyl-N'-nitro-N-nitrosoguanidine. Int J Cancer 56:124-128, 1994.

You WC, Blot WJ, Chang YS, Ershow AG, Yang ZT, An Q, Henderson B, Xu GW, Fraumeni JF, Jr, Wang TG: Diet and high risk of stomach cancer in Shandong China. Cancer Res 48:3518-3523, 1988.

Zhang L, Blot WJ, You W-C, Chang YS, Liu XQ, Kneller RW, Zhao L, Liu WD, Li JY, Jin ML, Xu GW, Fraumeni JF, Yang CS: Serum micronutrients in relation to precancerous gastric lesions. Int J Cancer 56:650-654, 1994.

Ziebarth D, Teichmann B: Nitrosation of orally administered drugs under simulated stomach conditions. IARC Scientif. Publ. No 31., 231-244, 1980.

Ziegler RG, Morris LE, Blot WJ, Pottern LM, Hoover R, Fraumeni JF, Jr: Esophageal cancer among black men in Washington, D.C. II. Role of nutrition. J Natl Cancer Inst 67:1199-1206, 1981.

BIOCHEMISTRY AND PHARMACOLOGY OF RETINOIDS

IN RELATION TO CHEMOPREVENTION OF CANCER

Donald L. Hill, Tzu-Wen Shih, Tsu-Han Lin, and
Y. Fulmer Shealy
Southern Research Institute
Birmingham, Alabama

In experimental animals dosed with carcinogens, retinoids, compounds related in structure to retinol and retinoic acid (RA), often have chemopreventive effects, particularly in models for mammary, bladder, and skin cancer (see 1,2). For natural and synthetic retinoids, their pharmacologic disposition, toxicity, and efficacy in the prevention of cancer vary with their structural features. Consideration of these factors can lead to a better understanding of the mechanism of action of retinoids and to the development of more effective chemopreventive compounds.

The metabolism of retinol and its esters has been extensively studied. The biochemical oxidation of retinol to RA is achieved in two reactions catalyzed by cytoplasmic, $NAD^+$-dependent enzymes, the first accomplishing the reversible conversion of retinol to retinal (3,4) and the second accomplishing the irreversible oxidation of retinal to RA (5,6). Another pathway for retinol metabolism is also known: in the presence of NADPH, an enzyme present in liver microsomes converts retinol to 4-hydroxyretinol, a product that can also be formed in a reconstituted monooxygenase system containing human liver P450IIC8 (7,8).

We recently noted a previously unreported activity: an NADPH-requiring enzyme present in rat liver microsomes that catalyzes the conversion of retinol to retinal (9). The enzyme activity is induced by 3-methylcholanthrene (MC). For the constitutive enzyme, the $K_m$ and $V_{max}$ values are 285 $\mu M$ retinol and 18 nmol/mg protein/hr, respectively; for the MC-induced activity, the corresponding values are 133 $\mu M$ retinol and 33 nmol/mg protein/hr. Neither the constitutive nor the induced activities are detectable in microsomes from seven other tissues; both are inhibited by citral, ketoconazole, SKF-525A, and α-naphthoflavone. The enzyme appears to be a retinol oxidase, distinct from the cytosolic enzyme that accomplishes the same reaction.

The oxidase pathway probably has limited significance in the physiological metabolism of retinol, since the $K_m$ values for both the constitutive and induced enzymes are higher than reported values for the hepatic concentration of retinol: 11-16 $\mu M$ for mice (10), 8 $\mu M$ for Wistar rats (11), and 21-30 $\mu M$ for Sprague-Dawley rats (12,13). Nevertheless, in rats dosed with pharmacologic amounts of retinol or retinol derivatives, this pathway could be important for metabolism of the high concentrations of retinol. Furthermore, the inducibility of the retinol-oxidizing enzyme may be related to the observation that exposure of animals to any of a variety of foreign compounds can deplete liver stores of vitamin A (14-16).

Some synthetic retinoids can be metabolized to retinol. Retinyl methyl ether (RME), which is as effective as, or more effective than, retinyl acetate in the prevention of mammary cancer in rats (17), is metabolically converted to retinol in intact rats (13,18). This reaction is accomplished by a hepatic mixed-function oxidase similar to other NADPH-requiring O-dealklases (19). The enzymatic activity is induced by MC but not by phenobarbital or RME itself. The methyl ether analog of etretinate is also a substrate for this enzyme, but retinyl butyl ether is not. The activity is not found in any of several other tissues. The demethylation of RME proceeds slowly in intact animals; for rats dosed orally with this compound, the terminal elimination half-life is 19 hr (20). High concentrations of RME are present in the adrenals and mammary glands (Table 1).

Accumulation of retinoids in mammary tissue may be related to their chemopreventive activity. RME, N-(4-hydroxy-phenyl)retinamide (4-HPR), and axerophthene (AXR), none of which is readily converted to a structure with a free carboxyl group, have activity in preventing breast cancer (17,21,22), and all accumulate (or total retinoids, as measured colorimetrically with trifluoroacetic acid, accumulate) in breast tissue (20,23,24,25) (Table 1). After a single dose of 40 mg/kg of RME to rats, its concentration in the tissue is about 10 $\mu g/g$ for several hours (20). In contrast, retinyl butyl ether (25) and retinoyl leucine (13) do not accumulate

Table 1

Accumulation in rat mammary tissue of retinoids active
in prevention of mammary cancer
(The values are for 24 hr after dosing.)

| Tissue or fluid | RME, 9 mg/rat, po, qd x1 | RME, 9 mg/rat, po, 3 x wk x 3 | RME, 10 mg/kg, po, qd x1 | RME, 40 mg/kg, po, qd x1 |
|---|---|---|---|---|
| | total retinoids (nmol/g)[a] | | RME (nmol/g or ml)[b] | |
| Liver, control | 370 | 530 | N/A[c] | N/A |
| Liver | 920 | 7380 | 1.0[d] | 1.0[d] |
| Breast, control | 5 | 9 | N/A | N/A |
| Breast | 60 | 710 | 6.7 | 26.7 |
| Plasma, RME | NM[c] | NM | 0.17[d] | 0.33[d] |

| Tissue or fluid | AXR, 9 mg/rat, po, 3 x wk x 3 | Tissue or fluid | 4HPR, 5 mg/kg, iv, qd x 1 |
|---|---|---|---|
| | total retinoids (nmol/g)[e] | | 4HPR (nmol/g or ml)[f] |
| Liver, control | 840 | Liver, control | N/A |
| Liver | 3220 | Liver, 4HPR | 0.40[d] |
| Breast, control | 4 | Breast, control | N/A |
| Breast | 295 | Breast, 4HPR | 1.06 |
| Serum, AXR | NM | Serum, 4HPR | 0.85[d] |

[a] Adapted from (25). [b] Adapted from (20).
[c] NM, not measured; N/A, not applicable.
[d] Decreases with time much faster than for breast tissue.
[e] Adapted from (23). [f] Adapted from (24).

in breast tissue; neither compound has appreciable activity in preventing mammary cancer (13). Further, in the mammary tissue of mice at 24 hr after dosing, the concentration of 4-HPR is no higher than that in liver (26); in contrast to the activity of this compound in rats, it is generally ineffective in preventing mammary cancer in mice (27).

To exert their activity, retinoids with chemopreventive activity in the mammary gland may not be converted to compounds with free carboxyl groups. RA and 13-cis-RA have little chemopreventive activity for mammary cancer (see 1). Furthermore, RA does not persist in tissues other than liver, fat, and brain. Following a nonexponential (linear) phase, plasma levels in mice and rats decrease rapidly to the endogenous concentration of about 2 ng/ml (28-32).

Retinoids with activity in preventing papillomas on the skin of mice have a side chain that possesses, or is readily convertible to, a free carboxylic acid group (13,33). Such a group appears to be necessary, but not sufficient, for chemo-preventive activity in the skin. A carboxyl group is also required for binding to cellular RA-binding protein (CRABP) (34), which apparently serves in the intracellular transport of RA, and for binding to the nuclear receptors (RARs) (35).

Apparently due to the induction of microsomal oxidases, the serum and tissue contents of RA are lower in mice dosed previously with this compound or with phenobarbital (36). This observation has clinical significance in that repeated dosing of patients with RA leads to lower plasma levels of this compound (37). Like retinol, RA is metabolized to 4-hydroxy and 4-oxo derivatives (38).

In contrast to RA, 13-cis-RA is eliminated from the serum of intravenously dosed mice in two or more exponential phases (29). Following oral doses to mice, serum levels of the compound rise for 15 min and then decline in an exponential fashion; absorption of 13-cis-RA from the gut is incomplete (39). Both the serum and tissue contents of 13-cis-RA are lower in mice previously dosed with phenobarbital or MC; they are not lower in mice dosed previously with 13-cis-RA (36).

13-cis-RA appears in the tissues of intact animals following pharmacologic doses of RA (31) and RA appears in animals dosed with 13-cis-RA (39). Interconversion of RA, 13-cis-RA, and 9-cis-RA is catalyzed nonenzymatically by compounds containing sulfhydryl groups (13,40). Dosing with either of these compounds gives rise, in tissues, to a mixture of all three. Thus, to some extent, the biological activities of the group should be shared.

The disappearance of N-(2-hydroxyethyl)retinamide (N-HOERA) from mouse serum following intravenous doses is biphasic and exponential (29), whereas a single exponential phase, with a half-life of 3.6 hr, is evident following oral doses (28). The compound persists in tissues longer than either RA or 13-cis-RA; of the tissues studied, it has the longest half-life in bladder. The absorption of N-HOERA following oral doses is considerably greater than that for 13-cis-RA, and no detectable intact compound is present in urine or feces (39). Prior dosing of mice with phenobarbital or MC reduces the serum and tissue levels of this amide (36).

4-HPR is slowly hydrolyzed to RA in rat tissues (41). This reaction is accomplished by an amidase present in rat liver microsomes (42). As substrates for this enzyme, the 13-cis and all-trans forms of N-ethylretinamide are most active; the all-trans form of 4-HPR is considerably more active than the 13-cis form. Retinoyl amino acids are poor substrates. Since 4-HPR (43) and other retinamides (all-trans- and 13-cis-N-ethylretinamide and 13-cis-N-HOERA) (44) have only slight teratogenic activity, it is unlikely that these amides are extensively hydrolyzed in intact animals.

If 4-HPR and other retinamides act as prodrugs to release RA, their efficacy would depend, not only upon sufficient hydrolysis, but also upon the presence of RA at the site of action. Although 4-HPR and its major metabolites distribute to the mammary gland and urinary bladder of both rats and mice, no RA derived from 4-HPR can be detected in these organs (24). The biological significance of the limited hydrolysis of retinamides remains to be determined.

Because 4-HPR and some other retinoids do not bind to CRABP or to the nuclear receptors and because they are not readily converted in intact animals to compounds that would bind to these proteins, other proteins may be involved in the transport and in the biological action of these retinoids. For retinamides not subject to hydrolysis, the known transport and receptor proteins cannot be involved in their biological activity. Perhaps a different class of receptors exists for retinoids without a terminal carboxyl group.

We propose that there are at least two classes of retinoids that are active in chemoprevention: one characterized by a terminal carboxylic acid group and activity in preventing skin cancer; the other, by a nonpolar terminal group and activity in preventing mammary cancer.

The rate of disappearance of retinoids from bladder tissue may be a factor in their chemopreventive potential. RA, 13-cis-RA, 4-HPR, and N-HOERA effectively prevent bladder cancer; in this tissue, they have, relative to other tissues, prolonged elimination half-lives (26,36,39) (Table 2). On the other hand, for chemoprevention of lung cancer, neither 13-cis-RA, N-HOERA, nor 4-HPR has appreciable activity; 13-cis-RA is likewise inactive in the prevention of colon cancer (see 2). Accordingly, there is relatively rapid loss of these compounds from the respective tissues (24,45).

Although 4-oxoRA is a catabolic product of RA (46), the compound retains biological activity in several systems. Such activity provides a rationale for synthesis of analogs of 4-oxoRA (see 47). Substituents at the 3-position might hinder further degradation. Several 3-substituted-4-oxo analogs and their corresponding methyl esters have activity on mouse skin, for inhibition of induction by 12-O-tetradecanoylphorbol 13-acetate (TPA) of ornithine decarboxylase activity (48). Concerning inhibition of induction of this enzyme, which is thought to correlate with inhibition of formation of skin papillomas (33), there is no substantial difference in the activities of the 4-oxoRA analogs and the corresponding methyl esters. The 3,3-dimethyl and 3-cinnamyl derivatives are among the most effective. In tests for inhibition of development of mouse-skin papillomas initiated by dimethylbenzanthracene and promoted by TPA, methyl 3,3-dimethyl- and methyl 3-cinnamyl-4-oxoretinoate are most effective (48).

We have now observed that the extent of accumulation in mouse skin of methyl RA, methyl 4-oxoRA, a group of methyl 3-substituted-4-oxoretinoates, and the corresponding retinoic acids, correlates with chemopreventive activity in this tissue. The details of these previously unpublished experiments are described below.

Retinoids were stored under argon at -70°C. Female CD-1 mice were purchased from Charles River Laboratories, Cambridge, MA. The dosing solutions were prepared by dissolving the retinoid in 0.9% NaCl, ethanol, and Tween 80 (96.5: 3.0: 0.5, v/v/v) and were given as single doses (10

Table 2
Retention in mouse tissues of retinoids active in
prevention of bladder cancer
(The mice were dosed po with 10 mg/kg.)

| Tissue or fluid | 13-<u>cis</u>-RA[a] $t_{1/2el}$[c] (min) | <u>N</u>-HOERA[a] $t_{1/2el}$ (hr) | 4-HPR[b] $t_{1/2el}$ (hr) |
|---|---|---|---|
| Serum | 19 | 2.9 | 4.3 |
| Liver | 19 | 2.9 | 4.3 |
| Lung | 15 | 3.3 | NM[d] |
| Sm. intestine | 11 | 2.1 | NM |
| Kidney | 15 | 2.5 | NM |
| Spleen | 17 | 3.0 | NM |
| Lg. intestine | 14 | 3.9 | NM |
| Fat | 15 | 3.2 | NM |
| Heart | 16 | 3.5 | NM |
| Brain | 16 | 4.7 | NM |
| Muscle | 17 | 4.5 | NM |
| Testes | 11 | 3.5 | NM |
| Bladder | 51 | 7.3 | 11.6 |

[a]   From (39). Used with permission.
[b]   Calculated from (26).
[c]   $t_{1/2el}$, half-life for elimination from serum or designated tissue.
[d]   NM, not measured.

mg/kg) intravenously <u>via</u> the tail vein. Mice were sacrificed at times ranging from 3 to 1440 min after dosing. At the time of sacrifice, blood samples were collected in Microtainer® tubes (Becton Dickinson and Co., Rutherford, NJ) containing the antiglycolytic agent, sodium fluoride, and the anticoagulant, potassium oxalate. The blood samples were centrifuged to prepare plasma, which, along with collected samples of skin, was stored frozen until analyzed.

Skin samples were homogenized in 5 volumes of saline. The homogenates were extracted with acetonitrile: methanol (4: 1, v/v), and the extracts were evaporated to dryness and reconstituted in the same solvent. Samples of plasma were extracted and reconstituted similarly.

Analysis of the retinoid esters and the corresponding free acids was accomplished with an HPLC system consisting of a solvent delivery Module 110B, an analog interface Module 406, a programmable detector Module 166 set at 340 nm, and an Autosampler 507 (Beckman Instruments, Inc., San Ramon, CA). Samples (40 $\mu$l) were injected onto a 4.6-mm i.d. x 250-mm Spherisorb ODS 5-$\mu$m column (Chromanetics, Williamstown, NJ). Elution was accomplished at a flow rate of 1 ml/min with 85% acetonitrile containing 20 mM ammonium acetate for methyl RA; 70% acetonitrile containing 0.3% acetic acid for methyl 4-oxoRA, methyl 3-methyl-4-oxoRA, and methyl 3,3'-dimethyl-4-oxoRA; and 80% acetonitrile containing 0.3% acetic acid for methyl 3-cinnamyl-4-oxoRA.

From the derived data, the following pharmacokinetic values were calculated: $t_{1/2ap}$, half-life for appearance in plasma or skin; $t_{1/2\alpha}$, half-life for the initial elimination phase; $t_{1/2\beta}$, half-life for the terminal elimination phase; AUC, area under the concentration-time curve; $T_{max}$, time at which the highest concentration is observed; $C_{max}$, the highest concentration observed; and CL, clearance.

Comparison of the pharmacokinetic values for the series of compounds (Tables 3-7) reveals several notable differences. For methyl 4-oxoRA in the plasma of mice, the values for $T_{1/2\beta}$ and AUC are lower than for any of the other compounds; the value for clearance is higher (Table 3, Figure 1). Although the maximum concentration of the free acid (8690 ng/ml) in plasma is higher and is reached sooner (32 min) than for the other compounds, its elimination half-life (37 min) is generally shorter. In the elimination of methyl 4-oxoRA from the skin of mice, the maximum concentration of the free acid

Table 3

Pharmacokinetic values for methyl 4-oxoRA (10 mg/kg) administered intravenously to mice

| Value | Units | Plasma | | Skin | |
|---|---|---|---|---|---|
| | | Parent ester | Free acid | Parent ester | Free acid |
| $t_{1/2ap}$[a] | min | N/A[b] | 15 | 10 | 12 |
| $t_{1/2\alpha}$ | min | 1 | N/A | N/A | N/A |
| $t_{1/2\beta}$ | min | 10 | 37 | 95 | 23 |
| AUC | ng-min/ml | $3.77 \times 10^4$ | $8.58 \times 10^5$ | $1.86 \times 10^5$ | $8.56 \times 10^4$ |
| $T_{max}$ | min | N/A | 32 | 26 | 23 |
| $C_{max}$ | ng/ml | N/A | 8690 | 1060 | 1270 |
| CL | ml/min | 331 | N/A | N/A | N/A |

Table 4

Pharmacokinetic values for methyl 3-cinnamyl-4-oxoRA (10 mg/kg) administered intravenously to mice

| Value | Units | Plasma | | Skin | |
|---|---|---|---|---|---|
| | | Parent ester | Free acid | Parent ester | Free acid |
| $t_{1/2ap}$[a] | min | N/A[b] | 22 | N/A | 78 |
| $t_{1/2\alpha}$ | min | 3 | N/A | N/A | N/A |
| $t_{1/2\beta}$ | min | 267 | 405 | 4280 | 344 |
| AUC | ng-min/ml | $1.04 \times 10^6$ | $2.40 \times 10^6$ | $7.34 \times 10^6$ | $1.59 \times 10^6$ |
| $T_{max}$ | min | N/A | 99 | N/A | 218 |
| $C_{max}$ | ng/ml | N/A | 3480 | 1190 | 2070 |
| CL | ml/min | 11 | N/A | N/A | N/A |

a    See the text for definition of the values derived.
b    N/A, not applicable or not observed.

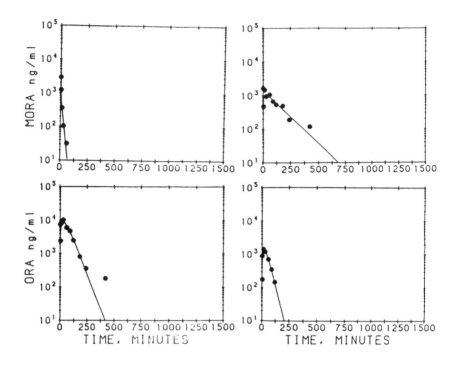

Figure 1.    Concentrations of methyl 4-oxoRA (MORA, top) and
4-oxoRA (ORA, bottom) in the plasma (left) and skin (right) of
mice dosed with methyl 4-oxoRA.

(1060 ng/g) is generally high. The elimination half-life (95 min) is short. Although the maximum concentration of the free acid (1270 ng/g) is generally high and is reached quickly (23 min), the AUC value (8.56 x $10^4$ ng-min/g) is low. These data indicate that methyl 4-oxoRA is rapidly hydrolyzed to the free acid and that its retention in the skin, either as the parent compound or as the free acid, is limited.

In contrast, for methyl 3-cinnamyl-4-oxoRA (Table 4, Figure 2) the values for $T_{1/2\beta}$ (267 min) and AUC (1.04 x $10^6$ ng-min/ml) are higher than for any of the other compounds; the value for clearance (11 ml/min) is lower. The $T_{1/2\beta}$ for the free acid (405 min) is long. In elimination from the skin of mice, the maximum concentration of the parent ester (1190 ng/g) is higher than for the other compounds. The elimination half-life (4280 min) is extremely long, and the AUC value (7.34 x $10^6$ ng-min/ml) is high. Similarly, the free acid shows generally high values for the elimination half-life (344 min), AUC (1.59 x $10^6$ ng-min/ml), $T_{max}$ (218 min), and $C_{max}$ (2070 ng/g). These data demonstrate that, following intravenous dosing, methyl 3-cinnamyl-4-oxoRA is slowly hydrolyzed to the free acid and that its retention in the skin, both as the parent compound and as the free acid, is prolonged.

The values for methyl RA (Table 5) are, in general, similar, but not quite as extreme, as those for methyl 3-cinnamyl-4-oxoRA; the values for methyl 3-methyl-4-oxoRA (Table 6) and methyl 3,3-dimethyl-4-oxoRA (Table 7) are, in general, intermediate between methyl 4-oxoRA and methyl RA.

These results show that some retinoid esters accumulate in the skin of mice and remain there for prolonged periods, gradually releasing the free acids, which are presumably the active forms of the drug. Thus, esters with bulky alkyl groups in the 3-position, may function as effective chemopreventive agents for skin cancers.

### Acknowledgement

The efforts related to generation of previously unreported data and to the synthesis and evaluation of analogs of 4-oxoretinoic acid were supported by Grant PO1 CA34968 from the National Cancer Institute, NIH, DHHS.

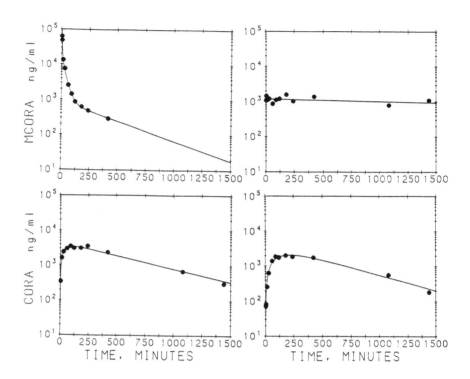

Figure 2. Concentrations of methyl 3-cinnamyl-4-oxoRA (MCORA, top) and 3-cinnamyl-4-oxoRA (CORA, bottom) in the plasma (left) and skin (right) of mice dosed with methyl 3-cinnamyl-4-oxoRA.

Table 5

Pharmacokinetic values for methyl RA (10 mg/kg)
administered intravenously to mice

| Value | Units | Plasma | | Skin | |
|---|---|---|---|---|---|
| | | Parent ester | Free acid | Parent ester | Free acid |
| $t_{1/2ap}$[a] | min | N/A[b] | 37 | 2 | 55 |
| $t_{1/2\alpha}$ | min | N/A | N/A | N/A | 80 |
| $t_{1/2\beta}$ | min | 36 | 63 | 3860 | 2340 |
| AUC | ng-min/ml | $2.78 \times 10^5$ | $4.37 \times 10^5$ | $3.30 \times 10^6$ | $3.26 \times 10^5$ |
| $T_{max}$ | min | N/A | 68 | 21 | 97 |
| $C_{max}$ | ng/ml | N/A | 2270 | 590 | 904 |
| CL | ml/min | 37 | N/A | N/A | N/A |

Table 6

Pharmacokinetic values for methyl 3-methyl-4-oxoRA
(10 mg/kg) administered intravenously to mice

| Value | Units | Plasma | | Skin | |
|---|---|---|---|---|---|
| | | Parent ester | Free acid | Parent ester | Free acid |
| $t_{1/2ap}$[a] | min | N/A[b] | 23 | 62 | 16 |
| $t_{1/2\alpha}$ | min | 1 | N/A | N/A | N/A |
| $t_{1/2\beta}$ | min | 32 | 36 | 166 | 44 |
| AUC | ng-min/ml | $1.37 \times 10^5$ | $2.67 \times 10^5$ | $2.68 \times 10^5$ | $3.95 \times 10^4$ |
| $T_{max}$ | min | N/A | 42 | 82 | 39 |
| $C_{max}$ | ng/ml | N/A | 2310 | 663 | 344 |
| CL | ml/min | 71 | N/A | N/A | N/A |

[a] See the text for definition of the values derived.
[b] N/A, not applicable or not observed.

Table 7
Pharmacokinetic values for methyl 3,3-dimethyl-4-oxoRA
(10 mg/kg) administered intravenously to mice

| Value | Units | Plasma | | Skin | |
|---|---|---|---|---|---|
| | | Parent ester | Free acid | Parent ester | Free acid |
| $t_{1/2ap}$[a] | min | N/A[b] | 20 | 223 | 11 |
| $t_{1/2\alpha}$ | min | 3 | N/A | N/A | N/A |
| $t_{1/2\beta}$ | min | 257 | 89 | 868 | 166 |
| AUC | ng-min/ml | $1.17 \times 10^5$ | $2.12 \times 10^5$ | $1.15 \times 10^6$ | $1.32 \times 10^5$ |
| $T_{max}$ | min | N/A | 54 | 302 | 46 |
| $C_{max}$ | ng/ml | N/A | 1070 | 618 | 456 |
| CL | ml/min | 83 | N/A | N/A | N/A |

[a] See the text for definition of the values derived.
[b] N/A, not applicable or not observed.

**References**

1. Moon, R.C.; McCormick, D.L.; Mehta, R.G. (1983). Inhibition of carcinogenesis by retinoids. Cancer Res. 43: 2469s-2475s.

2. Hill, D.L.; Grubbs, C.J. (1992). Retinoids and cancer prevention. Ann. Rev. Nutr. 12: 161-181.

3. Zachman, R.D.; Olson, J.A. (1961). A comparison of retinene reductase and alcohol dehydrogenase of rat liver. J. Biol. Chem. 236: 2309-2313.

4. Roberts, A.B.; Sporn, M.B. (1984). Cellular biology and biochemistry of the retinoids. In: "The retinoids" (Sporn, M.B.; Roberts, A.B.; Goodman, D.W., eds.), vol. 2, pp. 210-287. Academic Press, New York.

5. Dmitrovski, A.A. (1961). Oxidation of vitamin A aldehyde to vitamin A acid catalyzed by aldehyde oxidase. Biokhimiia 26: 109-113.

6. Futterman, S. (1962). Enzymatic oxidation of vitamin A aldehyde to vitamin A acid. J. Biol. Chem. 237: 677-680.

7. Leo, M.A.; Lieber, C.S. (1985). New pathway for retinol metabolism in liver microsomes. J. Biol. Chem. 260: 5228-5231.

8. Leo, M.A.; Lasker, J.M.; Raucy, J.L.; Kim, C-I., Black, M.; Lieber, C.S. (1989). Metabolism of retinol and retinoic acid by human liver cytochrome P450IIC8. Arch. Biochem. Biophys. 269: 305-312.

9. Shih, T.W.; Hill, D.L. (1991). Conversion of retinol to retinal by rat liver microsomes. Drug Metab. Dispos. 19: 332-335.

10. Brouwer, A.; van den Berg, K.J. (1984). Early and differential decrease in natural retinoid levels in C57BL/Rij and DBA/2 mice by 3,4,3',4'-tetra-chlorobiphenyl. Toxicol. Appl. Pharmacol. 73: 204-209.

11. Blomhoff, R.; Berg, T.; Norum, K.R. (1988). Distribution of retinol in rat liver cells: effect of age, sex, and nutritional status. Br. J. Nutr. 60: 233-239.

12. Alam, S.Q.; Alam, B.S. (1983). Lipid peroxide, α-tocopherol and retinoid levels in plasma and liver of rats fed diets containing β-carotene and 13-cis-retinoic acid. J. Nutr. 113: 2608-2614.

13. Hill, D.L.; Grubbs, C.J.; Shih, T.-W.; Shealy, Y.F. (1992). Unpublished results.

14. Lee, M.; Harris, K.; Trowbridge, H. (1964). Effect of the level of dietary protein on the toxicity of dieldrin for the laboratory rat. J. Nutr. 84: 136-144.

15.  Phillips, W.E.J. (1963). DDT and the metabolism of vitamin A and carotene in the rat. Can J. Biochem. 41: 1793-1802.

16.  Durham, S.K.; Brouwer, A. (1989). 3,4,3'4'-Tetrachlorobiphenyl-induced effect in the rat liver. I. Serum and hepatic retinoid reduction and morphologic changes. Toxicol. Pathol. 17: 536-544.

17.  Grubbs, C.J.; Moon, R.C.; Sporn, M.B.; Newton, D.L. (1977). Inhibition of mammary cancer by retinyl methyl ether. Cancer Res. 37: 599-602.

18.  Thompson, J.N.; Pitt, G.A.J. (1963). Conversion of retinyl methyl ether (vitamin A methyl ether) to retinol (vitamin A alcohol) in vivo. Biochim. Biophys. Acta 78: 753-755.

19.  Shih, T.W.; Shealy, Y.F.; Hill, D.L. (1991). Conversion of retinoid ethers to alcohols by enzymatic activity present in rat liver microsomes. Drug Metab. Dispos. 19: 336-339.

20.  McPhillips, D.M.; Lindamood, C. III; Heath, J.E.; Hill, D.L. (1988). The disposition and toxicology of retinyl methyl ether in rats dosed orally. Drug. Metab. Disposition 16: 683-689.

21.  Moon, R.C.; Thompson, H.J.; Becci, P.J.; Grubbs, C.J.; Gander, R.J.; Newton, D.L.; Smith, J.M.; Phillips, S.L.; Henderson, W.R.; Mullen, L.T.; Brown, C.C.; Sporn, M.B. (1979). N-(4-Hydroxyphenyl)retinamide, a new retinoid for prevention of breast cancer in the rat. Cancer Res. 39: 1339-1346.

22.  Thompson, H.J.; Becci, P.J.; Moon, R.C.; Sporn, M.B.; Newton, D.L.; Brown, C.C. (1980). Inhibition of 1-methyl-1-nitrosourea-induced mammary carcinogenesis in the rat by the retinoid axerophthene. Arzneim. Forsch. 30: 1127-29.

23.  Newton, D.L.; Frolik, C.A.; Roberts, A.B.; Smith, J.M.; Sporn, M.B.; Nurrenbach, A.; Paust, J. (1978). Biological activity and metabolism of the retinoid axerophthene (vitamin A hydrocarbon). Cancer Res. 38: 1734-1738.

24.  Hultin, T.A.; May, C.M.; Moon, R.C. (1986). N-(4-Hydroxyphenyl)-all-trans-retinamide pharmacokinetics in female rats and mice. Drug Metab. Dispos. 14: 714-717.

25.  Sporn, M.B.; Dunlop, N.M.; Newton, D.L.; Henderson, W.R. (1976). Relationships between structure and activity of retinoids. Nature 263: 110-113.

26.  Hultin, T.A.; McCormick, D.L.; May, C.M.; Moon, R.C. (1988). Effects of pretreatment with the retinoid N-(4-hydroxyphenyl)-all-trans-retinamide and phenobarbital on

the disposition and metabolism of N-(4-hydroxyphenyl)-all-trans-retinamide in mice. Drug Metab. Dispos. 16: 783-788.

27. Welsch, C.W.; DeHoog, J.V.; Moon, R.C. (1984). Lack of an effect of dietary retinoids in chemical carcinogenesis of the mouse mammary gland: inverse relationship between mammary tumor cell anaplasia and retinoid efficacy. Carcinogenesis 5: 1301-1304.

28. McPhillips, D.M.; Kalin, J.R.; Hill, D.L. (1987). The pharmacokinetics of all-trans-retinoic acid and N-(2-hydroxyethyl)retinamide in mice as determined with a sensitive and convenient procedure: solid-phase extraction and reverse-phase HPLC. Drug Metab. Dispos. 15: 207-211.

29. Wang, C.-C.; Campbell, S.; Furner, R.L.; Hill, D.L. (1980). Disposition of all-trans- and 13-cis-retinoic acids and N-hydroxyethylretinamide in mice after intravenous administration. Drug Metab. Dispos. 8: 8-11.

30. Swanson, B.N.; Frolik, C.A.; Zaharevitz, D.W.; Roller, P.P.; Sporn, M.B. (1981). Dose-dependent kinetics of all-trans-retinoic acid in rats. Plasma levels and excretion into bile, urine, and faeces. Biochem. Pharmacol. 30: 107-113.

31. Kalin, J.R.; Starling, M.E.; Hill, D.L. (1981). Disposition of all-trans-retinoic acid in mice following oral doses. Drug Metab. Dispos. 9: 196-201.

32. Shelley, R.S.; Jun, H.W.; Price, J.C.; Cadwallader, D.E. (1982). Blood level studies of all-trans- and 13-cis-retinoic acids in rats using different formulations. J. Pharm. Sci. 71: 904-907.

33. Verma, A.K.; Shapas, B.G.; Rice, H.M.; Boutwell, R.K. (1979). Correlation of the inhibition by retinoids of tumor promoter-induced mouse epidermal ornithine decarboxylase activity and of skin tumor promotion. Cancer Res. 39: 419-25.

34. Sani, B.P.; Hill, D.L. (1974). Retinoic acid: A binding protein in chick embryo metatarsal skin. Biochem. Biophys. Res. Comm. 61: 1276-1282.

35. Sani, B.P.; Singh, R.K.; Reddy, L.G.; Gaub, M-P. (1990). Isolation, partial purification and characterization of nuclear retinoic acid receptors from chick skin. Arch. Biochem. Biophys. 283: 107-113.

36. Kalin, J.R.; Wells, M.J.; Hill, D.L. (1984). Effects of phenobarbital, 3-methylcholanthrene and retinoid pretreatment on disposition of orally administered retinoids in mice. Drug Metab. Dispos. 12: 63-67.

37.  Rigas, J.R.; Francis, P.A.; Muindi, J.R.F.; Kris, M.G.;
     Huselton, C.; DeGrazia, F.; Orazem, J.P.; Young, C.W.;
     Warrell, R.P., Jr. (1993). Constitutive variability in
     the pharmacokinetics of the natural retinoid, all-trans-
     retinoic acid, and its modulation by ketoconazole. J.
     Natl. Cancer Inst. 85: 1921-1926.

38.  Frolik, C.A.; Roberts, A.B.; Tavla, T.E.; Roller, P.P.;
     Newton, D.L.; Sporn, M.B. (1979). Isolation and
     identification of 4-hydroxy- and 4-oxoretinoic acid. In
     vitro metabolites of all-trans-retinoic acid in hamster
     trachea and liver. Biochemistry 18: 2092-2097.

39.  Kalin, J.R.; Wells, M.J.; Hill, D.L. (1982).
     Disposition of 13-cis-retinoic acid and N-(2-
     hydroxyethyl)retinamide in mice following oral doses.
     Drug Metab. Dispos. 10: 391-398.

40.  Shih, T.-W.; Shealy, Y.F.; Strother, D.L.; Hill, D.L.
     (1986). Nonenzymic isomerization of all-trans- and 13-
     cis-retinoids catalyzed by sulfhydryl groups. Drug.
     Metab. Dispos. 14: 698-702.

41.  McCormick, A.M.; Patel, M.; Patrizi, V.B.; Fang, X.Z.
     (1985). Metabolism of 4-hydroxyphenylretinamide to
     retinoic acid in vivo and in cultured bladder carcinoma
     cells. Fed. Proc. 44: 1672.

42.  Shih, T.-W.; Shealy, Y.F.; Hill, D.L. (1988). Enzymatic
     hydrolysis of retinamides. Drug. Metab. Dispos. 16:
     337-340.

43.  Kenel, M.F.; Krayer, J.H.; Merz, E.A.; Pritchard, J.F.
     (1988). Teratogenicity of N-(4-hydroxyphenyl)-all-
     trans-retinamide in rats and rabbits. Teratog.
     Carcinog. Mutagen. 8: 1-11.

44.  Willhite, C.C.; Shealy, Y.F. (1984). Amelioration of
     embryotoxicity by structural modification of the
     terminal group of cancer chemopreventive retinoids. J.
     Natl. Cancer Inst. 72: 689-695.

45.  Swanson, B.N.; Zaharevitz, D.W.; Sporn, M.B. (1980).
     Pharmacokinetics of N-(4-hydroxyphenyl)-all-trans-
     retinamide in rats. Drug Metab. Dispos. 8: 168-172.

46.  Frolik, C.A. (1984). Metabolism of retinoids. In: "The
     retinoids" (Sporn, M.B.; Roberts, A.B.; Goodman, D.W.,
     eds.), vol. 2, pp. 177-208. Academic Press, New York.

47.  Shealy, Y.F. (1989). Synthesis and evaluation of some
     new retinoids for cancer chemoprevention. Prev. Med. 18:
     624-645.

48.  Shealy, Y.F.; Hosmer, C.A.; Riordan, J.M.; Wille, J.W.;
     Rogers, T.S.; Hill, D.L. (1994). Cancer chemo-
     preventive 3-substituted-4-oxoretinoic acids. J. Med.
     Chem., in press.

# INVOLVEMENT OF RETINOIC ACID NUCLEAR RECEPTORS IN TRANSCRIPTIONAL REGULATION OF TISSUE TRANSGLUTAMINASE, THE GENE INVOLVED IN APOPTOSIS

Ajit K. Verma and Mitchell F. Denning

Department of Human Oncology, Medical School,
University of Wisconsin Comprehensive Cancer Center
Madison, WI 53792 (AKV)
National Cancer Institute, Bethesda, MD 20892 (MFD)

## INTRODUCTION

Retinoic acid (RA), an active metabolite of dietary vitamin A (1,2), is essential to maintain normal growth and differentiation of epithelial cells (3,4). RA and certain of its analogs have also been used in experimental animals to prevent and treat cancers of a variety of epithelial tissues (4-9). The mode of action of RA remains speculative. Accumulating evidence indicate that RA mediates its effects through specific nuclear receptors (10-16). RA nuclear receptors belong to a super-family of steroid, thyroid and vitamin D receptors, the ligand-inducible transcriptional factors (10-12). Two major families of RA nuclear receptors (RAR and RXR) have been identified. The RAR ($\alpha$,$\beta$, $\gamma$) are activated by both all trans-RA and 9-cis-RA while RXR ($\alpha$, $\beta$, $\gamma$) are activated by 9-cis-RA only (16,17). Thus, RAR and RXR are distinct retinoid receptor subfamilies (16,17). RAR require co-regulators to bind effectively to RA responsive element (RARE) in a target gene. RXR functions as auxiliary receptor for RAR and related receptors (18). RXR$\beta$ forms heterodimers with RAR to increase its DNA binding and transcriptional activity (16,19). Other transcriptional factors such as COUP-TF can also modulate RAR activities (20). We determined the role that RAR plays in the signal transduction pathway leading to the expression of tissue transglutaminase (TG) by RA (21,22). Data indicating that vitamin A nutritional status in rats influences the expression of both RAR and tissue TG in certain tissues will be presented. The results that imply that the levels of RAR determine the magnitude of tissue TG induction by retinoic acid will also be summarized.

The gene encoding tissue TG is among the RA responsive genes. (21,22). TGs (EC 2.3.2.13) are a family of $Ca^{2+}$-dependent enzymes that catalyze the covalent cross-linking of proteins by the formation of $\epsilon-$ ($\gamma$-glutaminyl)-lysyl isopeptides bonds (23-25). Two members of the TG family, epidermal TG and tissue TG, are differentially regulated by RA. Epidermal TG (Type I or keratinocyte) is a membrane associated enzyme, while tissue TG is a cytosolic enzyme (24-30). The cDNAs for both tissue and epidermal TGs have been cloned (26,27). The epidermal TG shares only 49-53% homology with other TGs. Evidence, based on thermostability, chromatographic behavior, and kinetic characteristics, indicate that epidermal TG is distinct from tissue TG (23). Increased epidermal TG activity, altered cytokeratin expression, and cross-linked envelope formation are important components of squamous differentiation. RA treatment inhibits both the induction of epidermal TG and the formation of cornified envelopes in the tracheal cells (26). Epidermal TG is increased in the superbasal differentiating cells while tissue TG activity is increased preferentially in the basal epidermal cells. Epidermal TG is involved in the formation of cornified envelopes, the insoluble cross-linked proteins. Several substrates (involucrin, loricrin, keratolinin) of epidermal TG have been shown to be the components of cornified envelopes (30). Epidermal TG has a higher molecular weight (92 KD) than other TGs (50-72 KD). Epidermal TG is an essential component of the pathway to squamous differentiation while tissue TG has been shown to play a role in the programming of cell death, activation of macrophages, endocytosis, and cell growth (24,25). The mechanism underlying the induction of tissue TG by RA has been analyzed in murine peritoneal macrophages (24,25). The induction of tissue TG mRNA by RA was not due to an increase in its stability but was due to an increase in the rate of transcription. We analyzed the association of RAR with tissue TG gene expression both in vivo in intact rat tissue and in vitro in rat tracheal 2C5 cells and these results form the subject matter of this chapter.

## RESULTS

### A. Vitamin A Nutritional Status in Rats Regulates the Level of Expression of RAR and Tissue TG in Various Tissue.

Weanling male Sprague-Dawley rats, 3 weeks of age weighing ~ 35gm, were used to determine the influence of vitamin A nutritional status on the level of expression of RAR and tissue TG (21). Rats were randomly divided into groups of 15 rats, were allowed to have free excess to food and water, and were weighed weekly. The rats were kept in mesh-bottom cages (3 rats/cage) in a room with a constant air flow system, controlled temperature (21-23°C), and a 12-hr light: dark cycle. The rats were fed for 7 wk either a purified diet that was deficient in vitamin A (ICN Biochemicals, Cleveland, OH) or a control diet supplemented with retinyl acetate (24 mg/kg diet). Vitamin A deficiency was confirmed by analysis of tissue concentrations of retinol and retinyl plamitate. In a second experiment, weanling male Sprague-Dawley rats were fed the control or vitamin A-deficient diet for 7 wk. There were 24 rats per diet regimen (4 rats/cage). After vitamin A deficiency was established by comparative growth curves and analysis of liver retinol and reinyl palmitate, rats on each diet regimen were randomly separated into two groups (12 rats per group, 4 rats/cage). One group continued to receive its original diet; the other was fed the original diet supplemented with RA at a dose of 12 mg/kg diet. These animals were used for tissue analysis 4 wk after the start of RA supplementation.

Rats fed the vitamin A-deficient diet had significantly ($P<0.05$) lower body weight than the rats fed the control diet containing 24 mg/kg retinyl acetate. Rats on the vitamin A-deficient diet had depleted concentrations of retinol ($\leq 0.063 \pm 0.02$ nmol/g tissue) and retinyl esters ($\leq 0.37 \pm 0.15$ nmol/g tissue) in various tissues, including the liver. The vitamin A-deficient rats appeared healthy and did not exhibit infection or neurological signs or symptoms (21).

The effects of vitamin A nutritional status in rats on the levels of expression of RAR in various rat tissue were quantitated by the Northern blotting procedure (21). Fragments of human RAR cDNA used as probes for hybridization were as follows: RARα: 1.78 Kb EcoR1 RARα cDNA insert; RARβ: 652-and 615-bp EcoR1 RARβ cDNA inserts; RARγ: 1.6 Kb EcoR1 fragment of RARγø. Using these RAR probes, no cross-hybridization among RAR was observed (21).

RARα, RARβ and RARγ were differentially expressed in various rat tissues (Fig. 1A-1C). The lung had the highest level of RARα and RARβ while the trachea has the highest-level of RARγ among the various rat tissue analyzed (Fig. 1A-1C). Rats fed the vitamin A-deficient diet had 55-96% lower expression of RARβ in several tissues, including kidney, liver, intestine, lung, brain, bladder and trachea (Fig. 1D, 1E). RARγ message levels in the bladder, lung and trachea of vitamin A-deficient rats were 33, 47 and 78% lower respectively. The levels of RAR expression in vitamin A-deficient rats were 90% lower in the brain and 30, 60, 30 and 61% higher in the kidney, liver, intestine, and lung, respectively (Fig. 1D, 1E). Despite the fact that Haq et al. (31) used a different protocol to render rats vitamin A-deficient (32), their results are compatible with our findings. In accord with our findings (21), Haq et al. (31) detected two transcripts of RARα (3.7 and 2.8 kb), two RARβ mRNA species (3.3 and 3.0 kb) and a single 3.4-kb RARγ transcript in liver and lung. Retinol deficiency caused 70 and 65% lower levels of RRβ in liver and lung, respectively.

The expression of RARγ was also lower in the liver and lung of retinol-deficient rats (31).

The results of the effects of vitamin A-deficiency on the level of expression of tissue TG are also shown in Figure 1D and 1E. Clearly, the levels of tissue TG mRNA in the liver, lung, trachea and bladder were 81, 92, 72 and 43% lower, respectively in vitamin A-deficient rats. The alteration in RAR expression correlated with changes in tissue TG expression. A positive correlation between the levels of RAR (β and γ) and tissue TG was observed in the bladder, lung and trachea (Fig. 1D , 1E).

Vitamin A deficiency in rats has been shown to result in squamous differentiation of tracheal epithelium accompanied by expression of specific keratins (33). Kato et al. (34) reported that vitamin A nutritional status in rats modulated the level of the retinoid-binding proteins, cellular retinol-binding protein (CRBP) and cellular retinoic acid-binding protein. However, findings by Rajan et al. (35) indicate that the effects of dietary retinol on the levels of CRBP mRNA are highly tissue specific. Retinol deficiency did not alter the levels of CRBP mRNA in proximal epididymis, liver and kidney, but a substantial decrease in the levels of CRBP mRNA was observed in lung, testis, spleen and small intestine of retinol-deficient rats. Kim and Wolf (36) have shown that the physiological levels of vitamin A in rats determine the expression of fibronectin, which is involved in cell adhesion and differentiation. It is likely that the effects of vitamin A deficiency are the result of altered expressions of RAR.

The results presented here clearly indicate that dietary vitamin A levels modulate the expression of RAR and tissue TG (Fig. 1). Levels of expression of RARα and RARγ were consistently lower than normal in several tissues of vitamin A-deficient rats . A dramatic decrease in RARα expression occurred only in the brain tissue of vitamin A-deficient rats (Fig.1). The effect of vitamin A deficiency on the level of RAR expression was at least partially reversible. When vitamin A-deficient rats were switched to a vitamin A-repleted diet, the levels of expression of RARβ and RARγ were near normal (21). A possible interpretation of these results is that RA regulates the expression of its own receptors. RA has been shown to induce the expression of RARβ by regulation at the transcriptional level (37). However, evidence indicates that RARα and RARγ are not inducible and are expressed from relatively stable mRNA (37). Our results indicate that in certain rat tissues (trachea, lung and bladder) vitamin A regulates the levels of expression of both RARβ and RARγ (Fig. 1).

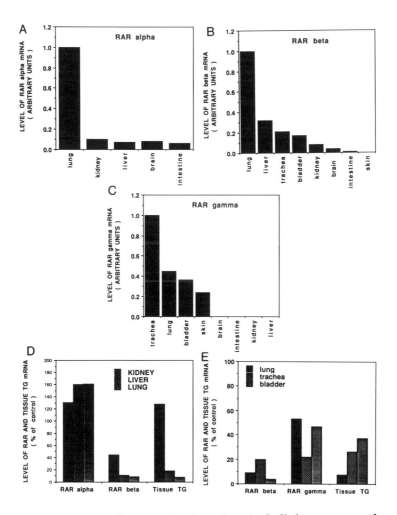

**Figure 1.** **The effects of vitamin A-deficiency on the expression of RAR and Tissue TG.** Male Sprague-Dawley rats were fed for 7 wk a control diet or vitamin A-deficient diet (21). Total or Poly (A+) RNA from the indicated tissues (1 g) obtained from pooled samples from 10 rats was isolated and the level of expression of RAR was determined by the Northern blot analyses. Autoradiograms were scanned using a laser densitometer, and all RAR values were normalized to the values of GAPDH. A,B,C indicate the expression of RAR in various tissue of rats on a control diet D,E indicate the changes in the levels of expression of RAR and Tissue TG in various tissue of rats on a vitamin A-deficient diet.

B.  Effects of RAR Levels on RA-Induced Tissue TG Gene Expression
in Rat Tracheal 2C5 Cells.

The results presented in the preceding section indicate that
vitamin A nutritional status in rats is associated with the level of
expression of both RAR and tissue TG. However, these results (Fig. 1)
do not provide evidence of a direct link between RAR level and the level
of expression of tissue TG. To test the hypothesis that RAR levels may
dictate the degree of expression of tissue TG by RA, we used a non-
tumorigenic rat tracheal 2C5 cell line (22, 38). 2C5 cells express low
levels of RARα, RARβ, RARγ and RXRα mRNA (Fig. 2) and
treatment of 2C5 cells with RA results in dramatic induction of tissue TG
activity (22). We altered the levels of RAR in 2C5 cells by transfecting
2C5 cells with RARα, RARβ or an RARγ expression vector (Fig. 3).

1.  Selection and characterization of RAR transfectants: Cells
were transfected with the expression vectors RAR-αø, RAR-βø,
RARγø, or RAR-Aαø plus pSV2-Neo (5:1 ratio) by the calcium
phosphate method as previously described (22). Transfectants were
grown and expanded in media containing 400 µg/ml G418 until they
were frozen. The RAR transfectants of 2C5 cells were characterized for
RAR DNA level by Southern blot analysis (22) and for the level of
mRNA by Northern blot analysis (22). The level of RAR protein from
the transfectants was determined by the separation of [$^3$H]RA-RAR
complex by high-performance size-exclusion chromatography (39).

As shown in Figure 4B, the DNA from several of the RAR-αø
transfectants contained a 618 bp Pst I fragment which hybridized to
RARα. This 618 bp fragment is the same size as the Pst I fragment
from the transfected expression vector and was absent from the Neol
transfectant. The RARα cDNA copy number was estimated by laser
beam densitometry and varied from 1 for RARα24 to approximately 60
for RARα23. The 2.9 kb band represented the endogenous RARα
gene. Southern blot analysis of the RAR-βø transfectants is shown in
Figure 4A. The 652 bp EcoRI fragment hybridized to RARβ was
present only in the RAR-βø transfectants and absent in the pSV2-Neo
transfectants. Figure 4C shows a Southern blot of EcoR1 digested
genomic DNA from various RARγ transfectants probed with a RARγ
probe. The high molecular weight band (>12 kb) is present in the pSV2-
Neo transfectant (Neo7) and the mock transfectant (Mock1) and is due to
endogenous RARγ sequences. The 1.6 Kb band is the same size as the
EcoR1 fragment containing the transfected RARγ cDNA and is visible in
RARAγ6 cells, RARγ8 cells, and RARγ2 transfectants.

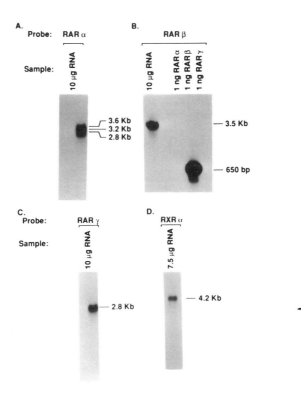

**Figure 2.   Expression of endogenous RARα, RARβ, RARγ, and RXRα mRNA in 2C5 cells.** The indicated amount of poly A⁺ RNA from 2C5 cells was analyzed for the expression of RAR and RXR by Northern blot analyses.    To check for cross hybridization between the RARs, the RARβ blot also contained 1 ng of EcoR1 inserts from RARα, RARβ, and RARγ cDNA.

The level of RAR expression in the transfectants was quantitated by Northern blot analysis.  As shown in Figure 5A, RARα was overexpressed in the transfectants RARα23 and RARα24.  The antisense transfectant RARAα10 was expressing very high levels of antisense RNA.  The RARα transcript sizes were 2.36 kb, 2.0 kb and 1.78 kb and may have resulted from differences in splicing and/or polyadenylation.

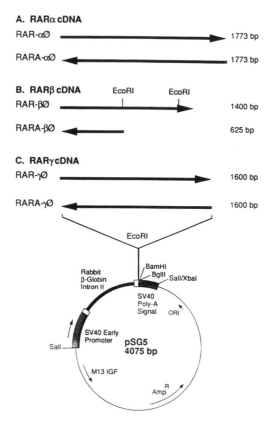

**Figure 3.    RAR expression vectors**. All RAR cDNAs were inserted into the EcoR1 site of the eukaryotic expression vector pSG5. The cDNAs are shown as thick arrows pointing in the sense or antisense direction.

Figure 5B illustrates that the RARβ transfectants RARβ10, RARβ13, RARβ14, and RARβ15 also overexpressed the transfected RAR. The sizes of the RARβ transcripts were 3.5 kb, 2.6 kb and 2.0 kb. The Northern blot analysis of RARγ transfectants in Figure 5C shows a 2.8 Kb band in all cells. This band corresponds in size to the endogenous RARγ transcript detectable in 2C5 cells (Figure 2). Several transfectants express additional RARγ hybridzing species of 1.9 Kb. The highest level of overexpression was observed in the sense transfectants RARγ2 and RARγ8 which expressed a 1.9 Kb message. The antisense transfectant RARAγ6 also expressed an antisense RARγ message (1.9 Kb) which hybridized to the double stranded probe.

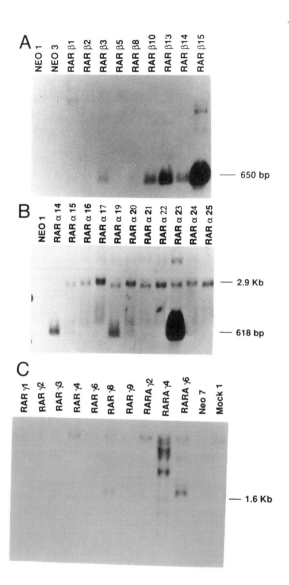

**Figure 4.    Southern blot analysis of RAR transfectants.**
10μg of DNA from the indicated RARβ (A), RARα (B), or RARγ (C)
transfectant was digested with Pst 1 (RARα) or ECoR1 (RARβ and
RARγ) and subjected to Southern blot analysis on a 1% agarose gel.

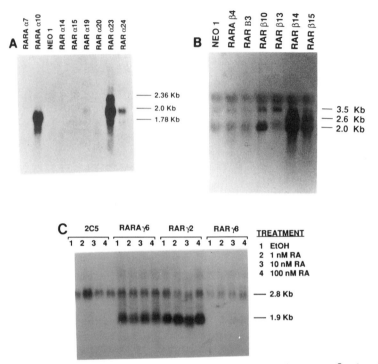

**Figure 5.    Northern blot analysis of RAR transfectants.**
10μg total RNA from the indicated RARα (A) RARβ (B) or RARγ (C)
transfectant was used for the Northern blot analysis.

Binding of [³H]RA to RAR from nuclear fractions from 2C5,
RARα, RARβ and RARγ transfectants was analyzed by chromatography
on a size-exclusion column (39). The nuclear extracts from 2C5 and
RARα23 contain a major [³H]-RA binding activity which can be
inhibited by a 200-fold excess of cold RA. This specific binding elutes
at a $M_r$ of 49 kD. The predicted molecular weight of all identified RARs
is approximately 50 kD. Specific binding in the 49 kD peak was 5855
dpm for 2C5 and 15,184 dpm for RARα23 cells. The nuclear [³H]-RA
binding activity of RARα24 cells eluted at a predicted $M_r$ of 49 kD and
contained 13,214 dpm of specific binding. The RARγ sense
transfectants (RARγ2 and RARγ8) had increased specific RA binding
activity as compared to parental 2C5 cells (9089 and 8936 dpm vs 4332
dpm). This increase in RA binding of ~2-fold corresponded to the
increase in RARγ mRNA (2 to 3-fold) for the RARγ2 and RARγ8
transfectants. This binding data is in agreement with RARγ being the
most abundant RAR in 2C5 cells. The antisense RARAγ6 transfectant
had a decreased RA binding activity (2354 dpm vs 4332 dpm).

2. The response of RAR transfectants to RA for tissue TG gene expression. Tissue TG was induced by RA in several of the transfectants to determine if the response to RA correlated with the level of RAR. Figure 6A shows the effect of RA on TG in RARα transfectants. While TG was induced ~34-fold by 100 nM RA in the parental 2C5 cells, the RARα over-expressing transfectants RARα23 and RARα24 induced TG activity 80- and 77-fold respectively. TG activity in the RARα antisense transfectant RARAα10 was increased by only 9-fold. The induction of TG activity in the pSV2-Neo transfectant Neo2 (25 fold) was similar to that of the parental (data not shown).

To determine if the increase in TG activity by RA was truly the result of increased gene expression and not a post-translational modification or activation of the enzyme, the level of TG mRNA was determined by Northern blot analysis. The induction of TG activity in RARα transfectants was accompanied by an increase in TG mRNA as shown in Figure 7A. RA treatment caused an increase in two tissue TG mRNAs of 3.2 kb and 2.2 kb, with the 3.2 kb message being approximately 5 times more abundant than the 2.2 kb message.

The induction of tissue TG by RA in RARβ over-expressing cells is shown in Figure 6B. In RARβ10 cells, TG activity was increased to a much greater extent at lower RA concentrations (1.0 nM and 10 nM) than parental 2C5 cells. RARβ14 cells were only marginally more responsive to 100 nM RA than 2C5 cells.

Figure 6C illustrates that the level of RARγ expression is also correlated with the induction of tissue TG by RA. TG was induced in RARγ2 cells 23-fold at 10 nM RA and 71-fold at 100 nM RA while only 6-fold and 52-fold induction was observed in 2C5 cells at 10 nM and 100 nM RA respectively. The antisense transfectant RARAγ6 was less responsive than 2C5 cells for RA-induced TG activity. TG was induced in RARγ8 cells to a similar extent as in 2C5 cells despite being a RAR-γø transfectant. RNA was analyzed by Northern blot to determine if RARγ8 cells were indeed over-expressing RARγ during this experiment. Figure 7B shows that RARγ expression in RARγ8 cells had reverted to the level of 2C5 cells. Both RARγ2 and RARAγ6 were still expressing the transfected RARγ cDNA. Figure 7B demonstrates that RA-induced tissue TG activity in 2C5 cells and the RARγ transfectants was accompanied by an increase in tissue TG mRNA. The mRNA induction by RA was dose dependent and correlated with tissue TG activity.

These results (Figs.6 and 7) present direct evidence indicating the involvement of RAR in RA-induced TG expression in 2C5 cells. The role of RARα levels in regulating the induction of TG by RA was strengthened by the finding that the antisense transfectant RARAα10

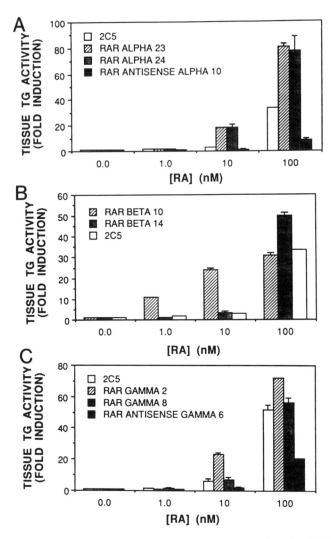

**Figure 6.** **Effect of RA on tissue TG activity in 2C5 cells and RAR transfectants.** The indicated RARα (A), RARβ (B), RARγ (C) transfectant or parental 2C5 cells were grown either in the presence of 0.1% ethanol ([RA] = 0.0) of the indicated concentration of RA. Tissue TG activity assayed after four days treatment. Fold induction was calculated by dividing the TG activity in the presence of RA by the TG activity in the absence of RA. Each value is the mean ± standard error of duplicate determinations from two culture dishes.

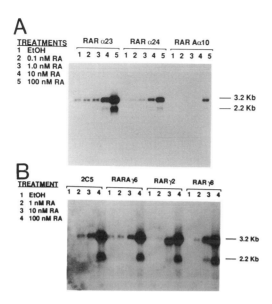

**Figure 7. Effect of RA on tissue TG mRNA levels in RAR transfectants.** Shown are the autoradiograms of Northern blot analyses of RNA from the indicated RAR transfectant. Cells were grown for four days in the presence of either 0.1% ethanol (EtOH) or different RA concentrations and then RNA was isolated. 10μg total RNA was loaded per lane and probed with the tissue TG cDNA.

was not as responsive as the parental and pSV-Neo transfectants. These results are consistent with the findings that the level of RARα determines tissue TG induction by RA (22). Both RARβ overexpressing transfectants (RARβ10 and RARβ14) were more responsive than parental 2C5 cells to RA for the induction of tissue TG. The expression of RARγ sense or antisense cDNA increased or decreased the induction of TG by RA respectively. The revertant RARγ8 transfectant returned to the parental level of induction as it no longer overexpressed RARγ. Northern blot analysis indicates that RARγ is the most expressed RAR in 2C5 cells and on this basis it could be postulated to be the most important RAR for the induction of tissue TG by RA.

The induction of tissue TG activity is accompanied by an increase in two TG mRNAs of 3.2 and 2.4 Kb in size. The induction of TG mRNA was correlated with an increase in TG activity caused by RA (r = 0.999). These results indicate that RA-induced TG activity is the result of increased TG gene expression.

## SUMMARY AND CONCLUSION

In summary, the results presented here indicate that vitamin A nutritional status differentially regulates the expression of RAR in rat tissues. A decrease in the expression of RARβ and RARγ paralleled a decrease in the expression of tissue TG in lung, trachea and bladder of retinol-deficient rats. Transfectants overexpressing RAR (α, β or γ) were more responsive than parental 2C5 cells to RA for the induction of tissue TG. For the regulation of tissue TG by RA, it appears that the levels of RARα, RARβ, and RARγ can all determine the magnitude of the induction. In tissues such as trachea where RARγ is the predominant RAR isoform, this isoform would be the major regulator of tissue TG expression and changes in nutritional status, such as vitamin A deficiency, which decrease RARγ levels, would subsequently decrease the induction of tissue TG by RA. It is likely that RA and a specific RAR complex interacts with the cis-acting elements (RARE) in the 5'-flanking region of tissue TG gene to confer increased transcription. RARE have been identified in a number of RA-responsive genes such as murine laminin B1 gene (40), human RARβ gene (41), murine complement factor H gene (42), alcohol dehydrogenase type I gene (43) and the gene for human osteocalcin (44).

## PERSPECTIVES

The alterations in the levels of retonoic acid nuclear receptors (RAR and RXR) and tissue TG may have implications in prevention and/or treatment of human cancer. Tissue TG, a unique member of the TG family of enzymes (23-25,45-46), is an essential component of the signal transduction pathway of programmed cell death (apoptosis) (47-50). Apoptosis is the normal physiological process of cell death that is involved in the control of eukaryotic cell population during embryogenesis, immune responses and in response to toxins. Apoptosis may be one of the ways to eliminate unwanted (preneoplastic) cell population. Tumor promoters such as 12-O-tetradecanoylphorbol-13-acetate (TPA) may promote tumor formation by inhibiting apoptosis (51,52). In this context, it is also noteworthy that TPA inhibits RA-induced tissue TG activity in mouse epidermis (23) and downregulates the expression of RAR and RXR (53). Epidemiological study and evidence from experimental animals indicate a close association between retinoic acid deficiency and enhanced susceptibility to chemical carcinogenesis of some organs such as lung and bladder (54,55).

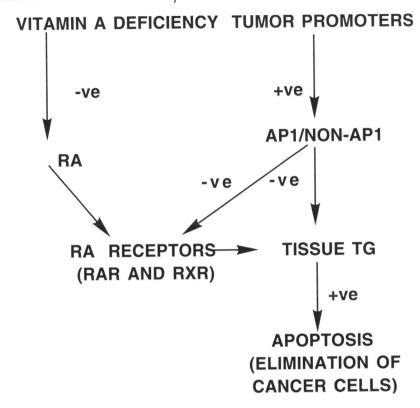

**Figure 8.** **Proposed Hypothesis** implicating tissue TG and RA nuclear receptors as targets for cancer prevention.

**+ve:** increase; **-ve:** decrease.

Vitamin A deficiency in rats accompanies decreased expression of RAR (RARβ and RARγ) and tissue TG in lung, trachea and bladder (21). Taken together, we propose that the retinoic acid nuclear receptors and tissue TG, in addition to ornithine decarboxylase (6-9, 56), may be critical molecular targets for chemoprevention of human cancer (Fig. 8).

**References**

1. DeLuca HF (1979) Retinoic acid metabolism. Fed Proc 38:2519-2523.
2. DeLuca LM. Bhat PV, Sasak W, Adama S (1979) Synthesis of phosphoryl and glycosyl phosphoryl derivatives of vitamin A in biological membranes. Fed Proc 38:2535-2539.
3. Walback SB, Howe PR (1925) Tissue changes following deprivation of fat-soluble vitamin A. J Exp Med 42:753-778.
4. Gudas LJ (1992) Retinoids, retinoid-responsive genes, cell differentiation, and cancer. Cell Growth & Differentiation 3:655-662.
5. Hill DL, Grubbs CJ (1992) Retinoids and cancer prevention. Annu. Rev. Nutr. 12:161-181.
6. Verma AK, Boutwell RK (1977) Vitamin A acid (retinoic acid), a potent inhibitor of 12-O-tetradecanoylphorbol-13-acetate-induced ornithine decarboxylase activity in mouse epidermis. Cancer Res. 37:2196-2201.
7. Verma AK, Rice HM, Shapas BG (1978) Inhibition of 12-O-tetradecanoylphorbol-13-acetate-induced ornithine decarboxylase activity in mouse epidermis by vitamin A analogues (retinoids).
8. Verma AK, Shapas BG, Rice HM, Boutwell RK (1979) Correlation of the inhibition by retinoids of tumor promoter-induced mouse epidermal ornithine decarboxylase activity and of skin tumor promotion. Cancer Res. 39:419-425.
9. Verma AK, Duvick L, Ali M (1986) Modulation of mouse skin tumor promotion by dietary 13-cis-retinoic acid and α-difluoromethylornithine. Carcinogenesis 7:1019-1023.
10. Mangelsdorf DJ, Ong ES, Dyck JA, Evans RM (1990) Nuclear receptor that identifies a novel retinoic acid response pathway. Nature 345:224-229.
11. Brand N, Petkovich M, Krust A, Chambon P, de The H, Marchio A, Tiollais P, Dejean A (1988) Identification of a second human retinoic acid receptor. Nature 332:850-853.
12. Benbrook D, Lernhardt E, Pfah M (1988) A new retinoic acid receptor identified from a hepatocellular carcinoma. Nature 333:669-672.
13. Zelent A, Krust A, Petkovich M, Kastner P, Chambon P (1989) Cloning of murine α and βretinoic acid receptors and a novel receptor γ predominantly expressed in skin. Nature 339:714-717.
14. Krust A, Kastner P, Petkovich M, Zelent A, Chambon P (1989) A third human retinoic acid receptor, hRAR-γ. Proc. Natl. Acad. Sci. USA 86:5310-5314.
15. Petkovich M (1992) Regulation of gene expression by vitamin A: the role of nuclear retinoic acid receptors. Annu. Reve. Nutr. 12:443-471.

16. Zhang X, Hoffmann B, Tran PB, Graupner G, Pfah M (1992) Retinoid X receptor in an auxiliary protein for thyroid hormone and retinoic acid receptors. Nature 355:441-446.
17. Thomas H, Bugge JP, Lonnoy O, Hendrik G, Stunnenberg H, (1992) RXRα, a promiscuous partner of retinoic acid and thyroid hormone receptors. EMBO J. 11:1409-1418.
18. Kliewer SA, Umesono K, Mangelsdorf DJ, Evans RM (1992) Retinoid X receptor interacts with nuclear receptors in retinoic acid, thyroid hormone and vitamin D3 signaling. Nature 355:446-449.
19. Marks MS, Hallenbeck PL, Nagata T, Segars JH, Appella E, Nikodem VM, Ozato K (1992) H-2RIIBP (RXRβ) heterodimerization provides a mechanism for combinatorial diversity in the regulation of retinoic acid and thyroid hormone-responsive genes. EMBO J. 11:1419-1435.
20. Kliewer SA, Umesono K, Heyman RA, Mangelsdorf DJ, Dyck JA, Evans RM (1992) Retinoid X receptor α COUP-TF interactions modulate retinoic acid signaling. Proc. Natl. Acad. Sci. USA 89:1;448-1452.
21. Verma AK, Shoemaker A, Simsiman R, Denning M, Zachman RA, (1992) Expression of retinoic acid nuclear receptors and tissue transglutaminase is altered in various tissues of rats fed a vitamin A-deficient diet. J. Nutr. 122:2144-2152.
22. Denning MF, Verma AK (1991) Involvement of retinoic acid nuclear receptors in retinoic acid-induced tissue transglutaminase gene expression in rat tracheal 2C5 cells. Biochem. Biophys. Res. Commun. 175:344-355.
23. Lichti U, Yuspa SH (1988) Modulation of tissue and epidermal transglutaminases in mouse epidermal cells after treatment with a 12-O-tetradecanoylphorbol-13-acetate/or retinoic acid *in vivo* and in culture. Cancer Res. 48:74-81.
24. Chiocca EA, Davies PJA, Stein JP (1988) The molecular basis of retinoic acid action. J Biol Chem 263:11584-11589.
25. Chiocca EA, Davies PJA, Stein JP (1989) Regulation of tissue transglutaminase gene expression as a molecular model for retinoid effects on proliferation and differentiation. J Cell Biochem 39:293-304.
26. Floyd EE, Jetten AM (1989) Regulation of type I (epidermal) transglutaminase mRNA levels during squamous differentiation: down-regulation by retinoids. Mol Cell Biol 9:4846-4851.
27. George MD, Volberg TM, Floyd EE, Stein JP, Jetten AM (1990) Regulation of transglutaminase type II transforming growth factor-B1 in normal and transformed human epidermal keratinocytes. J. Biol Chem 265:11098-11104.
28. Thacher SM (1989) Purification of keratinocyte transglutaminase in its expression during squamous differentiation. J. Invest Dermatol 92:578:584.

29. Nara K, Nakanishi KI, Hagiwara H, Wakita K, Kojima S, Hirose S. Retinol-induced morphological changes of cultured bovine endothelial cells are accompanied by a marked increase in transglutaminase (1989) J. Biol Chem 264:19308-19312.

30. Reibel J, Clausen H, Dale BA, Thacher SM (1989) Immunohistochemical analysis of stratum corneum components in oral squamous epithelia. Differentiation 41:237-244.

31. Haq RU, Pfahl M and Chytil R (1991) Retinoic acid affects the expression of nuclear retinoic acid receptors in tissues of retinol-deficient rats. Proc. Nat. Acad. Sci. USA 88:8272-8276.

32. Lamb AJ, Apiwatanaporn P and Olson JA (1974) Induction of rapid, synchronous vitamin A deficiency in the rat. J. Nutr. 104:1140-1148.

33. Jetten AM, George MA, Smits HL and Volberg TM (1989) Keratin 13 expression is linked to squamous differentiation in rabbit tracheal epithelial cells and down-regulated by retinoic acid. Exp. Cell Res. 182:622-634.

34. Kato M, Blaner WS, Mertz JR, Das K, Kato K and Goodman DS (1985) Influence of retinoid nutritional status on cellular retinol- and cellular retinoic acid-binding protein concentrations in various rat tissues. J. Biol. Chem. 260:4832-4838.

35. Rajan N, Blaner WS, Soprano DR, Suhara A & Goodman D S (1990) Cellular retinol-binding protein messenger RNA levels in normal and retinoid-deficient rats. J. Lipid Res. 31:821-829.

36. Kim, HY & Wolf G (1987) Vitamin A deficiency alters genomic expression for fibronectin in liver and hepatocytes. J. Biol. Chem. 262:365-371.

37. de The H, Vivanco-Ruiz M, del M, Tiollais P, Stunneneberg H and Dejean A (1990) Identification of a retinoic acid responsive element in the retinoic acid receptor beta gene. Nature (Lond.) 343:177-180.

38. Denning MF, Verma AK (1994) The mechanism of the inhibition of squamous differentiation of rat tracheal 2C5 cells by retinoic acid. Carcinogenesis 15:503-507.

39. Nervi C, Grippo JF, Sherman MI, George MD, and Jetten AM (1989) Identification and characterization of nuclear retinoic acid-binding activity in human myeloblastic leukemia HL-60 cells. Proc. Nat. Acad Sci USA 86:5854-5858.

40. Vasios GW, Gold JD, Petkovich M, Chambon, P, Gudas LJ (1989) A retinoic acid-responsive element is present in the 5'-flanking region of the laminin B1 gene. Proc. Natl. Acad. Sci. USA 86:9099-9103.

41. deThe, H, Vivanco-Ruiz MM, Tiollais P, Stunnenberg H, Dejean A. (1990) Identification of a retinoic acid responsive element in the retinoic acid receptor beta gene. Nature 3432:177-180.

42. Munox-Canoves P, Vik DP, Tack BF (1990) Mapping of a retinoic acid-responsive element in the promoter region of the complement factor H gene. J. Biol. Chem. 265-20065-20068.

43. Duester G, Shean ML, McBride MS, Stewart MJ (1991) Retinoic acid-responsive element in the human alcohol dehydrogenase gene ADH3: implications for regulation of retinoic acid synthesis. Mol. Cell Biol. 11:1638-1646.

44. Schule R, Umesono K, Mangelsdorf DJ, Bolado J, Pike JW, Evans RM (1990) Jun-Fos and receptors of vitamins A and D recognize a common response element in the human osteocalcin gene. Cell 61:497-504.

45. Gentile V, Davies PJ, Baldini A (1994) The human tissue transglutaminase gene maps on chromosome 2 by in situ fluorescence hybridization. Genomics 20:295-297.

46. Greenberg GS, Birckbichler PJ, Rice RH (1991) Transglutaminases: multifunctional cross-linking enzymes that stabilize tissues. FASEB Journal 5:3071-3077.

47. Tessitore L, Gostelli P, Sacchi G, Piacentini M, Baccino, FM (1993) The role of apoptosis in growing and stationary rat ascites hepatoma, Yoshida AH-130. Journal of Pathology 171:301-309.

48. Amendole A, Lombardi G, Oliverio S, Gelizzi V, Piacentini, M (1994) HIV-gp120 dependent induction of apoptosis in antigen-specific human T cell clones is characterized by 'tissue' translutaminase expression and prevented by cyclosporin A. FEBS Letters 339:258-264.

49. Fukuda K, Kojiro M, Chiu JF (1993) Induction of apoptosis by transforming growth factor-beta 1 in the rat hepatoma cell line mcA-RH7777: a possible association with tissue transglutaminase expression. Hepatology 18:945-953.

50. Szenda B, Schally AV, Lapis K (1991) Immunocytochemical demonstration of tissue translutaminase indicative of programmed cell death (apoptosis) in hormone sensitive mammary tumors. Acta Morphologica Hungarica 39:53-58.

51. Wright SC, Zhong J, Larrick JW (1994) Inhibition of apoptosis as a mechanism of tumor promotion. FASEB J. 8:654-660.

52. Wright SC, Zhong J, Zheng H, Larrick JW (1993) Nicotine inhibition of apoptosis suggests a role in tumor production. FASEB J. 7:1045-1051.

53. Kumar R, Shoemaker AR, Verma AK (1994) Retinoic acid nuclear receptors and tumor promotion: decreased expression of retinoic acid nuclear receptors by the tumor promoter 12-O-tetradecanoylphorbol-13-acetate. Carcinogenesis 15:701-705.

54. Nettesheim P (1980) Inhibition of carcinogenesis by retinoids. Can Med Assoc J 122:757-765.

55. Sporn MB, Dunlop NM, Newton DL, Smith JM (1976) Prevention of chemical carcinogenesis by vitamin A and its synethetic analogs (retinoids). Fed Proc 35:1332-1338.
56. Verma AK, (1992) Ornithine decarboxylase, a possible target for human cancer prevention. In: Cellular and Molecular Targets for Chemoprevention, Steele, Stoner, Boone, and Kelloff (eds.,) pp. 207-224, CRC Press, Inc., N.W., Boca Raton, Florida

# MECHANISMS OF DIETARY FAT-INDUCED COLON CANCER PROMOTION

Bandaru S. Reddy

American Health Foundation,

One Dana Road, Valhalla, New York, 10595

## INTRODUCTION

During the past several years, epidemiologic studies have indicated the influence of nutrition, diet and lifestyles on the development of certain forms of cancer and these findings have led several investigators to identify the ways in which these factors modulate the risk of cancer. Although the exact proportion of diet involvement in cancer causation is unknown, Wynder and Gori (1) and Doll and Peto (2) estimated that about 35% (range 10-70%) of all cancer mortality in the United States may be attributable to dietary factors. Since Wynder et al. (3) proposed in the late 1960's that colon cancer incidence is mainly associated with dietary fat, a substantial amount of progress has been made in understanding the relationship between dietary factors and the development of colon cancer in man. Recent population-based and case-control studies have demonstrated that the colon cancer risk enhances with increased intake of dietary fat (6,7). Continuing population studies revealed that the diets particularly high in total fat and low in certain dietary fibers are generally associated with an increased risk of developing colon cancer (7). Several case-control studies suggest a positive association between dietary fats, especially saturated fat (4,5). A recent prospective study in women provided evidence that a high intake of animal fat but not vegetable fat increases the risk of colon cancer (8).

EXPERIMENTAL STUDIES IN LABORATORY ANIMALS

Laboratory animal studies provided evidence that not only the amount but also the types of fat (differing in fatty acid composition) are important factors in determining the enhancing effect of this nutrient in colon tumor development (9). In addition, the stage of carcinogenesis at which the effect of dietary fat is exerted appears to depend on the fatty acid composition (9). In general, the overall evidence from the animal model studies is consistent with the epidemiological data.

Investigations were carried out to test the effect of high (23%) and low (5%) fat diets containing beef fat, corn oil or lard on colon carcinogenesis by a variety of carcinogens, 1,2-dimethyl-hydrazine (DMH), methylazoxymethanol (MAM) acetate, 3,2'-dimethyl-4-animobiphenyl (DMAB), or methylnitrosourea (MNU) which differ in metabolic activation (10-16). These studies indicate that, irrespective of colon carcinogens used, diets containing a high amount of beef fat, lard or corn oil fed to animals during initiation and postinitiation stages (before, during, and after carcinogen treatment) had a greater colon tumor enhancing effect than the diet low in fat (Table 1).

Studies were also conducted to evaluate whether the dietary fat, both type and amount, influences colon carcinogenesis during initiation or at postinitiation stage. Ingestion of a high fat diet containing beef tallow or corn oil during postinitiation stage increased the intestinal tumor incidence in rats, but not during the initiation stage suggesting that excess dietary fat acts at the postinitiation phase of colon carcinogenesis (17,18). When the animals were fed the diet containing high lard during the stage of initiation, there was an increase in the incidence of colon tumors (18) (Table 2). When the high corn oil or lard diets were fed during the postinitiation stage of carcinogenesis, there was a significant increase in colon tumor incidence compared with that of animals fed either the low corn oil or lard diet. The effect of high dietary fish oil during the initiation phase of AOM-induced colon carcinogenesis was also investigated in our laboratory (19). These results indicate a significant reduction in colon tumor incidence in animals fed the high fish oil diet as compared to those fed the high corn oil diet during the initiation phase of carcinogenesis. These results thus indicate that the modulating effect of colon carcinogenesis by the dietary fat during the initiation phase depends on the types of fat and their fatty acid composition.

The role of type and amount of dietary fat during the postinitiation phase of colon carcinogenesis has been studied in

**Table 1. Effect of type and amount of dietary fat both during initiation and postinitiation phases of colon carcinogenesis in F344 rats.**

| Experiment No./ Type & amount of dietary fat | Carcinogen | Male (M) or Female (F) | % animals with colon colon tumors |
|---|---|---|---|
| 1   5% Corn oil | DMH | F | 36[a] |
| 20% Corn oil | DMH | F | 64 |
| 5% Lard | DMH | F | 17[a] |
| 20% Lard | DMH | F | 67 |
| 2   5% Beef fat | DMH | M | 27[a] |
| 20% Beef fat | DMH | M | 60 |
| 5% Beef fat | MNU | M | 33[a] |
| 20% Beef fat | MNU | M | 73 |
| 5% Beef fat | MAM | M | 45[a] |
| 20% Beef fat | MAM acetate | M | 80 |
| 3   5% Beef fat | DMAB | M | 26[a] |
| 20% Beef fat | DMAB | M | 74 |
| 4   5% Corn oil | AOM, | F | 17[a] |
| 23.5% Corn oil | AOM | F | 46 |
| 5% Safflower oil | AOM | F | 13[a] |
| 23.5% Safflower oil | AOM | F | 36 |
| 5% Olive oil | AOM | F | 10 |
| 23.5% Olive oil | AOM | F | 13 |
| 23.5% Coconut oil | AOM | F | 13 |

[a] Significantly different from its respective high fat control at $p < 0.05$.

**Table 2. Effects of diets rich in omega-3 (fish oil) and omega-6 (corn oil) fatty acids fed during initiation or postinitiation phase of colon carcinogensis**

| Diets fed during Initiation | Postinitiation | % animals with colon tumors |
|---|---|---|
| Low corn oil | Low corn oil | 47[b,d] |
| Low corn oil | High corn oil | 97[c] |
| High corn oil | Low corn oil | 53[b] |
| High corn oil | High corn oil | 97[c] |
| High corn oil | High fish oil | 50[b] |
| High fish oil | High corn oil | 50[b] |
| High fish oil | High fish oil | 23[d] |

[a]Low corn oil, 5%; high corn oil, 23.5%; high fish oil, 5% corn oil + 18.52% Menhaden fish oil. [b-d]Values in the same column that do not share a common superscript are significantly different at $p < 0.05$.

our laboratory (19-21). The animals fed the diets containing high corn oil or high safflower oil had a higher incidence of AOM-induced colon tumors than did those fed the diets low in fat (Table 1). By contrast, diets high in coconut oil, olive oil or menhaden fish oil had no colon tumor-promoting effect compared with diets high in corn oil or safflower oil. Nelson et al. (22) demonstrated that DMH-induced colon carcinogenesis was significantly suppressed by dietary fish oil. Significant protection against AOM-induced colon neoplasia was also provided by dietary fish oil in CF1 female mice (23). In addition, dietary fish oil produced early protective effect in colonic mucosa as indicated by focal areas of dysplasia (FAD) and epithelial cell proliferation. A ratio of omega-6 to omega-3 fatty acids of approximately 1.0 prevented the development of an adenoma-type proliferative pattern, thereby reducing FAD numbers and subsequent tumor incidence.

In addition to menhaden oil, the inhibitory effect of eicosapentaenoic acid (EPA) and perilla oil rich in α-linolenic acid (c18:3, n-3) has been studied in colon carcinogenesis. Minoura et al. (24) demonstrated that dietrry EPA diet (4.7% EPA + 0.3% LA) significantly inhibited AOM-induced colon tumor incidence as compared to 5% linoleic (LA) acid diet. Narisawa et al. (25) and Hirosa et al. (26) demonstrated that dietary perilla oil inhibited MNU- and DMH-induced colon carcinogenesis.

In summary, laboratory animal studies have provided useful data for evaluating the role of dietary fat in the development of colon carcinogenesis. Majority of studies suggest that not only the amount but also the types of fat (differing in fatty acid composition) are important factors in determining the modulating effect of dietary fats in colon tumor development. The stage of carcinogenesis at which the effect of dietary fat is exerted appears to be mostly during the postinitiation phase of carcinogenesis; however, certain dietary fats such as lard or fish oil also act during the initiation phase of colon carcinogenesis.

## POSSIBLE MODE OF ACTION OF TYPES OF FAT IN COLON CARCINOGENESIS

Effect of Types and Amount of Dietary Fat on Bile Acids.

Although the mechanism of colon tumor-promoting effect of high dietary fat is incompletely understood, we and other (27) have shown that dietary fat increases the concentration of colonic (fecal) secondary bile acids namely deoxycholic acid and lithocholic acid as well as fatty acids. Metabolic epidemiologic studies demonstrated that populations who are at high risk for colon cancer excrete high levels of secondary bile acids (27). Laboratory animal model studies demonstrated that these secondary bile acids induce cell proliferation and act as promoters for cancer of the colon (27). In humans, individuals at increased risk for colon cancer have been bound to have abnormal patterns of cell proliferation including higher rates of DNA synthesis in normal appearing colorectal mucosa (28,29). These changes precede tumor development and therefore constitute a key step in colon carcinogenesis (28). It is important to note that high concentration of luminal secondary bile salts and fatty acids also increase colonic epithelial ODC activity and cell proliferation (28,30). Recent studies demonstrate that bile acids enhance the growth of aberrant crypt foci, putative neoplastic lesions of colon cancer, and increase the resistance to apoptosis (31).

### Effect of Types of Dietary Fat on Ornithine Decarboxylase and Tyrosine Phosphorylation During Colon Carcinogenesis

It is noteworthy that the AOM model for colon carcinogenesis has a characteristic multistep process in that the colonic mucosal ODC activity is elevated in a fashion similar to that seen in clinical samples. In addition, tyrosine-specific protein phosphorylation is now recognized as an important regulatory mechanism of cell proliferation in response to a number of processes, including the actions of several growth factors, growth factor receptors and oncogenes (32).

In view of the potential significance of ODC and TPK in tumorigenesis, and of differences in tumor-promoting effects of high dietary levels of corn and fish oils, we assessed the modulating effect of low-fat corn oil (LFCO), high-fat corn oil (HFCO), and high-fat fish oil (HFFO) diets on AOM-induced colonic mucosal ODC and TPK activities (33). The results of this study clearly demonstrate that the HFCO diet significantly increased ODC activity in colon mucosa compared with the LFCO diets, whereas the HFFO diet distinctly suppressed ODC activity compared with the HFCO diet (Table 3). Previous studies demonstrate that administration of secondary bile acids and unsaturated fatty acids such as arachidonic acid (AA) and linoleic acid (LA) and feeding diets high in LA-rich corn oil increase colonic mucosal ODC activity in rats (33-35). Although the mechanism by which the HFCO diet increases colonic ODC activity is not fully understood, we and others have shown that the HFCO diet increases the concentration of colonic secondary bile acids, namely deoxycholic acid and lithocholic acid (36), which have been shown to increase colon mucosal cell proliferation and ODC activity (37). Another possible explanation for ODC induction by the HFCO diet is based on the observation that feeding diets rich in LA, and precursor of AA, results in increased levels of AA metabolites, namely cyclooxygenase and lipoxygenase products which are involved in the induction of tissue ODC activity (37,38). It is also interesting to note that inhibitors of AA metabolism block the induction of ODC activity (38,39). It is possible that feeding diets rich in omega-3 (fish oil) fatty acids results in decreased levels of AA and its metabolites thereby inhibiting tissue ODC activity.

**Table 3. Effect of high-fat diets containing corn oil, olive oil and fish oil on azoxymethane-induced colonic mucosal ODC, TPK, and PGE$_2$ levels in F344 rats**

|  | Experimental Group | | |
| Type | Low-fat corn oil (LFCO) | High-fat corn oil (HFCO) | High-fat fish oil (HFFO) |
| --- | --- | --- | --- |
| Cystosolic ODC[a] | | | |
| Saline-treated | 8.1±1.6[b,c] | 16.5±2.6 | 7.7±1.2[c] |
| AOM-treated | 47.2±8.2[c] | 69.8±8.4 | 36.2±4.7[c] |
| Membrane TPK[a] | | | |
| Saline-treated | 25.2±5.1 | 30.5±6.5 | 19.9±4.1[c] |
| AOM-treated | 59.5±10.2[c] | 79.2±14.2 | 47.3±7.4[c] |
| Mucosal PGE$_2$[a] | | | |
| Saline-treated | | | |
| Basal | - | 0.52±0.07 | 0.31±0.05[c] |
| Ex Vivo | - | 1.81±0.2 | 0.71±0.1[c] |
| AOM-treated | | | |
| Basal | - | 0.86±0.14 | 0.51±0.06[c] |
| Ex Vivo | - | 3.10±0.52 | 1.24±0.38[c] |

[a] ODC (ornithine decarboxylase) activity expressed as pmol $^{14}CO_2$ released/mg protein/h; TPK (tyrosine protein kinase) activity expressed as pmol [$^{32}$p]ATP incorporating/mg protein/min; ng PGE$_2$/mg protein.
[b] Mean ± SD (n = 6).
[c] Significantly different from HFCO group, p < 0.05.

With regard to TPK activation, studies conducted in our laboratory indicate that carcinogen treatment significantly enhances colon mucosal TPK activity in male F344 rats (40). Thus, it is reasonable to suggest that an elevation or a drop in colon mucosal TPK activity is associated with an increase or decrease in tumorigenesis. HFCO diet enhanced intestinal TPK activity, whereas HFFO diet decreased the intestine mucosal TPK activity, suggesting that types of dietary fat differing in fatty acid composition also modulate tissue TPK activity (33). Although the exact mechanism by which types of dietary fat modulate TPK activity remains unclear, several studies suggest that bile acids, which are increased by feeding high levels of corn oil, are potent stimuli of proliferative activity, as well as, induce reactive oxygen species production (41). There is evidence to indicate that $H_2O_2$ enhances the TPK phosphorylation and induces hyperphosphorylation of various proteins on tyrosine residues, probably by suppressing tyrosine protein phosphatase activity (42). These results support a key role for TPK in mediation of the stimulatory action of bile acids on the proliferative activity of colonic mucosa ultimately leading to colon tumor promotion.

### Effect of Types of Fat on Arachidonic Acid Metabolism and Prostaglandins

Another possible explanation by which high dietary fat increases colon tumor promotion is through alteration of membrane phospholipid turnover and prostaglandin synthesis. One of the striking cellular actions of secondary bile salts which enhance proliferative activity of colonic epithelium is the rapid stimulation of membrane phospholipid turnover that may occur as result of bile salt activation of phospholipases (especially $A_2$), bile salt- or fatty acid-induced alterations of phospholipid substrates or both of these effects. As a result of increased phospholipid turnover and the release of free AA and other products of phospholipid breakdown, a number of biologically active moieties are generated locally in the colon that might alter cellular proliferative activity. AA is metabolized via cyclooxygenase pathway to a number of bioctive prostanoids. Recent studies demonstrated that carcinogen treatment significantly increased the basal levels and *ex vivo* production of $PGE_2$ and 6-keto $PGF_{1\alpha}$ in colon (33). The *ex vivo* production of $PGE_2$ and 6-keto $PGF_{1\alpha}$ was greater in animals fed the HFCO diet than in those fed the HFFO diet (Table 3). With regard to lack of colon tumor promoting effect of fish oil (or tumor inhibitory effect of fish oil compared to corn oil), omega-3 fatty acids present in fish oil namely DHA and EPA have been shown to inhibit the cyclooxygenase pathway as well as arachidonic acid metabolism for prostaglandin synthesis (43). Recently Narisawa et al. (35) demonstrated that deoxycholic acid treatment increased ODC activity of colonic mucosa by stimulating $PGE_2$ synthesis. These interesting observations suggest potential importance of secondary bile acids, AA metabolism, and PGs in modifying tumor promotion by dietary fish oil and corn oil in colon carcinogenesis.

### Effect of Types and Amount of Fat on Cellular Messenger System in Relation to Colon Tumor Promotion.

In recent years, there has been considerable interest in cellular messenger system which is activated as a consequence of increased membrane phosphoinositol turnover induced by hormones and other extracellular signals (44). Activation of phospholipase C by various stimuli results in transient increases in the cellular 1,2-Sn-diacylglycerol (DAG) content which is derived from the breakdown of inositol phospholipids (44). It has also been shown that deoxycholic acid increases the accumulation of DAG in colonic epithelial cells (41). DAG has been shown to activate protein kinase C (PKC) which has a critical role in signal transduction for a variety of biologically active substances that activate cellular functions and proliferation (44,45). This activation process involves translocation of cytosolic PKC to the plasma membranes which, in turn, leads to phosphorylation of target molecules, thereby influencing cell proliferation and/or differentiation. In addition to activation of PKC by DAG, bile acids especially deoxycholic acid activate colonic epithelial PKC as reflected by translocation from the soluble fraction to the particulate fraction of cells (45).

Recent studies conducted in the laboratory of Birt (46) suggest that diets restricted in calories from fat and carbohydrate reduce phosphotidylinositol turnover in mouse epidermis. It is possible that similar situation may exist in colon. Based on this, we predict that high dietary fat containing corn oil, lard or beef tallow may enhance phosphatidylinositol turnover and phosphorylated forms of phosphatidylinositol thereby increases the production or release of DAG by phospholipase C in the colonic mucosa. Studies by Donnelly et al. (47) and Birt et al. (46) demonstrated that high-fat diet containing corn oil elevated both particulate and soluble PKC activities in the epidermis of SENCAR mice as compared to those fed a low-fat diet. The effects of high-fat diet on epidermal-cell PKC correlate well with the effects of diet on skin tumorigenesis in SENCAR mice (46). These observations indicate the potential importance of DAG and PKC in modifying tumor promotion by high dietary fat.

Recent studies also demonstrated that dietary lipids and bile acids in the gut might act together to influence the production of DAG by bacterial phopholipase C present in colon (48). Thus, the levels of specific DAGs present in the colonic contents might be modulated by several factors namely dietary intake of types of fat. Also, phosphotidylinositol and phosphotidyl ethanolamine present in the lumen of colon serve as substrates for the production of DAG by the gut microflora (78). Furthermore, Craven et al. (41) showed that intracolonic instillation of DAG activates colonic epithelial PKC and induces ODC and cell proliferation in rats. Taken together, these results suggest an interplay between the consumption of high dietary fat and gut microflora, DG and DAG and colonic mucosal DAG and PKC activities that have been shown to play a role in tumor promotion.

### Molecular Basis for the Relationship Between the Dietary Fat and Colon Cancer.

The transforming proteins encoded by Ki- and H-ras genes are mutated versions of cellular homology of ras protooncogenes and have been implicated in the etiology of many human cancers including colon cancer (49,50). Specifically, mutations in the human K-ras have been reported to be as high as 50% in adenocarcinomas of the colon (51,52). In animal models, mutant ras alleles have also been detected in tumors and in preneoplastic colonic mucosa of rats treated with DMH (53) and AOM (54). Ras p21 is a regulatory protein anchored to the cytoplasmic face of plasma membrane and participates in transmembrane signalling events leading to DNA synthesis during cellular growth and differentiation (56). Its normal function appears to be subverted in the neoplastic process.

In analyzing the relationship between the amount and types of dietary and ras p21, it is interesting to note that the mevalonate which is an essential precursor for the biosynthesis of all isoprenoids including cholesterol and farnesol, is an important intermediate of dietary fat metabolism (57). It is known that the bulk product of mevalonate metabolism, cholesterol, is obtained from two sources namely endogenously by synthesis from acetyl-CoA through mevalonate and exogenously from receptor mediated uptake of plasma low-density lipoproteins (58). Mevalonate homeostasis is achieved through cholesterol-mediated repression of the genes for 3-hydroxy-3-methylglutaryl coenzyme A (HMG-CoA) reductase and posttranscriptional regulation of HMG-CoA reductase by one of the non-cholesterol isoprenoids (58). Interest in the regulatory importance of mevalonate was heightened recently by the discovery that growth-regulating ras p21 proteins (59) encoded by ras protooncogenes and oncogenes (60,61) are covalently attached to farnesyl residues which anchor them to cell membranes. In addition, inhibition of synthesis of mevalonate which is a precursor for cholesterol (which is involved in bile acid synthesis), prevents farnesylation of these ras proteins (62) and blocks cell growth (63). It is noteworthy that farnesylation of ras p21 is essential for expression of its oncogenic activity (59). Interestingly, it has been shown that non-processed, non-farnesylated mutants of oncogenic ras which cannot localize into the membrane are no longer transforming and display a dominant inhibitory phenotype to antagonize the activity of membrane bound oncogenic ras p21 (61). It is also noteworthy that selective inhibition of isoprenylation by lovastatin, a cholesterol biosynthesis inhibitor, has inhibited the growth of ras-transformed cells in nude mice (64). It is possible that amount and types of lipids can affect the farnesylation of ras p21 through cholesterol biosynthesis. High dietary fat intake may enhance the farnesylation of ras p21 leading to a shift towards increased membrane localization of ras p21 facilitating the induced expression of ras function. Studies are warranted to test this hypothesis.

## CONCLUSIONS

The role of nutritional factors, especially dietary fat in the etiology of cancer has become increasingly apparent. In recent years, scientific investigations have produced considerable information on the relationship between the dietary fat and cancer of the colon. The information base is sufficiently convincing with respect to an enhancing effect as a function of total fat intake and certain types of fat and a protective effect of certain sources of fat in colon cancer.

## REFERENCES

1.  **Wynder, E.L. and Gori, G.B.** Contribution of the environment to cancer incidence: an epidemiologic exercise. *J. Natl. Cancer Inst.*, 58, 825-832, 1977.
2.  **Doll, R. and Peto, R.,** The causes of cancer: Quantitative estimates of avoidable risks of cancer in the United States today. *J. Natl. Cancer Inst.*, 66, 1191-1308, 1981.
3.  **Wynder, E.L, Kajitani, T., Ishikawa, S., Dodo, H. and Takano, A.,** Environmental factors in cancer of cancer of colon and rectum. *Cancer,* 23, 1210-1220, 1969.

4.  World Health Statistics Annual, World Health Organization, Geneva, Switzerland, 1980.
5.  **Miller, A.B., Howe, G.R. and Jain, M.,** Food items and food groups as risk factors in a case-control study of diet and colon cancer. *Int. J. Cancer.,* 32, 155-166, 1983.
6.  **Graham, S., Marshall, J., Hanghey, B., Mittleman, A., Swanson, M, Zielexny, M., Byers, T., Wilkinson, G. and West, D.,** *Am. J. Epidemiol.,* 128, 490-503, 1988.
7.  **Reddy, B.S., Hedges,. A.T., Laakso, K. and Wynder, E.L.,** Metabolic epidemiology of large bowel cancer: Fecal bulk and constituents of high-risk North American and low-risk Finnish population. *Cancer,* 42, 2832-2838, 1978.
8.  **Willet, W.C., Stampfer, M.J., Colditz, G.A., Rosner, B.A. and Speizer, F.E.,** Relation of meat, fat, and fiber intake to the risk of colon cancer in a prospective study among women. *New Eng. J. Med.,* 323, 1664-1672, 1990.
9.  **Reddy, B.S.,** Diet and colon cancer: Evidence from human and animal model studies. In: Reddy BS, Cohen LA (eds) Diet, Nutrition, and Cancer: A Critical Evaluation, Vol. 1. CRC Press, Boca Raton, Florida, 1986, pp 47-65.
10. **Reddy, B.S., Watanabe, K. and Weisburger, J.H.,** Effect of high-fat diet on colon carcinogenesis in F344 rats treated with 1,2-dimethylhydrazine, methylazoxymethanol acetate and methylnitrosourea. *Cancer Res.,* 37, 4156-4159, 1977.
11. **Reddy, B.S. and Ohmori, T.,** Effect of intestinal microflora and dietary fat on 3,2'-dimethyl-4-aminobiphenyl-induced colon carcinogenesis in F344 rats. *Cancer Res.,* 41, 1363-1367, 1981.
12. **Nigro, N.D., Singh, D.V., Campbell, R.L. and Pak, M.S.,** Effect of dietary beef fat on intestinal tumor formation by azoxymethane in rats. *J. Natl. Cancer Inst.,* 54, 439-442, 1975.
13. **Howarth, A.E. and Pihl, E.,** High-fat diet promotes and causes distal shift of experimental rat colonic cancer-beer and alcohol do not. *Nutr. Cancer,* 6, 229-235, 1985.
14. **Reddy, B.S., Narisawa, T., Vukusich, D., Weisburger, J.H. and Wynder, E.L.,** Effect of quality and quantity of dietary fat and dimethylhydrazine in colon carcinogenesis in rats. *Proc. Soc Exp. Biol. Med.,* 151, 237-239, 1976.
15. **Sakaguchi, M., Hiramatsu, Y., Takada, H., Yamamura, M., Hioki, K., Sato, K. and Yamamoto, M.,** Effect of dietary unsaturated and saturated fats on azoxymethane-induced colon carcinogenesis in rats. *Cancer Res.,* 44, 1472-1477, 1984.
16. **Pence, B.C. and Buddingh, F.,** Inhibition of dietary fat-promoted colon carcinogenesis in rats by supplemental calcium or vitamin D3. *Carcinogenesis,* 9, 187-190, 1988.

17.   **Bull, A.W., Soullier, B.K., Wilson, P.S., Haydon, M.T., and Nigro, N.D.,** Promotion of azoxymethane-induced intestinal cancer by high-fat diets in rats. *Cancer Res.,* 39, 4956-4959, 1979.

18.   **Reddy, B.S. and Maruyama, H.,** Effect of different levels of dietary corn oil and lard during the initiation phase of colon carcinogenesis in F344 rats. *J. Natl. Cancer Inst.,* 77, 815-822, 1986.

19.   **Reddy, B.S., Burill, C. and Rigotty, J.,** Effect of diets high in omega-3 and omega-6 fatty acids on the initiation and postinitiation stages of colon carcinogenesis. *Cancer Res.,* 51, 487-491, 1991.

20.   **Reddy, B.S. and Maruyama, H.,** Effect of dietary fish oil on azoxymethane-induced colon carcinogenesis in male F344 rats. *Cancer Res.,* 46, 3367-3370, 1986.

21.   **Reddy, B.S. and Maeura, Y.,** Tumor promotion by dietary fat in azoxymethane induced colon carcinogenesis in female F344 rats: Influence of amount and source of dietary fat. *J. Natl. Cancer Inst.,* 72, 745-750, 1984.

22.   **Nelson, R.L., Tanure, J.C., Andrianopoulos, G., Souza, G. and Lands, W.E.M.,** A comparison of dietary fish oil and corn oil in experimental colorectal carcinogenesis. *Nutr. Cancer,* 11, 215-220, 1988.

23    **Deschner, E.E., Lytle, J.J., Wong, G., Ruperto, J.F. and Newmark, H.L.,** The effect of dietary omega-3 fatty acids (fish oil) on azoxymethane-induced focal areas of dysplasia and colon tumor incidence. *Cancer,* 66, 2350-2356, 1990.

24.   **Minoura, T., Takata, T., Sakaguchi, M., Hideho, T., Yamamura, M., Hioka, K. and Yamamoto, M.,** Effect of dietary eicosapentaenoic acid on azoxymethane-induced colon carcinogenesis in rats. *Cancer Res.,* 48, 4790-4794, 1988.

25.   **Narisawa, T., Takahashi, M., Kotanagi, H., Kusaka, H., Yamazaki, Y., Koyamo, H., Fukawra, Y., Nishizawa, Y., Kolsugeri, M., Isoda, Y., Hirano, J. and Tanidu, N.,** Inhibitory effect of dietary perilla oil rich in the n-polyunsaturated fatty acid à-linolenic acid on colon carcinogenesis in rats. *Jpn. J. Cancer Res.,* 82, 1089-1096, 1991.

26.   **Hirosa, M., Masuda, A., Ito, N., Kamano, K. and Okuyama, H.,** Effects of dietary perilla oil, soybean oil and safflower oil on 7,12-dimethylbenz[a]anthracene (DMAB) and 1,2-dimethylhydrazine (DMH)-induced mammary gland and colon carcinogenesis in female SD rats. *Carcinogenesis,* 11, 731-735, 1990.

27.   **Reddy, B.S.,** Animal experimental evidence on macronutrients and cancer. In: Micozzi MS, Moon TE (eds)

Macronutrients Investigating Their Role in Cancer. Marcel Dekker Inc, New York, 1992, pp 33-54.

28. **Lipkin, M.**, Biomarkers of increased susceptibility to gastrointestinal cancer: new application to studies of cancer prevention in human subjects. *Cancer Res.*, 48, 235-245, 1988.

29. **Deschner, E,E. and Maskens, A.P.**, Significance of labeling index and labeling distribution as a kinetic parameters in colorectal mucosa of cancer patients and DMH treated animals. *Cancer, 50,* 1136-1141, 1982.

30. **Takano, S., Matsushima, M., Erturk. E. and Bryan, G.T.**, Early induction of rat colonic epithelial ornithine and S-adenosyl-L-methionine decarboxylase activities by N-methyl-N'-nitro-N-nitrosoguanidine or bile salts. *Cancer Res.*, 41, 624-628, 1981.

31. **Magnuson, B.A., Shirtliff, N. and Bird, R.P.**, Resistance to aberrant crypt foci to apoptosis induced by azoxymethane in rats chronically fed cholic acid. *Carcinogenesis, 15,* 1459-1462, 1994.

32. **Cantley, L.C., Auger, K.R., Carpenter, C., Duckworth, B., Graziani, A., Kapeller, R. and Soltoff, S**, Oncogenes and signal transduction. *Cell* 64, 281-302, 1991.

33. **Rao, C.V. and Reddy, B.S.**, Modulating effect of amount and types of dietary fat on ornithine decarboxylase, tyrosine protein kinase and prostaglandins production during colon carcinogenesis. *Carcinogenesis, 14,* 1327-1333, 1993.

34. **Reddy, B.S. and Sugie, S.**, Effect of different levels of omega-3 and omega-6 fatty acids on azoxymethane-induced colon carcinogenesis in F344 rats. *Cancer Res.,* 48, 6642-6647, 1988.

35. **Narisawa, T., Takahashi, M., Niwa, M., Fukaura, Y. and Wakizaka, A.**, Involvement of prostaglandin E2 in bile acid caused promotion of colon carcinogenesis and anti-promotion by the cyclooxygenase inhibitor indomethacin. *Gann*, 78, 791-798, 1985.

36. **Reddy, B.S., Mangat, S., Sheinfil, A., Weisburger, J.H. and Wynder, E.L.**, Effect of type and amount of dietary fat and 1,2-dimethylhydrazine on biliary bile acids, fecal bile acids and neutral sterols in rats. *Cancer Res.*, 37, 2132-2137, 1977.

37. **DeRubertis, F.R., Craven, P.A. and Saito, R.**, Bile salt stimulation of colonic epithelial proliferation: evidence for the involvement of lipoxygenase products. *J. Clin. Invest.*, 74, 1614-1624, 1984.

38. **Nakadate, T., Yamamoto, S., Ishii, M. and Kato, R.**, Inhibition of 12-O-tetradecanoylphorbol-13-acetate-induced epidermal ornithine decarboxylase activity by phospholipase

A2 inhibitors and lipoxygenase inhibitor. *Cancer Res.*, 42, 2841-2845, 1982.

39. **Verma, A.K., Ashendel, C.L. and Boutwell, R.K.,** Inhibition by prostaglandin synthesis inhibitors of the induction of epidermal ornithine decarboxylase activity, the accumulation of prostaglandins, and tumor promotion caused by 12-O-tetradecanoyl-phorbol-13-acetate. *Cancer Res.*, 40, 308-315, 1980.

40. **Kumar, P.S., Roy, S.J., Tokumo, K. and Reddy, B.S.,** Effect of different levels of calorie restriction on azoxymethane-induced colon carcinogenesis in male F344 rats. *Cancer Res.*, 50, 5761-5766, 1990.

41. **Craven, P.A., Pfanstial, J. and DeRubertis, F.R.,** Role of activation of protein kinase C in the stimulation of colonic epithelial proliferation and reactive oxygen formation by bile salts. *J. Clin. Invest.*, 79, 532-541, 1987.

42. **Heffetz, D., Bushkin, I., Dror, R. and Zick, Y.,** The insulinomimetic agents H2O2 and vanadate stimulate protein tyrosine phosphorylation in intact cells. *J. Biol. Chem.*, 265, 2896-2902, 1990.

43. **Culp, B.R., Titus, B.J. and Lands, W.E.,** Inhibition of prostaglandin biosynthesis by eicosapentaenoic acid. *Prostaglandins Med.*, 3, 269-278, 1979.

44. **Nishizuka, Y., Takai, Y., Kishimoto, A., Kikkawa, U. and Kaibuchi K:** Phospholipid turnover in hormone actions. *Recent Prog. Horm. Res.*, 40, 301-345, 1984.

45. **Fitzer, C.J., O'Brian, C-A., Guillem, J.G. and Weinstein, B.I.,** The regulation of protein kinase C by chenodeoxycholate, deoxycholate and several structurally related bile acids. *Carcinogenesis*, 8, 217-220, 1987.

46. **Birt, D.F., Kris, E.S., Choe, M. and Pelling, J.C.,** Dietary energy and fat effects on tumor promotion. *Cancer Res.*, 52, 2035S-2039S, 1992.

47. **Donnelly, T.E., Birt, D.F., Sittlev, R., Anderson, C.L., Choe, M. and Julius, A.D.,** Benzoyl peroxide activation of protein kinase C activity in epidermal cell membranes. *Carcinogenesis*, 8, 1867-1870, 1987.

48. **Marotomi, M., Guillem, J.G., LoGerfo, P. and Weinstein, I.B.,** Production of diacylglycerol, an activator of protein kinase C, by human intestinal microflora. *Cancer Res.*, 50, 3595-3599, 1990.

49. **Bos, J.L.,** Ras oncogenes in human cancer: A review. *Cancer Res.*, 49, 4682-4689, 1989.

50. **Lacal, J.C. and Tronick, S.R.,** The ras oncogene. In: Reddy EP, Shalka AM, Curran T (eds) The Oncogene Handbook. Elsevier, New York, 1988, pp 535-550.

51.   Bos, J.L., Fearon, E.R., Hamilton, S.R., Verlaan-de Vries, M., van Boom, J.H., Van der Eb, A.J. and Vogelstein, B., Prevalence of ras mutations in human colorectal cancers. *Nature,* 327, 293-297, 1987.
52.   Vogelstein B, Fearon ER, Hamilton SR, Kern SE, Preisinger, A.C., Leppert, M., Nakamura, Y., White, R., Smits, A.M.M. and Bos, J.L., Genetic alterations during colorectal tumor development. *N. Engl. J. Med.,* 319, 525-532, 1988.
53.   Jacoby, R.F., Uor, X., Teng, B.B., Davidson, N.O. and Brasitus, T.A., Mutations in the K-ras oncogene induced by 1,2-dimethylhydrazine in preneoplastic and neoplastic rat colonic mucosa. *J. Clin. Invest.,* 87, 624-630, 1991.
54.   Singh, J., *Carcinogenesis*
56.   Feramisco, J.R., Gross, M., Kamata, T., Rasenberg, M. and Sweet, R.W., Microinjection of the oncogene form of the human H-ras (T-24) protein results in rapid proliferation of the quiescent cells. *Cell,* 38, 109-117, 1984.
57.   Rudney, H. and Sexton, R.C., Regulation of cholesterol biosynthesis. *Annual Rev. Nutr.,* 6: 245-271, 1986.
58.   Goldstein, J.L. and Brown, M.S., Regulation of the mevalonate pathway. *Nature,* 343, 425-430, 1990.
59.   Casey, P.J., Solsky, P.A., Der, C.J. and Bus, J.E., p21 ras is modified by a farnesyl isoprenoid. *Proc. Natl. Acad. Sci. USA,* 86, 8323-8327, 1989.
60.   Wolda, S.L. and Glomset, J.A., Evidence for modification of lamin B by a product of mevalonic acid. *J. Biol. Chem.,* 263, 5997-6000, 1988.
61.   Cox, A.D. and Channing, J.D., The ras/cholestrol connection: implications for ras oncogenecity. *Critical Reviews in Oncogenesis,* 3, 365-400, 1992.
62.   Hancock, J.F., Magee, A.I., Childs, J.E. and Marshall, C.J., All ras proteins are polyisoprenylated but only some are palmitoylated. *Cell,* 57, 1167-1177, 1989.
63.   Brown, M.S. and Goldstein, J.L., Multivalent feedback regulation of HMG CoA reductase, a control mechanism coordinating isoprenoid synthesis and cell growth. *J. Lipid. Res.,* 21, 505-517, 1980.
64.   Sebti, S.M., Thalcevic, G.T. and Jani, J.P., Lovastatin, a cholestrol biosynthesis inhibitor, inhibits the growth of human H-ras oncogene transformed cells in nude mice. *Cancer Communications,* 3, 141-147, 1991.

# CALORIES AND EXERCISE AS MODIFIERS OF CANCER RISK

E.B. Thorling & N.O. Jacobsen

Danish Cancer Society, Department of Nutrition and Cancer, Nørrebrogade 44, Bldg. 5, DK-8000 Aarhus C, Denmark, and Institute of Pathology, University Hospital of Aarhus, Nørrebrogade 44, Bldg. 18A, DK-8000 Aarhus C, Denmark

## INTRODUCTION

We can observe that a number of chronic diseases are associated with obesity and a fat-rich diet and we can observe that a sedentary lifestyle is associated with an increased risk of some cancers. But why are some people obese and some lean and muscular? Why do these people eat different diets and why do some people exercise and other people live a sedentary life? Weight loss induced by food restriction in animals seems to have a protective effect on the development of cancer, review given by Kritchevsky (1991). However, we do not know for sure about the mechanisms involved and the question of causality remains a guessing game in which we accumulate circumstantial evidence but where proofs are hard to come by.

The urge to exercise varies a great deal in between people and over time in the same person. This goes for man and for experimental animals as well. Individual rats of our own inbred strain of Fischer 344 rats will exercise to a very different extent when allowed to run a voluntary running wheel. L. Cohen has shown that female rats in his laboratory run up to 10 times the distance covered by males of the same age (Cohen et al., 1992). Our rats start out running increasing daily distances up to the age of 3-4 months after which the interest in the wheel appears to cease slowly with age. Why this urge to exercise in all healthy animals? What determines the extent of exercise and type of exercise chosen by the individual - from long distance running to javelin throwing, boxing, and chess? Is the actually observed exercise an indicator of "something deeper" which is the determining factor, responsible for the association to cancer and cardiovascular disease.

One of the most cited investigations on the effect of exercise is the "Harvard alumni studies" by i.a. Paffenbarger et al. (1992). Evidently, lifelong engagement in sports activities confer a lower risk for large bowel cancer and prostate cancer in man and for reproductive cancers in women (Frisch, 1985; Frisch, 1992). But again, why are some of the students engaged in sports activities and others not? This is the nagging question of "self-selected groups" in epidemiological studies - well known from e.g. studies in religious groups.

The latest published work on the association between exercise and cancer is from the "United Kingdom Testicular Cancer Study Group" led by David Forman (1994). They found (Figs. 1-2) that the odds ratio of

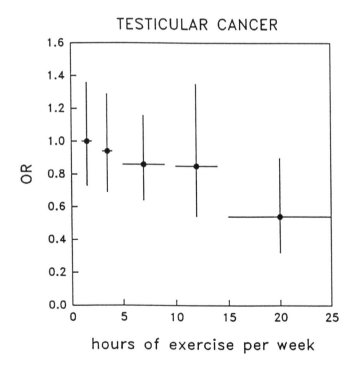

**Fig. 1**. Odds ratio for the development of testicular cancer as a function of hours of exercise per week. Figure based on table values given in reference No. 15.

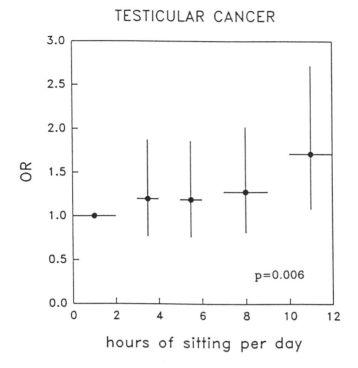

**Fig. 2.** Odds ratio for the development of testicular cancer as a function of hours of sitting per day. Figure based on table values given in reference No. 15.

testicular cancer was inversely related to the weekly hours of exercise and directly positively correlated to the daily hours of sitting. Again one wonders why some kids are actively engaged in exercise that apparently feels repulsive to the "sitting" group.

A number of studies have concerned themselves with the effect of giving a fat-rich diet to experimental animals and in most cases found a marked increase in the number of tumours after challenging with carcinogens. Various fat types have been used to possibly disclose a differential effect of the main groups of fatty acids, the saturated, the monoenes and the polyunsaturated. In the last case differences are being studied between the so-called "fish oils" - the omega 3 or n-3 fatty acids - as compared to the omega 6 or n-6 fatty acids. The picture is not yet entirely clear. Rats are smart enough to somehow "taste" the caloric content of the diet and consequently eat less of a fat-rich diet. This raises the question of comparability of supply of "other nutrients" when the animals on the fat-rich diet eat smaller quantities. This problem, of course, can be taken care of when realized, by balancing the diets for the experimental groups. In man, however, diet is not automatically balanced which means that people on a fat-rich diet tend to acquire less of the important nutrients from fruits and vegetables. This may actually be a key issue in these studies that deserves more attention.

We are still asking the question: Will fat people who slim appropriately acquire a diminished risk of getting cancer of e.g. colon? With minor revisions the question may be reformulated into: If one eats excess fat - but exercise accordingly - to avoid deposition of the fat (in which case it may not be excess?), will it still be harmful to our health - when cancer is considered - to say nothing about cardiovascular disease? Until recently this was the relative simple formulation but today we should add a further pertinent question. Are all fats equally evil? Disclosing, of course, that this may indeed not be the case.

## ANIMAL EXPERIMENTS

Animal experiments might conceivably be of some help, with all the precautions taken in the interpretation of these data and in transforming the results to human relevance. It should be remembered that most animals (all) have digestive systems that differ markedly from that of man in design and chemistry and of course in the preferred diet.

We have set up a model system in rats in which we have studied the effect of exercise on the azoxymethane-induced colon cancer.

## TREADMILLS

The treadmills were of the barrel type consisting of 4 barrels. The diameter was 63 cm giving a circumference of 2 meters. The length of the individual barrel was 80 cm allowing ample space in each barrel for up to 20 rats. The barrels - drums - were made of acrylic plastic with rungs 5 mm "high" glued to the inside of the barrel for every 15 cm to allow foothold for the rats. (On smooth surfaces rats would slide round in the barrel when rotated and the smooth surface evidently scared the rats). The "door" to the barrel was fitted with a stainless steel grid to allow faeces to drop out during the running periods. By the end of the day the barrels were cleansed with soapwater and wiped dry by letting towels "tumble" for half an hour.

The barrels were driven by a 1 horsepower three-phase electromotor with frequency modulator allowing for infinite regulation of the speed. After months of trial and error we found that a "belt speed" of 7 m per minute was reasonable, not stressing the rats unnecessary, allowing them to proceed at a quick walk/run, make short stops and to catch up in a brief run. They would exercise for 5 hours/day on weekdays corresponding to 10 km/week in a room with inversed light schedule 12 plus 12 hours. The belt speed is a critical point. Running schedule has varied in published papers on the effect of treadmill exercise. There are indications from these and other studies that there is an optimal amount of exercise - not well defined yet - above which "stress" is induced and where a beneficial effect on the development of cancer is no longer observed. In fact, as pointed out by Cohen (1991) promotion is found in mammary cancer.

## ANIMALS

Animals for breeding were Fischer 344 rats purchased from Zentralinstitut für Versuchstierzucht in Hannover, Germany, and a stock maintained in our lab.

To allow the animals to exercise during their physiologic activity period (the night) the animals were kept in rooms with an inversed light schedule 12 plus 12 hours.

The breeding animals were kept on a regular low-fat chow as prepared by Bomholtgård Breeding and Research Centre Ltd. Food and water would be available ad libitum except for periods of exercise in the treadmill.

## CARCINOGEN

At the age of 5 weeks (and a weight from 100-140 g) the rats were injected subcutaneously three times (with an interval of 3 days) with a dose of 15 mg per kg body weight of azoxymethane (Sigma) in saline. The solution was prepared fresh and injections completed within half an hour. Three days after the last injection the rats were randomized to the experimental groups.

This dose schedule was found well suited for the male rats resulting in the appearance of large bowel cancer in most of the rats after 38 weeks. Relatively few small bowel tumors and few other malignancies were observed. In females, however, the effect of azoxymethane was more unpredictable with few large bowel tumors and a number of different tumors in various organs. Increasing the dose resulted in increased acute lethality and was unapplicable. The carcinogenesis experiments were consequently conducted in male rats only.

## GENERAL EFFECT OF THE EXERCISE SCHEDULE

We have been most concerned about the regulation of the weight in relation to exercise. As demonstrated in Fig. 3 the growth curves show that exercising male rats put on weight at a slower rate than sedentary rats. As also found by others (Applegate et al., 1982) female rats do not loose weight when exposed to this kind of moderate exercise.

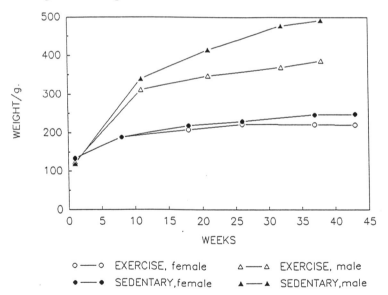

**Fig. 3.** Growth curves for exercised and sedentary males and females of Fischer 344 strain of rats. The rats were exercised for 5 hours daily on weekdays, running on average 10 km per week.

This fact would have made the female rats more ideal for our experiment since one of the questions we asked was whether exercise "per se" was responsible for the effect on tumor development, independent of the weight loss. Unfortunately, azoxymethane in the dose schedule used in our male rats was a poor colon carcinogen in the females of the Fischer 344 strain of rats.

From a physiological point of view, however, it is interesting that the males and the females react in different ways to moderate exercise. Male rats when exercised will eat more per animal and per g body weight, but not enough to compensate for the increased energy demand. Females, however, may compensate fully. Human experience points to similar mechanisms in man and women (Björntorp, 1989). A plausible, albeit teleological, explanation points to the need for adequate fat stores in case of pregnancy and nursing for the females - but the mechanisms are not known.

Fig. 4 shows the ratio fat content, lean body mass of exercised and sedentary rats after 168.5 and 317 km on a regular laboratory chow. The most remarkable observation is the very much lower fat content of the carcass from the exercised male rats. We also did some studies on the

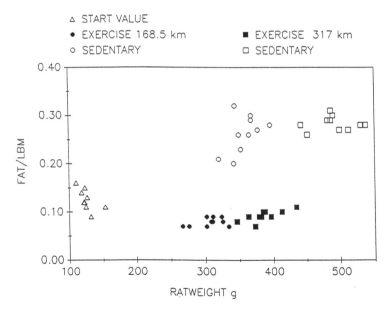

**Fig. 4.** Ratio fat mass to lean body mass in sedentary and exercised male Fischer 344 rats.

bones from these rats. Briefly, exercise leads to stronger bones and earlier flattening of the cartilage on the head of femur (Mosekilde et al., 1994; Søgaard et al., 1994).

These basic effects of exercise are also found in animals given a high fat diet. Fig. 5 shows the growth curves for male rats on two different diets containing either 23 per cent corn oil or a mixture of 21 per cent coconut oil and 2 per cent corn oil. Interestingly enough, the exercising as well as the sedentary rats on the coconut oil diet put on more weight than the rats on the corn oil diet although the two diets were "constructed" to be isocaloric. The difference in between these curves and the growth curves for rats on regular low fat diet is surprisingly small. Others have even found no difference in the growth rate for rats on diets with a varying fat content (Kristiansen et al., 1993).

It appears that on this point there is also a difference between rats and humans most of whom tend to become obese on a fat-rich diet.

In a third group of experiments we used sunflower oil 23 per cent and a similar diet in which 6 per cent of the sunflower oil was exchanged with a fish oil rich preparation high in omega 3 fatty acids.

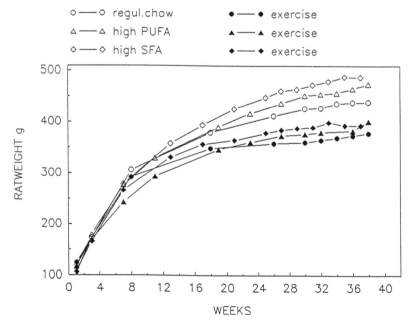

**Fig. 5.** Growth curves for sedentary and exercised male Fischer 344 rats on 3 different diets.

## ENDPOINTS AND PATHOLOGY

The extent to which the carcinogen had induced neoplasms in the experimental groups was estimated 38 weeks after injection of the carcinogen. Some animals, however, would develop tumors at an earlier state. A large weight loss or rectal bleeding was taken as an indication of the presence of tumor and the animals were removed from the experimental group for pathological examination. At the termination of the experiment a regular autopsy was performed and all organs scrutinized for the presence of tumors. The bowels were opened, flushed with saline and all suspect areas removed, fixed in formalin and prepared for microscopy. The neoplasms removed from the small and large bowel were tubular adenomas and adenocarcinomas. The adenomas showed proliferation of tubular structures composed of moderately or severe dysplastic intestinal epithelial cells. Adenocarcinomas were defined by their invasion beyond the muscularis mucosae. They were either typical intestinal adenocarcinomas growing in more or less well formed tubular structures or of a mucinous type usually with a component of signet ring cells. The kidney tumors were of a primitive mesenchymal pleomorphic type.

## EFFECT OF EXERCISE ON DEVELOPMENT OF NEOPLASIA

### First Series: Regular Low-fat Lab. Chow

Two groups of 32 male rats were started out as outlined above. One group was transferred to the treadmills for 5 hours on weekdays running 10 km a week.

The sedentary rats started to bleed from rectum slightly earlier than the running rats. By the end of the experimental period at 38 weeks after the injection of azoxymethane, 8 rats (25%) from the exercising group and 14 rats (44%) from the sedentary group had developed rectal bleeding and tumors of the colon.

The remaining rats were killed and autopsied in week 38. Most of the neoplasms were found in the distal half of the colon. All neoplasms are shown in Table 1.

**Table 1.** Number and types of neoplasias in male Fischer rats 38 weeks after exposure to azoxymethane (3 times 15 mg/kg).

|                                            | Exercise  | Sedentary |
|--------------------------------------------|-----------|-----------|
| Number of animals                          | 32        | 32        |
| Animals with neoplasia in colon            | 17 (53%)  | 25 (78%)  |
| Animals with tubular adenomas in colon     | 14 (44%)  | 23 (72%)  |
| Total number of tubular adenomas in colon  | 18        | 32        |
| Animals with invasive carcinomas in colon  | 5         | 5         |
| Total number of invasive carcinomas in colon | 6       | 7         |
| Small bowel tubular adenomas               | 4         | 3         |
| Duodenal carcinomas                        | 1         | 0         |
| Kidney carcinomas                          | 0         | 2         |
| Ear duct tumours                           | 0         | 1         |

Statistical analysis of the data after grouping of the tumors according to malignant properties showed significantly higher incidence of neoplasms of the colon in the sedentary group than in the exercising rats.

## Second Series: High-fat Diets

The intention of giving two different diets was, of course, to change the composition of the fat in the fatty tissues of the animals and to obtain two groups with major differences in the content of saturated and unsaturated fatty acids. A minor experiment was, therefore, interpolated to demonstrate to which extent and how fast the fatty acid pattern would change after a switch from the regular low-fat lab. chow to the experimental diets. Fig. 6 shows the changes in the major fat groups, each point representing the average of 3 rats. The new equilibrium was evidently reached in a few weeks, with the better part of the change completed already after one week.

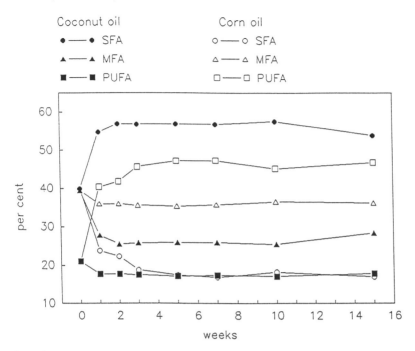

**Fig. 6.** Changes observed in saturated, mono-unsaturated and poly-unsaturated lipids in the omentum of male Fischer 344 rats after a switch to experimental diets high in coconut oil or high in corn oil.

As in series 1 the experiments were concluded after 38 weeks and all suspect neoplasms removed for microscopy. As apparent from Table 2, 10 sedentary rats in the corn oil group developed carcinomas in the colon (37%) and one animal developed a cecal carcinoma, whereas no tumors were observed in the exercising rats given the same diet (95% confidence interval for the difference 0.20-0.54%, $p < 0.001$). In the coconut oil group, the sedentary rats developed 6 malignant tumors in the colon (20%), whereas the exercising animals developed 3 tumors (10%) (95% confidence interval for the difference -0.08-0.26%, $p < 0.3$). Also the development of highly dysplastic adenomas was lower in the coconut oil group than in the corn oil group (sedentary: 18 coconut oil, 19 corn oil; exercise: 12 coconut oil, 19 corn oil). These differences were more pronounced when the total number of neoplasms was considered (sedentary: 22 coconut oil, 40 corn oil; exercise: 17 coconut oil, 32 corn oil).

**Table 2.** Number of neoplasms in the four experimental groups. Numbers in brackets indicate the number of rats in which the neoplasms were found.

| Localization | Corn oil group | | Coconut oil group | |
|---|---|---|---|---|
| | Exercise | Sedentary | Exercise | Sedentary |
| Number of rats | 30 | 30 | 30 | 30 |
| *Colon:* | | | | |
| Moderate dysplasia | 2 (2) | 3 (2) | 5 (5) | 3 (3) |
| Severe dysplasia | 32 (19) | 40 (19) | 17 (12) | 22 (18) |
| Carcinoma | 0 | 10 (10) | 3 (3) | 6 (6) |
| Coecum carcinoma | 0 | 1 (1) | 0 | 0 |
| *Small bowel:* | | | | |
| Moderate dysplasia | 0 | 0 | 0 | 0 |
| Severe dysplasia | 0 | 2 (2) | 1 (1) | 1 (1) |
| Carcinoma | 0 | 5 (5) | 2 (2) | 3 (3) |
| *Kidney:* | | | | |
| Mesenchymal tumours | 2 (2) | 4 (4) | 2 (2) | 6 (6) |
| Miscellaneous | 1 carcinoma with metastasis prostata? 2 earduct tumours | 1 liver carcinoma 1 stomach carcinoma | 1 earduct tumour | 1 lymphoma of the spleen |

The development of kidney tumors was not different for the two diets, but in both groups, the exercising rats developed only half as many tumors as the sedentary rats. Other tumors appear to be too rare to allow a meaningful statistical evaluation. The occurrence of tumors in the small bowel, however, showed trends similar to those in the colon.

The distribution of the neoplasms in colon exhibits some remarkable differences between the corn oil- and the coconut oil-fed rats (Fig. 7). Most of the neoplasms in the corn oil groups are localized in the distal half of the colon, with a maximum incidence rate about 15 cm from the ileocecal junction. In the coconut oil-fed rats, 4 of the 6 malignant tumors appeared in the proximal colon about 5 cm from the ileocecal junction, with most of the adenomas located in the distal part of the colon about 18 cm from the ileocecal junction. Exercise apparently did not alter this distribution in the groups, only the total number and the progression toward invasive growth.

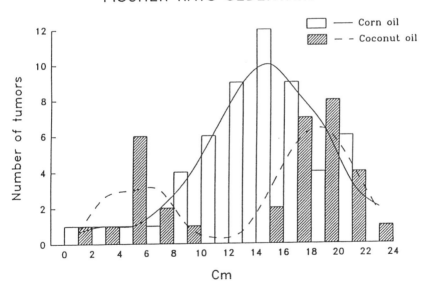

**Fig. 7.** Distribution in the colon of colon neoplasias in male Fischer 344 rats after 38 weeks on two different experimental diets. Bars indicate number of neoplasias observed in the given interval. Curves represent the results of calculations based on the exact position of the neoplasia with smoothing for stochastic variation over 3 points. The rats were given azoxymethane 15 mg/kg body weight at the age of 7 weeks.

A third series of experiments aimed at elucidating a possible influence of omega 3 fatty acids on the effect of a high-fat diet.

In spite of identical set-ups in our 3 series we do not feel completely happy about a direct comparison in between the experiments. Basic trends should hold water but several confounders might differ from series to series. To be fully comparable groups should have been randomized from the same population and given the same batch of carcinogen at the same time of the year etc. Our experiments were carried out over 3-4 years.

In our experiment 3 we found a faster development of the rectal bleedings and tumor appearance than in our first two series possibly due to stronger promotion by the sunflower oil or a stronger effect of the azoxymethane which is a very labile substance. We are not quite through the pathology yet, but so far it is apparent that the basic principles of a protective effect of exercise were re-established although to a lesser extent than in the previous experiments. Cohen et al. (1993) have shown similar dose effects in their experiments with DMBA and mammary cancer. The effect of exercise was obvious when a dose of 5 mg DMBA was given but the protective effect was overcome if the dose was increased to 10 mg. Evidently, a protective effect may be nullified if the carcinogenic stimulus is strong enough - which should surprise no one. In the group of rats given a diet in which 6 per cent of the sunflower oil was exchanged with a fish oil preparation fewer tumors were observed.

CONCLUSION

In summary, we have demonstrated that rats allowed to exercise to a moderate extent develop fewer neoplasms of the colon and kidney after azoxymethane than rats forced to live a sedentary life in "normal" animal cages. Our experiments were carried out in male rats who remained considerably slimmer during the exercise schedules than the sedentary rats in the control group. We are, therefore, not able to separate an effect of "pure" exercise from an effect due to reduced lipid stores of the body.

Our experiments are in line with epidemiological studies and other animal studies using different strains of rats and mice and different carcinogens. Much, however, has to be learned about a suitable amount of exercise and the relevance for humans. With modesty, however, it appears fair to conclude that the experiments suggest that moderate exercise might have a protective effect against certain cancers.

**P.S.:** Some part of this paper has been published in Europ. J. Cancer Prevention (1993) and Nutrition and Cancer (1994).

REFERENCES

1.    Applegate, E.A., Upton, D.E., and Stern, J.S. Food intake, body
      composition and blood lipids following treadmill exercise in male
      and female rats. Physiol. Behav., *28:* 917-920, 1982.
2.    Björntorp, P.A. Sex differences in the regulation of energy
      balance with exercise. Am. J. Clin. Nutr., *49:* 958-961, 1989.
3.    Cohen, L.A. Physical activity and cancer. Cancer Prevent. *June,*
      1-10, 1991.
4.    Cohen, L.A., Boylan, E., Epstein, M., and Zang, E. Voluntary
      exercise and experimental mammary cancer. In: Exercise,
      Calories, Fat, and Cancer, M.M. Jacobs (Ed.). Plenum Press,
      New York, 1992, pp. 41-59.
5.    Cohen, L.A., Kendall, M.E., Meschter, C., Epstein, M.A., Rein-
      hardt, J., and Zang, E. Inhibition of rat mammary tumorigenesis
      by voluntary exericse. In Vivo, *7:* 151-158, 1993.
6.    Frisch, R.E., Wyshak, G., Albright, N.L., Albright, T.E.,
      Schiff, I., Jones, K.P., Witschi, J., Shiang, E., Koff, E., and
      Marguglio, M. Lower prevalence of breast cancer and cancers of
      the reproductive system among former college athletes compared
      to non-athletes. Br. J. Cancer, *52:* 885-891, 1985.
7.    Frisch, R.E., Wyshak, G., Albright, N.L., Albright, T.E.,
      Schiff, I., and Witschi, J. Former athletes have a lower lifetime
      occurrence of breast cancer and cancers of the reproductive
      system. In: Exercise, Calories, Fat, and Cancer, M.M. Jacobs
      (Ed.). Plenum Press, New York, 1992, pp. 29-39.
8.    Kristiansen, E., Madsen, C. Meyer, O. Roswall, K., and Thorup,
      I. Effects of high-fat diet on incidence of spontaneous tumors in
      Wistar rats. Nutr. Cancer, *19:* 99-110, 1993.
9.    Kritchevsky, D. Caloric restriction and cancer: Search for the
      molecular mechanisms. In: Vitamins and Minerals in the Preven-
      tion and Treatment of Cancer, M.M. Jacobs (Ed.). CRC Press,
      Boca Raton, 1991, pp. 113-122.
10.   Mosekilde, L., Danielsen, C.C., Søgaard, C.H., and Thorling, E.
      The effect of long-term exercise on vertebral and femoral bone
      mass, dimensions, and strength - assessed in a rat model. Bone,
      *15:* 293-301, 1994.

11. Paffenbarger, R.S., Jr., Lee, I.M., and Wing, A.L. The influence of physical activity on the incidence of site-specific cancers in college alumni. In: Exercise, Calories, Fat, and Cancer, M.M. Jacobs (Ed.). Plenum Press, New York, 1992, pp. 7-15.

12. Søgaard, C.H., Danielsen, C.C., Thorling, E.B., and Mosekilde, L. Long-term exercise of young and adult female rats: Effect on femoral neck biomechanical competence and bone structure. J. Bone Mineral Res., *9:* 409-416, 1994.

13. Thorling, E.B., Jacobsen, N.O., and Overvad, K. Effect of exercise on intestinal tumour development in the male Fischer rat after exposure to azoxymethane. Europ. J. Cancer Prevent., *2:* 77-82, 1993.

14. Thorling, E.B., Jacobsen, N.O., and Overvad, K. The effect of treadmill exercise on azoxymethane-induced intestinal neoplasia in the male Fischer rat on two different high-fat diets. Nutr. Cancer, *22:* 31-41, 1994.

15. United Kingdom Testicular Cancer Study Group: Aetiology of testicular cancer: Association with congenital abnormalities, age at puberty, infertility, and exercise. Br. Med. J., *308:* 1393-1398, 1994.

POLYCYCLIC AROMATIC HYDROCARBON-DNA ADDUCTS IN

SMOKERS AND THEIR RELATIONSHIP TO MICRONUTRIENT LEVELS AND

GLUTATHIONE-S-TRANSFERASE M1 GENOTYPE

Ricardo A. Grinberg-Funes[1], Vishwa N. Singh[1],
Frederica P.Perera[2], Douglas A. Bell[3], Tie Lan Young[2],
Christopher Dickey[2], Lian W. Wang[2],
Regina M. Santella[2]

1 Hoffmann-La Roche, Nutley, NJ 07110, 2 Columbia
Presbyterian Cancer Center and Columbia School of
Public Health, N.Y., NY 10032, 3 National Institute
of Environmental Health Science, Research Triangle
Park, NC 27709

ABSTRACT

Sixty-three male cigarette smokers were entered into
a cross-sectional study to determine whether inverse
associations existed between polycyclic aromatic
hydrocarbon (PAH)-DNA adduct levels and intake/serum levels
of vitamin A, vitamin C and vitamin E. Associations
between PAH-DNA adducts and intakes of carotene as well as
serum levels of $\beta$-carotene were also determined. Fasting
blood samples were collected for assays of PAH-DNA adducts
in circulating mononuclear cells, plasma cotinine and serum
levels of vitamin A, $\beta$-carotene, vitamin C and vitamin E.
Since genetic deficiency in the detoxifying enzyme
glutathione S-transferase M1 (GSTM1) has been associated
with increased risk of lung cancer, GSTM1 genotype was also
determined. Analysis of PAH-DNA adducts by competitive
enzyme-linked immunosorbent assay (ELISA) indicated that
70% of the subjects had detectable adducts with a mean of
4.38 adducts/$10^8$ nucleotides (range 1.00-24.1/$10^8$).
Pearson's method was utilized to determine whether any
associations existed between the various host variables and
PAH-DNA adducts. Previously, no significant associations
were found between PAH-DNA adducts and cigarettes
smoked/day, pack-years, daily/lifetime tar exposures or

*191*

plasma cotinine levels [Carcinogenesis 13:2041,1992]. PAH-DNA adducts were inversely associated with serum cholesterol-adjusted vitamin E levels (r=-0.25, p≤0.05) and with smoking-adjusted vitamin C serum levels (r=-0.22, p≤0.09). Stratification by GSTM1 genotype indicated that these associations were limited to subjects with the null genotype. The relationship between adducts and serum cholesterol-adjusted vitamin E was significant in those of the null genotype (r=-0.38, p≤0.04) but not in those with the gene present (r=-0.12, p=0.5). Similarly, for smoking-adjusted vitamin C, the relationship with adducts was stronger in subjects with the null genotype (r=-0.35, p≤0.06) than in those with GSTM1 present (r=-0.05, p=0.77). These results are consistent with findings of prior epidemiological studies identifying significant inverse associations between antioxidant micronutrient status or GSTM1 genotype and the incidence of lung cancer. Additional studies should be conducted to confirm a possible protective role for vitamin E in PAH-DNA adduct formation and to explore further the possible roles of vitamin A, β-carotene and vitamin C in modulating adduct formation and lung cancer risk.


INTRODUCTION

Benzo(a)pyrene (BP) is one of a large number of polycyclic aromatic hydrocarbons (PAHs) formed by the pyrolytic process during cigarette smoking and is frequently used as a representative indicator of total PAH levels. A significant route of human exposure to BP during cigarette smoking is by deposition in the lower lung where it is readily absorbed (1). BP is then metabolically activated by the mixed function oxidases of various cells, including the lung epithelia, to an electrophilic, highly reactive form which can bind covalently to DNA [reviewed in (2)].

Peripheral white blood cell DNA has been used in a number of studies for measurement of PAH-DNA adducts following exposure to PAHs in cigarette smokers (3-5), foundry workers (6,7), coke-oven workers (8), and people living in highly polluted industrialized regions (9). PAH-DNA adducts have also been detected in peripheral white blood cells and lung tissue of lung cancer patients (10,11).

The results of several in vitro and in vivo studies have shown that vitamin A (and retinoids), β-carotene, vitamin C and/or vitamin E can influence BP metabolism, and DNA binding, as well as BP-induced mutagenesis, carcinogenesis and chromosomal aberrations (12-19). In addition, an association between these micronutrients and the incidence of human lung cancer has been found in a number of epidemiological studies (reviewed in (20)). However, no clinical studies have been conducted to determine associations between these micronutrients and PAH binding to human DNA.

This study investigated whether PAH-DNA adducts in smokers, detected in circulating lymphocytes and monocytes by competitive ELISA [utilizing a polyclonal antiserum that recognizes benzo(a)pyrene diol epoxide-I (BPDE-I)-DNA adducts], were inversely associated with micronutrient intake and blood levels. The antiserum cross reacts with structurally related PAH diol epoxide-DNA adducts and thus provides a relative measure of this class of adducts (21,22). In addition, genetic deficiency in the detoxifying enzyme glutathione S-transferase M1 has been associated with increased risk of lung (23-26) and bladder (27) cancer and increased PAH-DNA adducts (28). Thus, subjects were also analyzed for GSTM1 genotype by PCR. The PAH-DNA adduct data and comparison to a non-smoker population has been reported previously (5). Twenty two % of nonsmokers and 70% of smokers had detectable adducts with a mean in nonsmokers of $1.35\pm0.78/10^8$ nucleotides and $4.38\pm4.28/10^8$ in smokers (p<0.001).

MATERIALS AND METHODS

Study Subjects and Questionnaires

A total of 63 male cigarette smokers employed at Hoffmann-La Roche, Nutley, New Jersey, volunteered for this study. At the time of fasting blood collection, a questionnaire was administered eliciting information on current active and passive smoking, occupational, residential, familial cancer incidence history as well as dietary intake of charcoal-broiled foods over the past year.  Daily and lifetime tar intake were calculated utilizing data from the 1991 Federal Trade Commission report on tar, nicotine and carbon monoxide of cigarettes.  Although current tar levels are lower than in previous years, this information is a relative measure of tar exposure useful for comparing individuals.  Environmental tobacco smoke exposure was calculated based on questionnaire data.

The standardized self-administered diet assessment Harvard/Willett questionnaire (29) was also administered.  The micronutrient intake scores were computed by multiplying the vitamin content of a specific portion of food, as estimated from standard food consumption tables, by the consumption frequency of that food.  The vitamin content of each food or beverage item consumed was calculated and these were summed to provide an index of average daily dietary micronutrient intake for the prior year.

### Blood Sampling and Analysis

PAH-DNA Binding Assay.  Whole blood (40 ml) was collected into heparinized tubes and separated within 4 hours of sampling.  Mononuclear cells were separated by Ficoll (Sigma Chemical Co., St. Louis, Mo.) and washed twice with PBS.  Pelleted cells were frozen at -80°C until DNA isolation by standard phenol and chloroform/isoamyl alcohol extractions and RNase treatment.  DNA yields were > 200$\mu$g.  PAH diol epoxide-DNA adducts were analyzed by competitive ELISA essentially as described previously (30).  Briefly, 96 microwell black plates (MicroFLUOR 'B', Dynatech Laboratories, Alexandria, Va.) were coated with 0.2 ng BPDE-I-DNA (5 adducts/$10^6$ nucelotides).  A previously characterized rabbit antiserum (31,32) was used at 1:1.6x$10^6$ dilution.  A standard curve was constructed by mixing 50$\mu$l diluted antiserum with BPDE-I-DNA (1.5/$10^6$) in carrier non-modified calf thymus DNA such that 50$\mu$l contained 5-150 fmol BPDE-I-deoxyguanosine adduct in 50 $\mu$g of DNA.  Test samples were assayed at 50 $\mu$g/well after sonication and denaturation by boiling for 3 minutes and cooling on ice.  Goat anti-rabbit IgG-alkaline phosphatase (Boehringer Mannheim, Indianapolis, IN) was used at 1:400

dilution and the substrate was 4-methylumbelliferyl phosphate (100 $\mu$l, 50 $\mu$g/ml 0.1 M diethanolamine, pH 9.6). Fluorescence was read on a Microfluor reader (Dynatech Laboratories). Samples were run in triplicate and median values were used for determination of % inhibition. For analytical purposes, those samples with < 15% inhibition were considered non-detectable and were assigned a value of 1 adduct/$10^8$ nucleotides, an amount midway between the lowest positive value and zero.

Vitamin and Cotinine Assays. Whole blood (10 ml) was collected in red stopper tubes in subdued light. Serum was transferred into cryotubes which were stored in the dark at -80°C prior to analysis for vitamin A, vitamin E ($\alpha$-tocopherol), $\beta$-carotene and cotinine. Other cryotubes containing equal volumes of serum (0.8 ml) and 10% metaphosphoric acid were also stored at -80°C prior to the analysis for vitamin C. Standard procedures were utilized for the analyses of vitamin A, vitamin E, $\beta$-carotene (33,34) and cotinine (35) by Dr. Ed Norkus, Our Lady of Mercy Hospital, Bronx NY.

GSTM1 Genotype. GSTM1 genotype was determined by PCR essentially as described previously (27). ß-Globin and interferon $\gamma$ were coamplified with GSTM1 as internal standards.

Statistical Analysis. Adduct and vitamin data were log-normally distributed and showed a large variance. The data were therefore $\log_{10}$-transformed prior to analysis. There was a significant relationship between serum levels of cholesterol and vitamin A ($r=0.28$, $p=0.02$) but not vitamin E ($r=0.13$, $p=0.28$ or $\beta$-carotene ($r=0.05$, $p=0.68$). In addition previous studies have adjusted serum vitamin E for cholesterol or total lipids (29,36,37). For these reasons, vitamin A, E and $\beta$-carotene serum levels were adjusted by divided by individual serum cholesterol levels. Although a prior study has observed an increase in plasma lipid levels with smoking (38), there was no association in the subjects in this study ($r=0.08$, $p=0.5$). Student's T-test was used to describe the difference in the level of PAH-DNA adducts by GSTM1 genotype. The relationship between PAH-DNA adduct levels and each of a number of variables (smoking history, GSTM1 genotype, vitamin intake and serum levels) was initially described by Pearson's Correlation coefficients. This analysis as well as historical data revealed the necessity to further adjust vitamin C and $\beta$-carotene intake and serum levels by cigarettes smoked per day (39). Multiple linear regression analysis was used to control for cigarette smoking variables as well as GSTM1 genotype in further analysis of the effect of vitamin levels on DNA adducts.

## RESULTS

The mean age of smokers was 47.6 ± 8.0 years (range 27-74 years). Approximately 90% of all subjects were smoking at least 20 cigarettes/day (average 26.4 ± 16.0 ;range 10-50 cigarettes/day). Pack-years ranged from 15 to 100 with a mean of 38.1 ± 16.6. Mean plasma cotinine levels were 286 ± 90 $\mu$g/L (range 130-500 $\mu$g/L). Seventy percent of subjects had detectable PAH-DNA adducts in mononuclear cells (lymphocytes plus monocytes) with a mean of 4.38 ± 4.29/$10^8$ (range 1 - 24.1/$10^8$). We previously reported that there were no significant correlations between PAH-DNA adducts and cigarettes smoked/day, pack-years, daily/lifetime tar exposures, plasma cotinine levels or dietary intake of charcoal-broiled foods (5).

Data from the dietary history questionnaire indicated that 85% of subjects had average daily vitamin A intakes above or equal to the recommended daily allowance (RDA) of 5,000 I.U./day with a mean in all subjects of 12,100±8,100 I.U./day (Table 1). Ninety-five percent of the subjects had vitamin C intakes greater than or equal to the RDA of 60 mg/day with a mean in all subjects of 314±368 mg/day. The 10 mg/day RDA for vitamin E was met by 40% of subjects. All subjects had serum vitamin A levels that fell within the normal range (Table 1). Eighty nine percent of subjects had serum vitamin C levels that were within the normal range of 0.31-2.1 mg/dL. Normal serum vitamin E levels (≥0.8 mg/dL) were detected in 67% of subjects and serum levels of ß-carotene (≥10 $\mu$g/dl) in 62%.

Vitamin E intake was significantly associated with serum cholesterol-adjusted vitamin E levels (r = 0.40, p ≤ 0.001). Vitamin C intake was also significantly correlated with serum vitamin C levels (r = 0.51, p≤0.001). Significant correlations were not detected between carotene intake and serum cholesterol-adjusted β-carotene levels and between vitamin A intake and cholestererol-adjusted serum vitamin A levels.

PAH-DNA adducts were not significantly associated with vitamin A intake (r=0.026), smoking-adjusted vitamin C intake (r=-0.044), vitamin E intake (r=-0.19) or smoking-adjusted carotene intake (r=0.026). PAH-DNA adducts were inversely associated with serum cholesterol-adjusted vitamin E levels (r=-0.25, p≤0.05) and with smoking-adjusted vitamin C serum levels (r=-0.22, p≤0.09) (Table 2). There was no association between adducts and either serum cholesterol and smoking-adjusted β-carotene (r=-0.048) or serum cholesterol-adjusted vitamin A (r=-0.058).

GSTM1 was present in 32 of the 63 subjects (51%). There was no significant difference in PAH-DNA adducts in subjects with one or both GSTM1 alleles (4.01±3.38/10$^8$) compared to those without GSTM1 (4.75±5.09/10$^8$) (Figure 1). The 2 subjects with the highest adduct levels were of the null genotype. The relationhsip between PAH-DNA adducts and serum vitamin levels was then analyzed after stratification on GSTM1 genotype. Only in those subjects with the null genotype was there an association between serum vitamin levels and adducts (Table 2). In subjects with the null genotype there was a significant association between adducts and cholesterol-adjusted serum vitamin E (r=-0.38, p≤0.04) but not in those with GSTM1 present (r=-0.12, p=0.5, Figure 2A). Similarly, a stronger relationship was found between smoking adjusted vitamin C levels and adducts in subjects with the null genotype (r=-0.35, p=0.06) compared to those with the GSTM1 present genotype (r=-0.05, p=0.78, Figure 2B). No association by genotype was found between serum levels of adjusted β-carotene or vitamin A and PAH-DNA adducts (Table 2).

## DISCUSSION

Inverse associations were found between PAH-DNA adduct levels and serum cholesterol-adjusted vitamin E and serum smoking-adjusted vitamin C. Of these, only the relationship between PAH-DNA adducts and cholesterol-adjusted serum vitamin E was statistically significant. Controlling for cigarettes smoked per-day, a possible confounder for vitamin intake and serum levels, strengthened these associations. No relationship was observed with vitamin A or β-carotene serum levels. Since normal vitamin A and C levels were present in 90-100% of participants, there may have been inadequate variability to observe a significant estimate of their correlation with DNA adducts. In contrast, only 67% of subjects had normal vitamin E serum levels which may have helped demonstrate the significant relationship with this vitamin.

In agreement with prior studies in a similar ethnic population, GSTM1 was present in 51% of the subjects (27). Although mean adduct levels were higher in individuals with the null genotype, the results were not significant. When subjects were stratified by GSTM1 genotype (Table 2), the inverse relationships between PAH-DNA adducts and adjusted serum levels of vitamin E and C were found only in those subjects with the null genotype. These results suggest that serum levels of antioxidant vitamins may be more important in inhibiting PAH-DNA adduct formation in individuals lacking GSTM1. GST can catalyze the conjugation reaction between glutathione and substrates bearing hydrophobic and electrophilic sites, thereby enhancing detoxification and elimination of various carcinogens. Perhaps only when this detoxification enzyme is lacking do antioxidants play an important role in preventing adduct formation. Another study has observed a positive association between the null genotype and PAH-DNA adducts in lung, measured by $^{32}$P-postlabeling (28). In addition, sister chromatid exchanges in smokers who are GSTM1 positive were lower than in those with the null genotype (40).

The results of several cross-sectional (41-45) and cohort studies (44,45) have shown an inverse association between blood vitamin E levels and lung cancer. However, other researchers have reported non-significant associations between blood vitamin E and lung cancer incidence (46,47). A few cross-sectional studies focusing on the association between calculated intake of vitamin E and the risk of lung cancer did not reveal a statistically significant protective effect of vitamin E (42,48). A role for vitamin E in prevention of initiation in chemical carcinogenesis has been demonstrated by its inhibition of the binding of BP to rat liver nuclei (49). Covalent binding of labeled BP metabolites to exogenous DNA has been reported to increase with microsomes from trout fed a vitamin E deficiency diet (50). In *vivo* and in *vitro* studies have suggested that vitamin E can enhance GST activity (51) and also increase P-450 levels in certain tissues (50,52).

Several studies have reported a possible modest protective effect of dietary vitamin C (53-55) or blood vitamin C levels (56) against lung cancer. A large cohort study (57) and a case-control study (58) found that high dietary vitamin C intakes were significantly related to reduced risks of lung cancer. In other studies, intake of vitamin C higher than the 60 mg/day R.D.A. had a protective effect against lung cancer (59). It is important to note that cigarette smoking is associated with both high lung cancer risk and low vitamin C status (60). Vitamin C can affect the metabolic activation of BP by inhibiting cytochrome P-450 (61) including microsomal aryl hydrocarbon hydroxylase activity in vitro (62). Shah et al. (12) reported decreased in vitro BP binding to DNA when BP was activated with a rat liver microsome preparation in the presence of vitamin C.

As reported previously, no significant correlations were observed between PAH-DNA adducts and cigarettes/day, pack-years and plasma cotinine (5). These results are consistent with the large interindividual variation in adduct levels that have been measured in workers with similar exposures (7). Differences in genetic capacity for the metabolism and detoxification of carcinogens are very important factors that determine interindividual variation in adduct formation (25,63). For example, correlations have been found between in vivo DNA adducts [measured by immunoaffinity purification followed by [32]P-postlabelling in lung tissue (64) or synchronous fluorescence spectroscopy in placenta (65)] and aryl hydrocarbon hydroxylase activity in the same tissues measured in vitro.

If antioxidant vitamins can decrease PAH-DNA adducts in smokers, such vitamins may also be protective against adduct formation related to other environmental, occupational and dietary exposures to PAHs. Prospective, randomized well-controlled clinical trials should be conducted in smokers and other high-risk groups for lung cancer to assess the roles of vitamin A, C, E and β-carotene in modulating both PAH-DNA adduct formation and cancer incidence.

REFERENCES

1.  Rom WN: "Environmental and occupational medicine."
    Little Brown and Co.,Boston, MA, 1992.

2.  Grunberger D, Singer B: "Molecular Biology of
    Mutagens and Carcinogens." New York: Plenum, 1983

3.  Perera FP, Santella RM, Brenner D, Poirier MC,
    Munshi AA, Fischman HK, VanRyzin J: DNA adducts,
    protein adducts and SCE in cigarette smokers and
    nonsmokers. J Natl Cancer Inst 79:449-456, 1987.

4.  Jahnke GD, Thompson CL, Walker MP, Gallagher JE,
    Lucier GW, DiAugustine RP: Multiple DNA adducts in
    lymphocytes of smokers and nonsmokers determined by
    [$^{32}$P]-postlabeling analysis. Carcinogenesis
    11:205-211, 1990.

5.  Santella RM, Grinberg-Funes RA, Young TL, Dickey C,
    Singh VN, Wang LW, Perera FP: Cigarette smoking
    related polycyclic aromatic hydrocarbon-DNA adducts
    in peripheral mononuclear cells. Carcinogenesis
    13:2041-2045, 1992.

6.  Shamsuddin AKM, Sinopoli NT, Hemminki K, Boesch RB,
    Harris CC: Detection of benzo[a]pyrene: DNA adducts
    in human white blood cells. Cancer Res 45:66-68,
    1985.

7.  Perera FP, Hemminki K, Young TL, Santella RM,
    Brenner D, and Kelly, G: Detection of polycyclic
    aromatic hydrocarbon-DNA adducts in white blood cells
    of foundry workers. Cancer Res 48:2288-2291, 1988.

8.  Harris CC, Vahakangas K, Newman MJ, Trivers GE,
    Shamsuddin A, Sinopoli N, Mann DL, Wright WE:
    Detection of benzo[a]pyrene diol epoxide-DNA adducts
    in peripheral blood lymphocytes and antibodies to the
    adducts in serum from coke oven workers. Proc Natl
    Acad Sci USA 82:6672-6676, 1985.

9. Perera FP, Hemminki K, Grzybowska E, Motykiewiez G, Santella RM, Young TL, Dickey C, Brandt-Rauf P, DeVivo I, Blaner B, Tsai W, Chorazy M: Molecular damage from environmental pollution in Poland. Nature (London) 360:256-258, 1992.

10. Perera FP, Mayer J, Jaretzki A, Hearne S, Brenner D, Young TL, Fischman HK, Grimes M, Grantham S, Tang MX, Tsai W-Y, Santella RM: Comparison of DNA adducts and sister chromatid exchange in lung cancer cases and controls. Cancer Res 49:4446-4451, 1989.

11. van Schooten FJ, Hillebrand MJX, van Leeuwen FE, van Zandwijk N, Jansen HM, den Engelse L, Kriek E: Polycyclic aromatic hydrocarbon-DNA adducts in white blood cells from lung cancer patients: no correlation with adduct levels in lung. Carcinogenesis 13:987-993, 1992.

12. Shah GM, Bhattacharya RK: Inhibition by 1-ascorbate of binding to DNA of benzo(a)pyrene and its metabolites. Indian J Biochem & Biophysics 17:96-98, 1980.

13. Nomi S, Matsuura T, Ueyama H, Ueda K: Effect of vitamin A compounds on the covalent binding of benzo(a)pyrene to nuclear macromolecules. J Nutr Sci Vitaminol 27:33-41, 1981.

14. Raina V, Gurtoo HL: Effects of vitamins A, C and E on aflatoxin B1 (AFB1) and benzo[a]pyrene (BP)-induced mutagenesis in Salmonella typhimurium TA-98 and TA-100. Proc Am Assoc Cancer Res 22:112, 1982.

15. Smalls R, Patterson RM: Reduction of benzo[a]pyrene induced chromosomal aberrations by DL-Alpha tocopherol. Eur J Cell Biol 28:92-97, 1982.

16. Rocchi P, Arfellini G, Capucci A, Grilli MP: Effect of vitamin A palmitate on mutagenesis induced by polycyclic aromatic hydrocarbons in human cells. Carcinogenesis 4:245-247, 1983.

17. Dogra SC, Khanduja KL, Gupta MP: The effect of vitamin A deficiency on the initiation and postinitiation phases of benzo[a]pyrene-induced lung tumorigenesis in rats. Br J Comm 52:931-935, 1985.

18. Kallistratos G, Fasske E: Inhibition of benzo[a]pyrene carcinogenesis in rats with vitamin C. J Cancer Res Clin Oncol 97:91-96, 1980.

19. McCarthy DJ, Lindamood III C, Hill DL: Effects of retinoids on metabolizing enzymes and on binding of benzo(a)pyrene to rat tissue DNA. Cancer Res 47:5014-5020, 1987.

20. Block G, Patterson B, Subar A: Fruit, vegetables, and cancer prevetion: A review of the epidemiological evidence. Nutr Cancer 18:1-29, 1992.

21. Santella RM, Gasparro FP, Hsieh LL: Quantitation of carcinogen-DNA adducts with monoclonal antibodies. Prog Exp Tumor Res 31: 63-75, 1987.

22. Weston A, Trivers G, Vahakangas K, Newman M, Rowe M: Detection of carcinogen-DNA adducts in human cells and antibodies to these adducts in human sera. Prog Exp Tumor Res 31:76-85, 1987.

23. Seidegard J, Pero RW, Miller DG, Beattie EJ: A glutathione transferase in human leukocytes as a marker for the susceptibility to lung cancer. Carcinogenesis 7:751-753, 1986.

24. Zhong S, Howie AF, Ketterer B, Taylor J, Hayes JD, Beckett GJ, Wathen CG, Wolf CR, Spurr NK: Glutathione S-transferase mu locus: use of genotyping and phenotyping assays to assess association with lung cancer susceptibility. Carcinogenesis 9:1533-1537, 1991.

25. Kihara M, Kihara M, Noda K, Okamoto N: Increased risk of lung cancer in Japanese smokers with class mu glutathione S-transferase gene deficiency. Cancer Lett 71:151-155, 1993.

26. Nazar-Stewart V, Motulsky AG, Eaton DL, White E, Hornung SK, Leng Z-T, Stapleton P, Weiss NS: The glutathione S-transferase μ polymorphism as a marker for susceptibility to lung carcinoma. Cancer Res 53:2313-2318, 1993.

27. Bell DA, Taylor JA, Paulson DF, Robertson CN, Mohler JL, Lucier GW: Genetic risk and carcinogen exposure: a common inherited defect of the carcinogen-metabolism gene glutathione S-transferase M1 (GSTM1) that increases susceptibility to bladder cancer. J Natl Cancer Inst 85:1159-1164, 1993.

28. Shields PG, Bowman ED, Harrington AM, Doan VT, Weston A: Polycyclic aromatic hydrocarbon-DNA adducts in human lung and cancer susceptibility genes. Cancer Res 53:3486-3492, 1992.

29. Willet WC, Stampfer MJ, Underwood BA, Speizer FE, Rosner B, Hennekens CH: Validation of a dietary questionnaire with plasma carotenoid and α-tocopherol levels. Am J Clin Nutr 38:631-639, 1983.

30. Santella RM, Weston A, Perera FP, Trivers GT, Harris CC, Young TL, Nguyen D, Lee BM, Poirier MC: Interlaboratory comparison of antisera and immunoassays for benzo(a)pyrene-diol-epoxide-I-modified DNA. Carcinogenesis 9 1265-1269, 1988.

31. Poirier MC, Santella R, Weinstein IB, Grunberger D, Yuspa SH: Quantitation of benzo[a]pyrene-deoxyguanosine adducts by radioimmunoassay. Cancer Res 40:412-416, 1980.

32. Poirier MC: Development of Immunoassays for the Detection of Carcinogen-DNA Adducts. In Molecular Dosimetry and Human Cancer: Analytical Epidemological, and Social Considerations, Groopman JD, Skipper PL, (ed). CRC Press, Boca Raton, 211-230, 1991.

33. Craft NE, Brown ED, Smith JC: Effects of storage and handling on concentrations of individual carotenoids, retinol, and tocopherol in plasma. Clin Chem 34:44-48, 1988.

34. Roe JH, Keuther CA: The determination of ascorbic acid in whole blood and urine through the 2,4-dinitrophenylhydrazine derivative of dehydroascorbic acid. J Biol Chem 147:399, 1943.

35. Machacek DA, Jiang NS: Quantitation of cotinine in plasma by liquid chromatography. Clin Chem 32: 979-982, 1986.

36. Longnecker MP, Martin-Moreno JM, Knekt P, Nomura AMY, Schober SE, Stahelin HB, Wald NJ, Gey F, Willett WC: Serum $\alpha$-tocopherol concentration in relation to subsequent colorectal Cancer: pooled data from five cohorts. J. Natl. Cancer Inst 84:430-435, 1992.

37. Willet WC, Polk BF, Underwood BA, Stampfer MJ, Pressel S, Rosner B, Taylor JO, Schnider K, Hames, CG: Relation of serum vitamins A and E and carotenioids to the risk of cancer. N Engl J Med 310: 430-434, 1984.

38. Craig WY, Palomaki GE, Haddow JE: Cigarette smoking and serum lipid and lipoprotein concentrations: an analysis of published data. Br Med J 298:784-8, 1989.

39. Shectman G: Estimating ascorbic acid requirements for cigarette smokers. Ann NY Acad Sci 686:335-345 1993.

40. van Poppel G, Verhagen H, van't Veer P, van Bladeren PJ: Markers for cytogentic damage in smokers: associations with plasma antioxidants and glutathione S-transferase $\mu$. Cancer Epi Biomark Preven 2:441-447, 1993.

41. Miyamoto H, Araya Y, Ito M, Isobe H, Dosaka H, Shimizu T, Kishi F, Yamamato I, Honma H, Kawakami Y: Serum selenium and vitamin A concentrations in families of lung cancer patients. Carcinogenesis, 60: 1159-1162, 1987.

42. Lopez SA, LeGardeur BY: Vitamins A, C and E in relation to lung cancer incidence. Am J Clin Nutr 35:851, 1982.

43. Rougereau A, Person O, Rougereau G: Retinol, β-carotene and α-tocopherol status in a French population of healthy subjects. Int J Vitam Nutr Res 57:31-35, 1987.

44. Menkes MS, Comstock GW, Vuilleumier JP, Helsing KJ, Rider AA, Brookmeyer R: Serum B-carotene, vitamins A and E, selenium, and the risk of lung cancer. N Engl J Med 315: 1250-1254, 1986.

45. Kok FJ, van Duijn CM, Hoffman A, Vermeeren R, De Bruijn AM, Valkenburg HA: Micronutrients and the risk of lung cancer. Am J Clin Nutr 316:1416, 1987.

46. Atukorala S, Basu TK, Dickerson JWT, Donaldson D, Sakula A: Vitamin A, zinc and lung cancer. Carcinogenesis 40:927-31, 1979.

47. Nomura AMY, Stemmermann GN, Heilbrun LK, Salkeld RM, Vuilleumier JP: Serum vitamin levels and the risk of cancer of specific sites in men of Japanese ancestry in Hawaii. Cancer Res 45:2369-72, 1985.

48. Byers TE, Grahma S. Haughey BP, Marshall JR, Swanson MK: Diet and lung cancer risk: Findings from the Western New York Diet Study. Am J Epidemiol 125: 351-6, 1987.

49. Matsuura T, Ueyama H, Nomi S, Ueda K: Effect of α-tocopherol on the binding of benzo[a]pyrene to nuclear macromolecules. J Nutr Sci Vitaminol 25: 495-504, 1979.

50. Williams DE, Carpenter HM, Buhler DR, Kelly JD, Dutchuk M: Alterations in lipid peroxidation antioxidant enzymes, and carcinogen metabolism in liver microsomes of vitamine E-deficient trout and rat. Toxicol Appl Pharmacol 116: 78-84, 1992.

51. Chen LH, Shiau CC: Induction of glutathione-S-transferase activity by antioxidants in hepatocyte culture. Anticaner Res 9:1069-72, 1989.

52. Chen Y-T, Ding H-H: Vitamins E and K induced aryl hydrocarbon hydroxylase activity in human cell cultures. Biochem. Biophys Res Commun 143:863-871, 1987.

53. Shekelle RB, Lepper M, Liu S, Maliza C, Raynor WJ, Rossof AH: Dietary vitamin A and risk of cancer in the Wester Electric Study. Lancet 2:1185-90, 1981.

54. Kvale G, Bejelke E, Gart JJ: Dietary habits and lung cancer risk. Intl J Cancer 31:397-405, 1983.

55. Hinds MW, Kolonel LN, Hawkin JH, Lee J: Dietary vitamin A, carotene, vitamin C and risk of lung cancer in Hawaii. Am J Epidemiol 199:227-37, 1984.

56. Staehelin HB, Gey KF, Brubacher G: Plasma vitamin C and cancer death: The prospective basel study. Ann NY Acad Sci 498:124-31, 1987.

57. Long-De W, Hammond EC: Lung cancer, fruit, green salad and vitamin pills. Chin Med J 98:206-210, 1985.

58. LeMarChand L, Yoshizawa CN, Kolonel LN, Hankin JH, Goodman MT: Vegetable consumption and lung cancer risk: A population based case-control study in Hawaii. J Natl Cancer Inst 81: 1158-1164, 1989.

59. Kromhout D: Essential micronutrients in relation to carcinogenesis. Am J Clin Nutr 45:1361-1367, 1987.

60. Hoefel OS: Smoking: An important factor in vitamin C deficiency. Int J Vitam Nutr Res Suppl 24:121-124, 1983.

61. Belvedere G, Miller H, Vatsis KP, Coon MJ, Gelboin HV: Hydroxylation of benzo[a]pyrene and binding of (-)-trans-7,8-dihydroxy-7,8-dihydrobenzo{a}pyrene metabolites to deoxyribonucleic acid catalyzed by purified forms of liver microsomal cytochrome P-450. Biochem Pharm 29:1693-702, 1980.

62. Kiyohara C, Omura M, Hirohata T: In vitro effects of L-ascorbic acid (vitamin C) on aryl hydrocarbon hydroxylase activity in hepatic microsomes of mice. Mutat Res 251:227-32, 1991.

63. Nebert DW: Role of genetics and drug metabolism in human cancer risk. Mutat Res 247:267-281, 1991.

64. Geneste O, Camus A-M, Castegnaro M, Petruzzelli S, Macchiarine P, Angeletti CA, Giuntini C, Bartsch H: Comparison of pulmonary DNA adduct levels, measured by $^{32}$P-postlabelling and aryl hydrocarbon hydroxylase activity in lung parenchyma of smokers and ex-smokers. Carcinogenesis 12:1301-1305, 1991.

65. Manchester DK, Bowman ED, Parker NB, Caporaso NE, and Weston A: Determinants of polycyclic aromatic hydrocarbon-DNA adducts in human placenta. Cancer Res 52:1499-503, 1992.

TABLE 1
DAILY DIETARY VITAMIN INTAKES AND
SERUM VITAMIN LEVELS

|  | INTAKE | SERUM LEVEL |
|---|---|---|
| Vitamin A |  |  |
| Mean ± S.D. | 12100 ± 8100 IU | 65.2 ± 14.1 $\mu$g/dL |
| Range | 1080 - 29600 | 36.7 - 99.6 |
| Vitamin C |  |  |
| Mean ± S.D. | 314 ± 368 mg | 1.04 ± 0.56 mg/dL |
| Range | 18.9 - 1610 | 0.14 - 2.63 |
| Carotene |  |  |
| Mean ± S.D. | 8860 ± 6820 IU | 10.7 ± 9.89[a] $\mu$g/dL |
| Range | 860 - 29600 | 0.3 ± 41.7 |

[a] serum levels of β-Carotene

## TABLE 2
### CORRELATIONS BETWEEN PAH-DNA ADDUCTS AND ADJUSTED SERUM VITAMIN LEVELS

| | All Subjects n=63 | | GSTM1 -/- n=31 | | GSTM1 +/+, +/- n=32 | |
|---|---|---|---|---|---|---|
| | Regression Coefficient | p | Regression Coefficient | p | Regression Coefficient | p |
| Vitamin E[a] | -0.25 | ≤0.05 | -0.38 | ≤0.04 | -0.12 | 0.50 |
| Vitamin C[b] | -0.22 | ≤0.09 | -0.35 | 0.06 | -0.05 | 0.77 |
| β-Carotene[a,b] | -0.048 | 0.71 | -0.05 | 0.78 | -0.06 | 0.75 |
| Vitamin A[a] | -0.058 | 0.65 | -0.10 | 0.58 | -0.03 | 0.89 |

209

# ASPECTS OF COMMERICAL DEEP-FAT FRYING OF FALLAFEL AND ITS RELATION TO LIVER TUMOR.

I.A. Sadek, Department of Zoology, Faculty of Science, Alexandria University, Alexandria, Egypt.

S.S.A. Zeyadah, Department of Nutrition (Food Analysis), High Institute of Public Health, Alexandria University, Alexandria, Egypt.

H.M. Ismail, Department of Nutrition (Food Analysis), High Institute of Public Health, Alexandria University, Alexandria, Egypt

S.I. Saleh, Central Laboratory for Food and Feed, Ministry of Agriculture, Alexandria, Egypt.

## ABSTRACT

Experimental animals, Bufo regularis, fed 0.2 mg N-nitrosomorpholine (NNM)/toad, 3 times/week for 3 months induced hepatocellular carcinoma in 11 out of 50 cases. Enhancement of liver tumor incidences (14 out of 50 cases) by NNM at the same level dose plus commercial vegetable oils used for deep fat frying of fallafel 0.2 ml/toad, 3 times/week for 3 months. Tumor incidences were detected in toads fed commercial vegetable ils used for deep fat frying of fallafel alone 0.2 ml/toad, 3 times/week for the same period (5 out of 50 cases). Tumors were not detected in toads which were fed with 0.2 ml/toad of unheated commercial vegetable oils, 3 times/week for 3 months.

## INTRODUCTION

Marked variations in dietary habits among populations of different cultures and lifestyles have been associated with a risk for the development of cancer. Among the dietary habits, dietary fat has received considerable attention as a risk factor in the etiology of colon and mammary cancer (1, 12). Dietary fats are often heated during processing and food preparation, and this can lead to oxidative changes that may influence their effect on tumorigenesis.

The fried products absorb a considerable amount of oil, which becomes a part of our diet. The nutritional consequences of ingesting deteriorated oils include a variety of symptoms ranging from an allergy of the digestive tract, growth depression and enlarged organs, to biochemical lesions (3). Furthermore, it was reported taht highly oxidized oils may produce polycyclic aromatic hydrocarbons which have a carcinogenic effect (14).

During the past few decades, a considerable amount of research has been devoted to frying oils. Some authors studied the physical and chemical changes occurring in oils (5), while others were mainly concerned with the fractionation of the oxidation products formed during frying (6). However, thermallly oxidized oils apparently have not been tested for their effects on tumor promotion in animal models.

Toads have been used as models to assay the development of tumors in relation to carcinogens (8), co-carcinogens (9), and vitamins (10). It is worth mentioning that similarities in cytological characteristics between tumors in frogs and human beings have been documented (11).

In Egypt, vegetable oils are used for cooking and frying. Vegetable patties known as "fallafel" are commonly deep-fried in vegetable oils (cottonseed and sunflower seed) by street vendors. It was, therefore, of interest to examine the effect of commercial vegetable oils used for deep fat frying of fallafel on liver tumor induced by N-nitrosomorpholine (NNM) in Egyptian toad.

## MATERIALS AND METHODS

### Samples

Eight oil samples were collected from several fast food outlets in Alexandria, Egypt after varying periods of usage between 15-25 hrs. These Alexandrian samples (cotton and sunflower oil) were collected at random from street vendors of fallafel. Oil samples were homogenized/mixed and stored at refrigerated temperature until used.

### Analytical Procedures

Refractice index. viscosity, smoke point, peroxide value (determined iodometrically), acid value, and iodine value were determined by the AOCS (12) procedures. P-anisidine

Table 1. Comparison between physical and chemical composition of commercial oils (cottonseed and sunflower oil) used in deep frying of fallafel in Alexandria city and control.

| Sample | Refractive Index | Viscosity (Min) | Smoke Point (C) | Peroxide Value mEQ/kg | Acid value (% g olicacid) | Iodine value (WiJ's) | P-anisidine value | Polymers content (%) | Total oxidation value |
|---|---|---|---|---|---|---|---|---|---|
| Treated (heat-ed) oil | 1.47 + 0.0 | 10.61 + 4.52 | 197.55 + 12.71 | 5.94+0.72 | 0.91+0.28 | 106.27+ 13.23 | 8.89 + 2.40 | 3.26+0.28 | 20.77 + 5.60 |
| control (un-heated) oil | 1.47+0.0 | 15.93+3.31 | 205.90+ 20.03 | 4.92+0.69 | 0.43+0.23 | 113.30+ 4.69 | 6.90+0.09 | 4.43+0.53 | 16.92+0.58 |

Each value in this table represents mean value of triplicate analysis mean + SD value was determined by IUPAC (13) procedures.  While polymer content was detected as described before (14).

## Toads

Sexuallly mature male and female toads, Bufo regularis, were used.  The experimental animals were collected by a regular supplier from El-Nozha district, Alexandria.  The average weight per experimental animal was 40 g.

## Dietary Treatment

The experimental animals were divided into 4 groups (50 toads/group) and treated as follows:

1.     The first group of animals were fed N-nitrosomorpholine (NNM) as a carcinogen (Sigma Chemical Company, St. Louis, MO, USA) at a dose level of 0.2 mg/toad, 3 times/week for 3 months.

2.     The experimental animals of group 2 were fed the same dose level of NNM and 0.2 ml commercial vegetable oils used for deep fat frying of fallafel from market, 3 times/week for the same period.

3.     Toads of group 3 were treated with 0.2 ml/toad of commercial vegetable oils used for deep-fat frying of fallafel alone, 3 times/week for 3 months.

4.     Animals of group 4 were fed with 0.2 ml/toad of unheated commercial vegetable oils, 3 times/week for 3 months.

5.     The last group of animals were not treated with anything and were used as control.

## Growth and Histopathological Observations

At the end of the 3 months, all animals were killed and the organs were examined by the naked eye.  It has been noticed that tumors appeared in the liver of some animals.  These tumors are small nodules, greyish-white in color.  For histological evaluation, the liver was fixed in Boiun and embedded in paraffin.  The sections were stained with hematoxylin and eosin.

## Statistical Analysis

Student t-test was performed to determine the level of significant differences between tumor incidence in toads treated with NNM alone when compared with toad treated with NNM and oil need for deep-fat frying of fallafel. Also, diffferences in physical and chemical composition between control oil (unheated oil) and heated oil were compared for significance. The values are given as the mean + SD.

## RESULTS

It has been shown that the dose of 0.2 mg NNM/toad, 3 times/week for 3 monoths given to toads of group 1 induced liver tumors in 11 out of 50 cases (Table 2). The liver tumor was diagnosed as hepatocellular carcinoma.

Toads of group 2 which were given the same dose of NNM and fed commercial vegetable oils (cotton and sunflower oil) used for deep-fat frying of fallafel 0.2 ml/toad, 3 times/week for 3 months, showed a significant increase in liver tumor incidence (14 out of 50 cases) according to the student t-test.

However, tumor incidences were detected in toads of gorup 3 which were fed commercial vegetable oils used for deep-fat frying of fallafel alone 0.2 ml/toad, 3 times/week for 3 months (5 out of 50 cases). Also, the liver neoplasm was diagnosed as hepatocellular carcinoma.

In contrast, no tumor incidences were detected in toads of group 4 which were fed with 0.2 ml/toad of unheated commercial vegetable oils, 3 times/week for 3 months. Tumors were not detected in toads of control group (group 5).

## DISCUSSION

Dietary components such as fat have been shown to affect tumorigenesis in several animal models (15). For example, increasing dietary levels of plant derived polyunsaturated fatty acids rich in the essential fatty acid linoleate (18:2, n-6) has been shown to enhance the development in chemically induced marine mammary carcinogenesis (16). Sakaguchi et al (17) also found that a semipurified diet containing 5% N-6 fat as linoleic acid caused more tumors than a 5% saturated fat diet made up largely with stearic acid.

The present results demonstrate the cocarcinogenicity of commercial vegetable oils used for deep-fat frying of fallafel. On the other hand, specific oxidation products of

Table 2. Liver tumor incidence in the toad, Bufo regularis, treated with NNM, commercial deep-fat frying of fallafel or both.

| Treatment Group | Dose/toad | Number of Autopsied Toads | Toads with Liver Tumors |
|---|---|---|---|
| NNM | 0.2 mg | 50 | 11 |
| NNM + Heated Oil | 0.2 mg + 0.2 ml | 50 | 14 |
| Heated Oil | 0.2 ml | 50 | 5 |
| Unheated Oil | 0.2 ml | 50 | 0 |
| Control | 0 | 50 | 0 |

polyunsaturated fatty acids may be mediators of the effects of dietary fat on carcinogenesis. Linoleic acid, the major polyunsaturated fatty acid in most vegetable oils, can be converted into arachidonic acid (7). Increased all membrane arachidonic acid in rats fed 5 adn 20% saturated fat diets has been shown by Nicholson et al (17, 18). This fatty acid can in turn be transformed into a variety of biologically-active products tghrough teh action of a number of different lipoxygenases or cyclooxygenase. These products include prostaglandins, thromboxane, prostacyclin and leukotrienes (19). Arachidonic acid is the immediate precursor of the series-2 prostaglandins, which have a very short half-life and are, therefore, synthesized locally. Minoura et al (20) demonstrated increased levels of prostaglandin $E_2$ in experimental colorectal tumors compared to mucosa. Another possible explanation by which high dietary levels of fat modulate colon carcinogenesis is associated with increased concentrations of secondary bile acids in the colon (21). These secondary bile acids increase colon epithelial ornithine decarboxylase (DDC) activity and cell proliferation and act as colon tumor promoters (22).

Of interest is that the toads fed commercial vegetable oils used for deep fat frying of fallafel alone induced liver tumors. This suggests that the products of commercial vegetable oils which are subjected to extensive heat abuse may include malonaldehyde and oxygen radicals that are capable of causing widespread tissue damage (23).

It is concluded that extensive heating of vegetable oils which are used for cooking and frying by street vendors may act not only as a co-carcinogen but also as a carcinagen.

## REFERENCES

1.    Miller AB, Howe GR, Jain M: Food items and food groups as risk factors in a case-control study of diet and colon cancer. Int. J. Cancer 32: 155-162, 1983.
2.    Reddy BS: Diet and colon cancer: evidence from human and animal model studies. In Reddy B.S. and Cohen, L. A. (eds), Diet, Nutrition and Cancer: A Critical Evaluation. CRC Press, Boca Raton, pp. 47-65, 1986.
3.    Perkins EG, Kummerow FA: The effect of polymers isolated from thermally oxidized corn oil. J. Nutr. 68:101-104, 1959.
4.    Dickens F, Jones HEH, Further studies on the carcinogenic action of certain lactones and related substances in the rat and mouse. Cancer 19:392-403, 1965.
5.    Min DB, Schweizer DQ: Lipid oxidation in potato chips. J. Am. Oil Chem. Soc. 60:1662-1665, 1983.

6. Waltking AE, Wessels H: Chromatographic separation of polar and non-polar components of frying fats. J. Associat. Official Analytical Chemists 64:1329-1332, 1981.
7. Carroll KK: Genetic Toxicology of the Diet. "Lipid oxidation and carcinogenesis" 1986; pp. 237-244. Alan R. Liss, Inc. Carroll, KK.
8. El-Mofty MM, Sadek IA, Soliman A, Mohamed A, Sakre, S: Alpha-ecdysone, a new bracken fern factor responsible for neoplasm induction in the Egyptian toad, Bufo regularis. Nutr Cancer 9:103-107, 1987.
9. Sadek IA: Effect of cholic acid on tumor in the Egyptian toad. Oncology 43:268-270, 1986.
10. Sadek IA: Vitamin E and its effects on skin papilloma (Prasad, KN, ed). Vitamins, Nutrition and Cancer. pp. 118-122, 1984; S. Karger, Basel.
11. Deyree WR, Long ME, Taylor HC Jr., Mckelway WP, Ehzman RL: Human and amphibian neoplasms compared tumors in frogs and human beings are strickingly similar in cytological characteristics. Science 131:276-280, 1960.
12. AOCS: Official and tentative methods of the American Oil Chemist's Society, Champaign, Illinois, USA, 3rd edition, 1983.
13. IUPAC: Standard methods for analysis of oils, fats and derivatives (Paquot, C., Ed), IUPAC. App. Chem. Div. Comm. on Oils, Fats and Derivatives, 6th edition, 1979.
14. Peled, M, Gutfinger T, Letan J: Effects of water and BHT on stability of cottonseed oil during frying. J. Sci. Food Agric. 26:1655-1666, 1975.
15. Ip, C, Birt DF, Rogers AE, Mettlin C: Dietary Fat and Cancer, Alan R. Liss, New York, 1986.
16. Ip, C, Carther CA , IP MM: Requirement of essential fatty acid for mammary tumorigenesis in the rat. Cancer Res. 45: 1997-2001, 1985.
17. Nicholson ML, Neoptolemos JP, Clayton HA, Talbot IC, Bell PRF: Increased arachidonic acid in experimental colorectal tumors. Br. J. Surg. 76:1337, 1989 (Abstract).
18. Nicholson ML, Neoptolemos JP, Clayton HA, Talbot IC, Bell PRF: Inhibition of experimental colorectal carcinogenesis by dietary N-6 polyunsaturated fats. Carcinogenesis 11:2191-2197, 1990.
19. Yamamoto S: Enzymes in the arachidonic acid cascade. In Pace-Asciak C, Granstrom E (Eds): New Comprehensive Biochemistry, Vol 5, Prostaglandins and Related Substances, Elsevier: Amsterdam, pp. 171-202, 1983.
20. Minoura T, Takata T, Sakaguchi M, Takada H, Yamamura H, Hioki K, Yamamoto M: Effect of dietary feicosapentaenoic acid on azoxymethane-induced colon carcinogenesis in rats. Cancer Res. 48: 4790-4794, 1988.
21. Weissburger JH, Fiala ES: Experimental colon carcinogens and their mode of action. In Autrup H and

Williams GM (eds) Experimental Colon Carcinogenesis. CRC Press, Boca Raton, pp. 27-50, 1983.
22.   Wade AE, Norred WP: Effect of dietary lipid on drug-metabolizing enzymes. Fed. Proc. 35: 2475-2479, 1976.
23.   Ames BN: Dietary carcinogens and anticarcinogens. Science 221: 256-264, 1983.
24.   Sakaguchi M, Hiramatsu Y, Takada H, Yamamura M, Hioki K, Saito K and Yamamoto M: Effect of dietary unsaturated and saturated fats on azoxymethane-induced colon carcinogenesis in rats. Cancer Res. 44:1472-1477.

# PART III

# Cancer Prevention Studies: Human Studies

# ANTIOXIDANT VITAMINS AND CANCER:   THE PHYSICIANS' HEALTH STUDY AND WOMEN'S HEALTH STUDY

Julie E. Buring, ScD
Charles H. Hennekens, MD
Brigham and Women's Hospital
Harvard Medical School
900 Commonwealth Avenue East
Boston, MA 02215

## INTRODUCTION

The possibility that antioxidant vitamins may prevent cancer has been the focus of considerable attention in recent years, both among the scientific research community and the general public. With respect to the major causes of death, in the United States and most developed countries, cancer accounts for about one-sixth of all deaths. For this reason, even the most plausible small to moderate benefits of antioxidant vitamins -- risk reductions of 20-30% -- could have a substantial public health impact. At present, however, antioxidant vitamins represent a promising, but unproven, means to prevent cancer. This paper reviews current evidence on antioxidants and cancer and describes ongoing large-scale randomized trials that will provide needed additional data on this question.

## LINES OF EVIDENCE

With respect to the causes of cancer, diet has long been hypothesized to play an important role in etiology. Tobacco and alcohol are the two leading avoidable causes of cancer, responsible for approximately 30% and 3% of all cancer deaths, respectively. However, in their 1981 review, Doll and Peto suggested that as much as 35% of all malignancies may be related to dietary practices (1).

223

The antioxidant vitamins beta-carotene, vitamin E and vitamin C are among the constituents of diet postulated to play a preventive role in cancer. Evidence pointing toward a possible role of antioxidant vitamins in cancer has accumulated from basic research, which has outlined plausible mechanisms by which they may exert chemopreventive effects, descriptive epidemiologic studies, which have raised the possibility that geographic differences in cancer incidence might be explained by regional variations in intake of antioxidant vitamins, and analytic epidemiologic studies among individuals, which have demonstrated inverse associations between either dietary intake or blood levels of antioxidant vitamins and risks of cancer. In addition, data are now available from two large-scale randomized trials testing antioxidant vitamins in cancer prevention, one in a well-nourished and another in a poorly-nourished population.

## Observational Evidence

The relationship of dietary intake of antioxidant vitamins with cancer risk has been the subject of a large number of observational analytic studies, using both case-control and prospective cohort designs. While findings from the two types of studies are largely consistent, case-control data are subject to selection bias (2). This review will therefore include only those studies of dietary intake or antioxidant blood levels that have used prospective cohort designs.

Dietary Intake Studies of Beta-Carotene. A large number of prospective dietary studies have assessed intake of beta-carotene in relation to subsequent cancer. Beta-carotene, or provitamin A, is a lipid-soluble nutrient principally found in yellow, orange and green leafy vegetables and certain fruits. In the body, dietary beta-carotene is converted to preformed vitamin A, or retinol, in the presence of retinol-deficiency. It could, therefore, indirectly play a role in cancer prevention if very low retinol levels are related to carcinogenesis. In well-nourished populations, however, most dietary carotene is absorbed directly from the intestine without undergoing transformation to retinol. As with other antioxidant vitamins, the hypothesized cancer chemopreventive benefit of beta-carotene is derived from the possibility that it may prevent tissue damage by trapping organic free radicals

and/or deactivating excited oxygen molecules, a by-product
of many metabolic functions (3).

In prospective dietary studies, subjects are classified
according to their reported intake of the nutrient of
interest, and subsequent cancer rates among those in the
highest and lowest intake category are then compared.  By
far the largest observational study of dietary beta-carotene
and caner is that conducted by Hirayama and colleagues in
Japan (4).  Statistically significant inverse associations
were seen between beta-carotene intake and cancer risk, with
relative risks in the highest intake category of 0.76 and
0.87 for men and women, respectively.  This cohort included
over 250,000 individuals, in whom more than 14,000 incident
cancers were diagnosed during a 17 year follow-up.  Three
other dietary studies have also reported significant inverse
associations between beta-carotene intake and cancer risk
(5-7).

A problem in interpreting observational dietary intake
studies is the possibility that the exposure of interest may
only be a marker for the true causal agent.  For example,
those with high beta-carotene intake may smoke less or have
other dietary or lifestyle practices associated with a
decreased risk of cancer.  Alternatively, the protection
afforded by consumption of a particular food may be
multifactorial, with several components of the food having
chemopreventive effects.  In this regard, two additional
studies have reported decreased risks of lung (8) and
prostate (9) cancer among those with high intake of
vegetables and fruits rich in both beta-carotene and vitamin
C.  Six prospective cohort studies have found no significant
association between dietary beta-carotene intake and
subsequent overall cancer (10) as well as cancer of the
colon and rectum (11) prostate (12) breast (13), lung (14),
and pancreas (15).

While most dietary intake studies distinguish between
vitamin A intake from beta-carotene and retinol, one of the
earliest analytic studies of diet and cancer related cancer
risk to total vitamin A intake from all sources.  The
initial five-year follow-up in this cohort of 8,278
Norwegian men reported a statistically significant
protective effect of high vitamin A intake on subsequent
lung cancer (16).  A subsequent report from this cohort
(17), which included an additional 5,480 men as well as

2,929 women, confirmed the earlier finding.  A recent report
on breast cancer from the Nurses' Health Study, a
prospective cohort investigation of more than 120,000 US
women, also found a statistically significant decreased
cancer risk among women with the highest level of intake of
total vitamin A (13).

    Blood-Based Studies of Beta-Carotene.  In blood-based
studies, blood samples are generally drawn and frozen at
baseline from a population free of cancer.  The study
participants are followed for the subsequent development of
cancer, and baseline levels of antioxidant vitamins among
incident cancer cases are then compared with levels in
matched controls who remained free of cancer.  Although
these studies are referred to as nested case-control
studies, they are regarded methodologically as prospective
studies, since they gather exposure information at baseline
and follow subjects forward for the development of disease.

Six blood-based studies have reported significantly lower
cancer risks for those in the upper category of serum or
plasma beta-carotene (18-23).  The most consistent pattern
relates to lung malignancies, with four blood-based studies
(18-20,23) showing similar findings of an approximate
halving of risk among those in the highest compared to
lowest category.  All of these studies controlled for the
possible effects of cigarette smoking.  Eight blood-based
studies have not found statistically significant
associations between beta-carotene levels and lower cancer
risk (24-31).

    Dietary Studies of Vitamin E.  Vitamin E, which also
has strong antioxidant properties, has been studied in
relatively few dietary intake studies.  Vitamin E is lipid-
soluble nutrient found in certain vegetable oils, and in egg
yolks, nuts, green plants, milk fat, liver and cereal grain.
Just three prospective cohort studies have assessed dietary
vitamin E intake and subsequent cancer (7,11,13), with none
reporting a significant association.

    Blood-Based Studies of Vitamin E.  In contrast, 18
blood-based studies of vitamin E have been conducted (18-
19,22-39).  Although many of these have found lower vitamin
E levels in cases than in controls, only five have found
statistically significant inverse associations between

vitamin E levels and subsequent cancer risk (19,22,33,35-36).

Dietary Studies of Vitamin C. Vitamin C is a water-soluble nutrient with antioxidant properties that is derived in the diet primarily from citrus fruits and some vegetables. Although the possible health benefits of vitamin C have been widely investigated, it has been the subject of relatively few prospective cancer studies. Three prospective dietary intake studies of vitamin C intake and subsequent cancer have reported statistically significant protective effects. In a study in Finland, a significant effect on lung cancer was seen in non-smokers but not in smokers (7). The two other studies reported decreased risks of colon (11) and lung (14) cancer among those with high dietary vitamin C intake. As noted earlier in the discussion of beta-carotene, two studies have examined cancer risk in relation to intake of fruits and vegetables rich in both vitamin C and beta-carotene, with both reporting a significant inverse association between cancer risk and high intake of these foods (8-9). Three studies have found no relation of dietary vitamin C intake and cancer risk (5,13,17).

Blood-Based Studies of Vitamin C. With respect to blood-based studies of vitamin C, plasma ascorbic acid can only be measured reliably in fresh blood specimens or those stored at very low temperatures (-70c) after being chemically stabilized. For this reason, the Basel Study, the only large-scale prospective investigation that has assessed prediagnostic vitamin C levels and cancer risk, tested fresh specimens from all 2,974 men taking part in the study's 1971-1973 follow-up exam. There was no significant risk reduction for total cancer associated with high plasma vitamin C levels, though there were significant associations for gastrointestinal and stomach cancer among older subjects (23).

Limitations of Analytic Observational Studies. While the prospective observational evidence concerning antioxidant vitamins and cancer is generally compatible with possible benefits of these agents on cancer risk, the available data are not all consistent. Additional observational data would certainly be a valuable contribution to the totality of evidence. But regardless of the number or sample size of such investigations or even the

consistency of their findings, observational studies are
unable to control for potential effects of confounding
variables not known to the investigator or not collected.
It may be, for example, that greater dietary intake of
antioxidant vitamins, measured by blood levels or a diet
assessment questionnaire, is only a marker for some other
dietary practices that are truly protective.  It is
certainly plausible that intake of antioxidant-rich foods is
indeed protective, but that the benefits may result not from
their antioxidant properties, but other components these
foods have in common.  It is also possible that intake of
antioxidant vitamins from food or supplements is correlated
with other unmeasured or unknown non-dietary lifestyle
behaviors.  Thus, when searching for small to moderate
effects the amount of uncontrolled confounding in all
observational studies is likely to be as large as the most
plausible alternative hypothesis (2).  Because of these
limitations inherent in all observational studies, only
randomized trials of sufficient sample size, dose and
duration of treatment and follow-up can address conclusively
whether antioxidant vitamins actually decrease cancer risk.


                          Randomized Trials

Only one large-scale randomized trial has been completed
testing antioxidant vitamins in cancer prevention among a
well-nourished population (40).  The recently published
Alpha-Tocopherol/Beta-Carotene (ATBC) Cancer Prevention
Study involved 6 years of randomized treatment with 20 mg of
beta-carotene and/or 50 mg of vitamin E daily in 29,133
Finnish male smokers, aged 50 to 69.  There was no
protective effect on lung cancer observed for either of the
two vitamins.  In fact, those assigned to beta-carotene had
a statistically significant 18% higher risk of lung cancer,
a finding greatly at variance with the totality of other
evidence suggesting a possible benefit.  For vitamin E,
there was a lower risk of prostate cancer.  The chief
limitation of the Finnish trial is the relatively short
duration of treatment and follow-up, which may have been
inadequate to yield a detectable reduction in cancer, which
is a multistage process that often proceeds over several
decades (41).  In addition, while the dose of beta-carotene
increased blood levels of participants receiving this
supplement by more than 10-fold, the low dose of vitamin E,

which was in a synthetic form with low bioavailability, only increased vitamin E blood levels by about one-third, far less than the doubling of blood levels achieved by regular supplement users in observational studies. Nevertheless, the results of the Finnish trial suggest that some benefits of antioxidant vitamins seen in prior observational studies may have been overestimates, and that there may even be some previously undetected harmful effects of these vitamins.

Only one other large-scale randomized trial has been completed assessing antioxidant vitamins in cancer prevention. The Chinese Cancer Prevention Trial randomized 29,584 residents of four communities in Linxian, a rural county in north-central China (42). This region suffers from one of the world's highest rates of esophageal and gastric cancer, and dietary intake of several micronutrients is very low. Nine different agents were tested (retinol, zinc, riboflavin, niacin, vitamin C, molybdenum, beta-carotene, vitamin E and selenium), with trial participants assigned at random to one of 8 different vitamin/mineral supplement combinations. For subjects receiving the combined treatment of beta-carotene, vitamin E and selenium, total mortality was 9% lower than among those not receiving this combination, with a significant 21% decrease in gastric cancer deaths. Because nutrients were studied in combined groups, it is impossible to distinguish the relative contributions of beta-carotene, vitamin E and selenium to any observed finding. Moreover, vitamin supplementation may well have effects in a poorly nourished population that it would not have among those with adequate intake of the vitamins and minerals tested.

Conclusive evidence on the balance of benefits and risks of antioxidant vitamins in cancer prevention will emerge from several large-scale randomized trials that are now ongoing among well-nourished populations. Ongoing trials of antioxidants include the "CARET" study, which is testing beta-carotene among 18,000 individuals at high risk for lung cancer due to heavy cigarette smoking history or occupational asbestos exposure, and the SU.VI.MAX study, which is testing beta-carotene, vitamin E, and vitamin C, as well as zinc and selenium in healthy French men and women.

Two ongoing trials are being conducted among US health professionals. The Physicians' Health Study, which began in 1982, is testing beta-carotene (50 mg on alternate days in

the form of Lurotin, supplied by BASF AG) among over 22,071
US male physicians (43). This trial will have an average
duration of treatment and follow-up of approximately 12.5
years at its scheduled termination in late 1995, and should
therefore provide particularly reliable evidence on the
potential role of beta-carotene in the primary prevention of
cancer. The Women's Health Study, which began in 1992, will
randomize approximately 40,000 apparently healthy US women,
using a 2x2x2 factorial design, to evaluate the benefits and
risks in cancer and cardiovascular disease of beta-carotene
(50 mg on alternate days, in the form of Lurotin, supplied
by BASF AG), vitamin E (600 IU on alternate days, supplied
by the Natural Source Vitamin E Association), and low-dose
aspirin (100 mg on alternate days, supplied by Miles Inc.)
(44).

## CONCLUSION

In summary, currently available data raise the possibility
that antioxidant vitamins may decrease risks of cancer. At
present, however, the message is not one for the general
public or even for health care providers, but rather for
researchers: namely, that antioxidant vitamins represent a
promising, but as yet unproven, means to reduce risks of
several chronic diseases, which should be tested in large-
scale randomized trials of sufficient sample size, dose, and
duration of treatment and follow-up. Evidence from such
large-scale trials, including the Physicians' Health Study
in men and Women's Health Study in women, will contribute
reliable data to a totality of evidence on antioxidant
vitamins which will permit appropriate clinical
recommendations for individual patients as well as rational
public health policy for the population as a whole.

## REFERENCES

1.    Doll R, Peto R.  The causes of cancer.  JNCI 1981;
      66:1191-1308.
2.    Hennekens CH, Buring JE.  Epidemiology in Medicine.
      Boston:  Little, Brown and Company, 1987.
3.    Peto R, Doll R, Buckley JD, Sporn MB.  Can dietary
      beta-carotene materially reduce human cancer rates?
      Nature 1981; 290:201-09.
4.    Hirayama T.  A large scale cohort study on cancer

risks by diet - with special reference to the risk reducing effects of green-yellow vegetable consumption. In: Diet, Nutrition and Cancer, Y Hayashi et al (eds). Japan Scientific Societies Press, Tokyo, pp. 41-53, 1986.

5.  Shekelle RB, Lepper M, Liu S, Maliza C, Raynor WJ, Rossof AH, Paul O, Shryock AM, Stamler J. Dietary vitamin A and risk of cancer in the Western Electric Study. Lancet 1981; 2:1185-90.

6.  Colditz GA, Branch LG, Lipnick RJ, Willett WC, Rosner B, Posner BM, Hennekens CH. Increased green and yellow vegetable intake and lowered cancer deaths in an elderly population. Am J Clin Nutr 1985; 41:32-36.

7.  Knekt P, Jarvinen R, Seppanen R, Rissanen A, Aromaa A, Heinonen OP, Albanes D, Heinonen M, Pukkala E, Teppo L. Dietary antioxidants and the risk of lung cancer. Am J Epidemiol 1991; 134:471-79.

8.  Long-de W, Hammond EC. Lung cancer, fruit, green salad and vitamin pills. Chin Med J 1985; 98:206-10.

9.  Mills PK, Beeson L, Phillips RL, Frasser GE. Cohort study of diet, lifestyle, and prostate cancer in Adventist men. Cancer 1989; 64:598-604.

10. Paganini-Hill A, Chao A, Ross RK, Henderson BE. Vitamin A, beta-carotene, and the risk of cancer: A prospective study. JNCI 1987; 79:443-48.

11. Heilbrun LK, Nomura A, Hankin JH, Stemmermann GN. Diet and colorectal cancer with special reference to fiber intake. Int J Cancer 1989; 44:1-6.

12. Hsing AW, McLaughlin JK, Schuman LM, Bjelke E, Gridley G, Wacholder S, Chien HTC, Blot WJ. Diet, tobacco use, and fatal prostate cancer: Results from the Lutheran Brotherhood Cohort Study. Cancer Res 1990; 50:6836-40.

13. Hunter D, Stampfer MJ, Colditz G, Manson J, Rosner B, Hennekens C, Speizer FE, Willett W. A prospective study of the intake of vitamins C, E, and A and the risk of breast cancer. N Engl J Med 1993; 329:234-40.

14. Kromhout D. Essential micronutrients in relation to carcinogenesis. Am J Clin Nutr 1987; 45:1361-67.

15. Mills PK, Beeson WL, Abbey DE, Fraser GE, Phillips RL. Dietary habits and past medical history as related to fatal pancreas cancer risk among Adventists. Cancer 1988; 61:2578-85.

16. Bjelke E. Dietary vitamin A and human lung cancer. Int J Cancer 1975; 15:561-65.

17. Kvale G, Bjelke E, Gart JJ. Dietary habits and lung

cancer risk.  Int J Cancer 1983; 15:397-405.

18.   Nomura AMY, Stemmermann GN, Heilbrun LK, Salkeld RM,
      Vuilleumier JP.  Serum vitamin levels and the risk of
      cancer of specific sites in men of Japanese ancestry
      in Hawaii.  Cancer Res 1985; 45:2369-72.

19.   Menkes MS, Comstock GW, Vuilleumier JP, Helsing KJ,
      Rider AA, Brookmeyer R.  Serum beta-carotene, vitamins
      A and E, selenium, and the risk of lung cancer.  NEJM
      1986; 315:1250-54.

20.   Wald NJ, Thompson SG, Densem JW, Boreham J, Bailey A.
      Serum beta-carotene and subsequent risk of cancer:
      Results from the BUPA Study.  Br J Cancer 1988;
      57:428-33.

21.   Knekt P, Aromaa A, Maatela J, Aaran R-K, Nikkari T,
      Hakama M, Hakulinen T, Peto R, Teppo L.  Serum vitamin
      A and subsequent risk of cancer:  cancer incidence
      follow-up of the Finnish Mobile Clinic Health
      Examination Survey.  Am J Epidemiol 1990; 132:857-70.

22.   Knekt P, Aromaa A, Maatela J, Alfthan G, Aaran R-K,
      Nikkari T, Hakama M, Hakulinen T, Teppo L.  Serum
      micronutrients and risks of cancers of low incidence
      in Finland.  Am J Epidemiol 1991; 134:356-61.

23.   Stahelin HB, Gey KF, Eichholzer M, Ludin E, Bernasconi
      F, Thurneysen J, Brubacher G.  Plasma antioxidant
      vitamins and subsequent cancer mortality in the 12-
      year Follow-up of the Prospective Basel Study.  Am J
      Epidemiol 1991; 133:766-75.

24.   Wald NJ, Boreham J, Hayward JL, Bulbrook RD.  Plasma
      retinol, beta-carotene and vitamin E levels in
      relation to the future risk of breast cancer.  Br J
      Cancer 1984; 49:321-24

25.   Willett WC, Polk BF, Underwood BA, Stampfer MJ,
      Pressel S, Rosner B, Taylor JO, Schneider K, Hames CG.
      Relation of serum vitamins A and E and carotenoids to
      the risk of cancer.  N Engl J Med 1984; 310:430-34.

26.   Burney PGJ, Comstock GW, Morris JS.  Serologic
      precursors of cancer:  serum micronutrients and the
      subsequent risk of pancreatic cancer.  Am J Clin Nutr
      1989; 49:895-900.

27.   Connett JE, Kuller LH, Kjelsberg MO, Polk BF, Collins
      G, Rider A, Hulley SB.  Relationship between
      carotenoids and cancer.  The Multiple Risk Factor
      Intervention Trial (MRFIT) Study.  Cancer 1989;
      64:126-34.

28.   Helzlsouer KJ, Comstock GW, Morris SJ.  Selenium,
      lycopene, alpha-tocopherol, beta-carotene, retinol,

and subsequent bladder cancer. Cancer Res 1989; 49:6144-48.

29. Hsing AW, Comstock GW, Abbey H, Polk BF. Serologic precursors of cancer. Retinol, carotenoids, and tocopherol and risk of prostate cancer. JNCI 1990; 82:941-46.

30. Schober SE, Comstock GW, Hesling KJ, Salkeld RM, Morris JS, Rider AA, Brookmeyer R. Serolologic precursors of cancer. I. Prediagnostic serum nutrients and colon cancer risk. Am J Epidemiol 1987; 126:1033-41.

31. Comstock GW, Helzlsouer KJ, Bush TL. Prediagnostic serum levels of carotenoids and vitamin E as related to subsequent cancer in Washington County, Maryland. Am J Clin Nutr 1991; 53:260S-4S

32. Fex G, et al. Low plasma selenium as a risk factor for cancer death in middle-aged men. Nutr Cancer 1987; 10:221-29.

33. Kok FJ, van Duijn CM, Hofman A, Vermeeren R, de Bruijn AM, Valkenburg HA. Micronutrients and the risk of lung cancer. (Letter) N Engl J Med 1987; 316;1416.

34. Wald NJ, Thompson SG, Densem JW, Boreham J, Bailey A. Serum vitamin E and subsequent risk of cancer. Br J Cancer 1987; 56:69-72.

35. Knekt P, Aromma A, Maatela J, Aaran R-K, Nikkari T, Hakama M, Hakulinen T, Peto R, Saxen E, Teppo L. Serum vitamin E and risk of cancer among Finnish men during a 10-year follow-up. Am J Epidemiol 1988; 127:28-41

36. Knekt P. Serum vitamin E level and risk of female cancer. Int J Epidemiol 1988; 17:281-88.

37. Russell MJ, Thomas BS, Bulbrook RD. A prospective study of the relationship betwen serum vitamins A and E and risk of breast cancer. Br J Cancer 1988; 57:213:15.

38. Salonen JT, Salonen R, Lappetelainen R, Haenpaa PH, Alfthan G, Puska P. Risk of cancer in relation to serum concentrations of selenium and vitamins A and E: matched case-control analysis of prospective data. Br Med J 1985; 290:417-20.

39. Wald NJ, Nicolaides-Bouman A, Hudson GA. Plasma retinol, beta-carotene and vitmain E levels in relation to the future risk of breast cancer. (Letter) Br J Cancer 1988; 57:235.

40. Alpha-Tocopherol, Beta Carotene Cancer Prevention Study Group. The effect of vitamin E and beta

carotene on the incidence of lung cancer and other cancers in male smokers. N Engl J Med 1994; 330:1029-1035.

41.    Hennekens CH, Buring JE, Peto R.  Antioxidant vitamins - benefits not yet proved.  N Engl J Med 1994; 330:1080-81.

42.    Blot WJ, Li J-Y, Taylor PR, et. al.  Nutrition intervention trials in Linxian, China: Supplementation with specific vitamin/mineral combinations, cancer incidence, and disease-specific mortality in the general population.  J Natl Cancer Inst 1993; 85:1483-92.

43.    Hennekens CH, Eberlein K.  A randomized trial of aspirin and beta-carotene among U.S. physicians.  Prev Med 1985; 14:165-8.

44.    Buring JE, Hennekens CH, for the Women's Health Study Research Group.  The Women's Health Study:  Summary of the study design.  J Myocardial Ischemia 1992; 4:27-29.

**BETA-CAROTENE AND ANTIOXIDANT NUTRIENTS**

**IN ORAL CANCER PREVENTION**

Harinder Garewal, M.D., Ph.D.

University of Arizona and VA Medical Center

Hematology/Oncology (111D)
3601 S. 6th Ave.
Tucson, AZ   85723

## ABSTRACT

Lack of toxicity and easy availability make beta-carotene and vitamin E excellent agents to test for cancer preventive activity.  Since intervention trials actually using cancer incidence as the endpoint in the general population are logistically and practically impossible for oral cavity cancer, as is the case for most types of cancer, evidence for chemoprevention must necessarily be indirect: laboratory and animal models, epidemiologic surveys, trials showing reversal of premalignant lesions or cancer prevention in usually high risk groups.  In several animal models, beta-carotene and other antioxidant nutrients strongly inhibit oral carcinogenesis.  Epidemiologic studies consistently correlate low intake with high cancer risk. Smokers have lower beta-carotene levels in plasma and oral mucosal cells than non-smokers.  Beta-carotene and vitamin E produce regression of oral leukoplakia, as has now been found in 8 clinical trials, 5 with beta-carotene alone, 1 with vitamin E and 2 that used a combination.  The design and limitations of such chemoprevention studies in oral leukoplakia is discussed.  All available evidence supports a very significant disease-preventive role for antioxidant nutrients in oral cancer.

## INTRODUCTION

Oral cavity cancer is a common, lethal disease, with very high rates being encountered in developing countries[1].  In the U.S. there are about 42,000 new cases of and 12,000 deaths from head and neck cancer annually [2].  Tobacco, either smoked or chewed, is responsible for more

than 75% of cases.  Alcohol is the other main causative
agent and acts synergistically with tobacco.  Since tobacco
contributes significantly to other major diseases, like lung
cancer and heart disease, its cessation will have an impact
on many life-threatening diseases, including oral cancer.
Similarly, other prevention modalities, such as antioxidant
agents, may also be beneficial for a number of diseases
linked by common etiologies.

Success in reducing morbidity and mortality from oral
cancer will depend on its prevention.  Although treatment of
established cancer has improved from the standpoint of
reduced morbidity and disfigurement, this has not resulted
in better survival or cure rate.  Even for early disease
patients, who can be cured of their primary lesion, the
occurrence of second primary malignancies leads to a dismal
5 year survival rate (4).  The "field cancerization"
hypothesis probably explains this trend towards multiple
primaries in the same individual (5).  Cessation of tobacco
use is undoubtedly of major importance in oral cancer
prevention.  Additionally, there is now considerable
evidence suggesting a preventive role for nutritional
agents, particularly the antioxidants beta-carotene and
vitamin E.

Without doubt or controversy, the best proof of cancer
preventive activity is demonstration of an actual reduction
in incidence via a properly designed clinical trial.  Proper
design means paying attention to a number of important
aspects including adequate duration, correct endpoint (i.e.
cancer), blinded design and maintenance of the blind,
inclusion of a placebo arm that can and must remain blinded,
and conduct in a population that is representative of the
one to which the results are to be applied.  Such
considerations, however, make a perfect trial virtually
impossible for most cancers because of logistical and
practical considerations arising from the fact that most
individual types of cancer are infrequent events in an
otherwise healthy population.  Thus conclusions regarding
putative chemopreventive activity must be arrived at by
evaluating data from all other available indirect lines of
evidence.

Table I lists the various lines of evidence supporting
a role for beta-carotene and vitamin E in oral cancer
prevention.  Less work has been completed with vitamin E.
Nevertheless, vitamin E shows equal promise in preclinical
work, a finding being borne out by the results of early
clinical trials.

**EPIDEMIOLOGIC EVIDENCE**

A low intake of carotenoids has been associated with
increased risk of cancer, including that of the oral cavity.

## Table I

## BETA-CAROTENE AND VITAMIN E IN ORAL CANCER PREVENTION

1.  Epidemiology:  Risk correlations with diet, blood levels and use of supplements.
2.  Inhibition of cellular transformation in vitro.
3.  Inhibition of carcinogenesis in animal models, such as the hamster cheek pouch.
4.  Pharmacology:  Low levels in plasma and oral mucosal cells in high risk groups, e.g. smokers vs non-smokers.
5.  Beta-carotene supplementation decreases micronucleated cells in very high risk groups.
6.  Beta-carotene and vitamin E can reverse oral leukoplakia, a premalignant lesion of the oral cavity.
7.  Can the incidence of second primary cancers be reduced by beta-carotene and/or vitamin E supplementation?

In fact, as reviewed by Block et. al. (6), if one considers all studies that report relative risk data, then all 4 of 4 studies in laryngeal cancer and 9 of 9 in oropharyngeal cancer have found a protective effect.  Although publication bias in favor of positive studies is a consideration, such unanimity is quite compelling and provides persuasive evidence in support of a genuine preventive role.

Because of the difficulty in quantitating dietary vitamin E, fewer studies with this antioxidant have been reported, but they also suggest protection (7,8).  Recent studies also suggest that use of **supplemental** vitamin E is associated with the greatest protection (8).

Tobacco users, at increased risk of oral cavity cancer, have lower plasma levels of carotenoids and beta-carotene than non-smokers.  Stich, et. al., and more recently Peng, et. al., have further shown that oral mucosal cell levels of beta-carotene are also lower in smokers vs non-smokers (9,10).  This difference exists despite similar dietary intakes and the magnitude of the difference is apparently too large for smokers to achieve non-smoker levels simply by diet modification (10).

### LABORATORY EVIDENCE

The carotenoids have antimutagenic and transformation inhibition properties in bacterial and cell culture systems (11).  Their capacity to block genotoxic damage in Chinese Hamster Ovary cells caused by oral carcinogens, such as extracts of areca nut, is of direct relevance to inhibition of oral carcinogenesis (12).  An animal model of significance to oral cavity cancer is the hamster cheek

pouch model in which precancerous and cancerous lesions are
produced after application of the carcinogen, 7,12-
dimethylbenz(a)anthracene.  Beta-carotene and vitamin E,
alone or together, are very active in inhibiting the
formation of cancerous lesions in this system (13,14).

Increased frequency of micronucleated cells reflects
genotoxic damage produced by carcinogens.  Stich and
colleagues have shown that beta-carotene, alone or in
combination with vitamin A, can decrease the incidence of
micronucleated cells in exfoliated oral mucosal cells from
populations at very high risk for oral cancer (15,16).
Preliminary results from our own and other studies in the
West, where the lesion is mainly from smoking, rather than
chewing, tobacco, have shown a much lower initial frequency
of micronucleated cells than in the trials by Stich, et. al.
No results on changes with treatment have yet been reported
in such "non-chewing" subjects and may be difficult to
demonstrate because of the low pretreatment frequency.

### BETA-CAROTENE AND VITAMIN E REVERSE ORAL CAVITY PREMALIGNANCY

Premalignant lesions are usually the first clinically
identifiable clues that allow recognition of a
carcinogenesis- affected mucosa.  Thus their reversal or
suppression is an important strategy in cancer prevention
studies.  Most oral cavity premalignant lesions are
categorized as leukoplakia, defined as a white mucosal patch
or plaque that cannot be rubbed off and is not attributable
to another disease entity.  In general, as is the case with
most epithelial premalignant lesions, leukoplakia has a
rather low malignant potential (17).  Sub-types, such as
erythroplakia and speckled leukoplakia, have a higher transformation rate, but are relatively rare lesions (17,18).
Similarly, the presence of severe histologic dysplasia
carries a higher risk (17).

The objectives of intervention trials involving
premalignant lesions, including leukoplakia, must always be
kept in mind when selecting agents for chemoprevention
studies.  If the objective is to develop new treatments for
the small minority of patients with erythroplakia and/or
high grade dysplasia that are not amenable to standard
treatments, then some treatment toxicity may be acceptable.
In this category are toxic agents such as topical bleomycin,
high dose vitamin A and synthetic retinoids like 13-cis-
retinoic acid.  These agents have been known to be active
for over two decades, but their toxicity precludes serious
consideration of their use for oral cancer prevention (19-
22).  If the objective is to develop agents for more
widespread use for prevention of oral cancer, then such
agents have no role, while the non-toxic antioxidants, such
as beta-carotene and vitamin E, are highly suited.

Beginning in the 1980's, a series of trials have shown that these antioxidant nutrients can reverse oral leukoplakia (Table II). Stich, et. al. conducted a series of trials in India using vitamin A and beta-carotene, alone or in combination (15). This study population differs from the other trials in that the lesion in India is caused primarily by chewing of betel nuts and other noxious substances, a very intense carcinogen exposure. A degree of vitamin A deficiency may also have been present at baseline. As shown in the Table, these investigators reported complete remission rates only which were compared with a 3% complete remission rate in a placebo group. The appearance of new lesions was also strongly inhibited in the treatment groups.

### Table II
### BETA-CAROTENE AND VITAMIN E LEUKOPLAKIA TRIALS

| Senior Author - Country (ref) | Agent | CR% | PR% | OR% |
|---|---|---|---|---|
| Stich - India (15) | BC | 15 | NS | NS |
| Garewal - USA (23) | BC | 8 | 63 | 71 |
| Toma - Italy (26) | BC | 33 | 11 | 44 |
| Malaker - Canada (24) | BC | 28 | 22 | 50 |
| Garewal - USA (27) | BC | NA | NA | 55 |
| Benner - USA (29) | E | 23 | 23 | 46* |
| Stich - India (15) | BC + A | 27 | NS | NS |
| Brandt - USA (25) | BC + E + C | NA | NA | 60 |

BC = beta-carotene, A = vitamin A, E = vitamin E, C = vitamin C, CR = complete response, PR = partial response, OR = overall response, NS = not stated, NA = not available in reported abstract.

*Response rate was 65% if based on 31 "evaluable" patients rather than all subjects entered.

Studies with beta-carotene in Western populations have been more recent. We conducted a pilot trial of beta-carotene alone, given at a daily dose of 30 mg/day for 3-6 months, with a response rate of 71% (95% confidence interval 53% - 89%) in 24 patients (23). In a carefully conducted cross-over phase II trial by Malaker, et. al. in Canada, patients were initially treated with beta-carotene for 6 - 9 months, with non-responders then receiving 13-cis-retinoic acid. A response rate of about 50% was noted with beta-carotene (24). Another study using a combination of antioxidant agents, including beta-carotene, was conducted by Kaugars and colleagues in Virginia. Subjects were supplemented with a non-toxic combination of beta-carotene, alpha-tocopherol and vitamin C. A 60% response rate was recently reported from this trial (25). Toma, et. al. from Italy have reported a response rate of 44% in 18 evaluable subjects treated with beta-carotene alone at a dose of 90mg/day (26).

We have recently completed accrual to a multi-institution trial, involving the University of California (Irvine), the University of Connecticut (Farmington) and the University of Arizona (27). Subjects are treated with beta-carotene, 60 mg/day for 6 months, and responding subjects are randomized in a blinded fashion to either continue beta-carotene or placebo for another 12 months. A response rate of 55% has been observed in a preliminary analysis of this study, thereby confirming the activity of this agent in a multi-institution setting (27).

Adopting a somewhat different strategy in a population-based, prospective, placebo-controlled, randomized trial conducted in men only, Zaridze and colleagues found a significant reduction in the prevalence of oral leukoplakia in a treatment group that received beta-carotene (40mg/day), retinol (100,000 IU/week) and vitamin E (80mg/week) for 6 months (28). Use of nass, a mixture of tobacco, ash, cotton oil and lime placed in the mouth, is a major cause of the lesion and oral cancer in Uzbekistan (Central Asia) where this trial was conducted. Although it is difficult to separate the effect of beta-carotene from retinol and vitamin E, the results of a secondary blood level analysis, and the once a week dosing schedule for retinol and vitamin E, suggested that beta-carotene was the primary agent producing the reduced lesion frequency.

Clinical intervention trials with single agent vitamin E are more recent. Benner, et. al. recently reported a multi-center study showing a response rate of 46% (95% confidence interval 32 - 61%) in 43 subjects treated with 400 IU of vitamin E twice daily for 24 weeks (29). The response rate for this study was 65% if calculated on the basis of evaluable subjects, of which there were 31.

## ORAL LEUKOPLAKIA TRIALS:   PROBLEMS AND CRITIQUES

Although oral leukoplakia studies involve clinical trials conducted in human beings, they must still be considered as comprising one additional approach to gather indirect evidence for cancer preventive activity, since even this is not the same as showing a reduction in cancer incidence. In order to critically interpret and better design future oral leukoplakia trials, and place them in their proper context relative to other lines of evidence, it is important to be familiar with some fundamental issues relevant to this approach.

## Choice of Agents

Oral leukoplakia is not cancer or a lethal disease by itself. It's behavior is similar to other premalignant lesions, for example colonic polyps. The majority of such lesions will not transform with the more serious lesions (large villous polyps or severely dysplastic leukoplakia) being relatively rare. In general, chemoprevention studies that target preneoplastic lesions have as their final goal the prevention of cancer rather than simply producing "responses" in the premalignant lesion. Thus the toxicity profile of the intervention agent must be addressed prior to conducting such studies. Only those agents can be justifiably tested which have a potential for use as preventive modalities. This is why high dose vitamin A and its synthetic analogs, the retinoids, are not suitable agents. Their toxicity is prohibitive for use in the low risk situation represented by the usual leukoplakia. To continue the analogy, the equivalent situation would be patients with a sporadic colonic polyp, whose risk of cancer is similar to the usual leukoplakia, and in whom any agent with toxicity would be unacceptable.

## Is Leukoplakia Response Linked to Reduction in Cancer?

Preneoplastic lesions are essentially another group of "intermediate markers". Although theoretically very plausible, the linkage between preneoplasia "response" and cancer incidence reduction, however appealing it may be, remains a hypothesis for now.

## Clinical Assessment of Response

Although several groups have attempted to use two-dimensional measurements of the lesion to judge response by standard reduction in size criteria, it is becoming increasingly clear that this cannot be reliably applied to most leukoplakic lesions. Clearing of leukoplakia does not always occur in a "reduction in dimensions" manner. Not infrequently, lesions clear in the middle or have multiple spots of improvement visible throughout. Oral photography, although helpful, is difficult to apply consistently, particularly in a multi-center setting (29). There is general consensus that photographs cannot be used for measurement of lesions, because of variations in technique. Thus, in our experience, response is best based on lesion evaluation by two examiners independently agreeing on a category. Photographs are helpful as an adjunct. Although this approach is seemingly more "subjective", in actual practice the tendency has been to be very careful and conservative in calling a response, due to the fact that the issue of "subjectivity" is uppermost in most evaluators' minds.

One approach that has been advocated as "the solution" is inclusion of a placebo arm in all such studies. Although this superficially sounds profoundly scientific, serious consideration of this suggestion reveals that a placebo is not quite the holy grail that will cure all problems. <u>A placebo arm is of value only if the agent being tested dose not have obvious and easily identifiable side effects in order to be effectively blinded</u>. Clearly, 13-cis-retinoic acid or similar retinoids, that produce marked mucocutaneous and other symptomatic toxicity (headaches, flushing, etc.), not to mention marked laboratory changes, cannot be kept blinded. In our own experience, based on numerous trials, patients taking high-dose 13-cis-retinoic acid, for example, can be recognized within 1 - 2 weeks of starting treatment. This is impossible to "hide" from the evaluator, since the toxicity is readily visible and the patient is often complaining spontaneously, well before any "suggestive" toxicity questions are asked! Similarly, for beta-carotene, the recognition rate can be very high, especially at doses exceeding 30mg/day. In our latest study, that used 60 mg/day, an independent observer was asked to simply look at the subject and guess whether they were on placebo or beta-carotene. The correct guess rate exceeds 75%. Consequently, simply adding a placebo arm does not resolve the issue of proper response assessment. It does double the size of the study, which is a very serious demand, since accrual to these trials has been a major problem. For certain agents, such as vitamin E, where there is no easily recognizable change or toxicity, inclusion of a placebo arm would be reasonable.

## Evaluation of histology and "histologic response"

Biopsy(s) and histologic evaluation of lesions at baseline is clearly indicated not only to confirm the absence of some other disease entity, but also to better delineate the seriousness of the lesion. Clinical responses observed with use of a chemopreventive agent can then be correlated with initial severity of the lesion.

Problems arise with a so-called "histologic response" category, usually based on comparing two biopsies separated by a treatment period of 3 - 6 months, as has been reported in some recent studies (30). This approach is almost certainly erroneous and generally unacceptable to most oral pathologists. Firstly, in leukoplakia the distribution of dysplasia or other histologic change is usually "patchy". Other examples of preneoplasia include ulcerative colitis, gastric intestinal metaplasia or Barrett's esophagus and in no case is this approach considered acceptable, i.e. evaluation of two biopsies and a response categorization based on that comparison. Although proponents of the "histologic response" category state that the second biopsy is done "as close to the initial site as possible", this does not solve the problem since two adjacent biopsies done at the same sitting can have different readings! Furthermore, it creates a whole new set of problems originating from the effect of injury at the first biopsy site, followed by it's healing, and the known impact of this on histology. Consequently, the only justifiable role of histologic evaluation after a treatment period is limited to confirmation of a clinical complete response when a biopsy may confirm whether normalization has occurred at the microscopic level also.

### Effect of Habit Changes on Response

Although major habit changes, such as total discontinuance of tobacco for the duration of the trial, are unusual, the effect of even temporary reduction in habits on response needs to be monitored closely. Recent experience has suggested that leukoplakic lesions will improve much more rapidly if exposure to an identifiable inciting agent, usually tobacco, is reduced.

### What About the Non-Responders?

In most recent, large trials, the response rate has been about 50 - 60%. Consequently, there are a substantial number of subjects, 40 - 50%, who do not respond to the intervention agent, and who need to be studied further. Recent studies, including our own experience, have indicated that there appears to be a higher percentage of "non-smoker" lesions in the non-responders (24). However, no single study is large enough to prove this with statistical significance.

### Study Duration

A treatment duration of at least 6 months should be planned since responses can occur late, i.e. 3 - 6 months, after beginning treatment.

### CONCLUSIONS AND FUTURE DIRECTIONS

In conclusion, numerous lines of evidence suggest a potential role for beta-carotene and other antioxidants in preventing oral cavity malignancy, deriving from a wide range of specialties, including epidemiology, laboratory studies, pharmacology and clinical intervention trials.

Another important group of subjects that are suitable for testing chemopreventive approaches are those who have had an early primary head and neck cancer that is considered cured. As mentioned earlier, these patients have a high risk for developing a second primary cancer of the aerodigestive tract (4,31). It is reasonable to speculate that these agents may be active in reversing the "field cancerization" defect thought to underlie this increased incidence of second cancers. Non-toxic agents are again preferred in this setting, inasmuch as prolonged treatment is anticipated and many of these patients will have received radiation treatment to the oral cavity resulting in chronic mucosal injury. Hence, they may be unable to tolerate the mucocutaneous toxicity associated with agents such as the retinoids.

A small, initial study, involving subjects with all stages of cancer and using high dose 13-cis-retinoic acid, found a reduction in second primary cancers (32). However, toxicity was very significant and no survival advantage could be demonstrated. More recently, the negative results of a larger, prospective, randomized, placebo-controlled European trial involving 316 evaluable subjects with earlier stage disease have been reported, with no effect on survival or second primary cancers (33). This trial used etretinate, a synthetic retinoid somewhat less toxic than 13-cis-retinoic acid. Nevertheless, retinoid toxicity was still a serious problem. Multicenter trials using beta-carotene have recently begun to test whether the incidence of second primaries can be reduced with this non-toxic agent.

Finally, it is important to consider these results in the context of the ability of these agents to prevent other life-threatening, chronic diseases, particularly cardiovascular disease. The results of recent studies are indeed very encouraging (34-36). The unifying mechanism underlying these diseases is accumulating oxidative damage, thereby providing a theoretical basis for the potential of antioxidants to prevent several seemingly unrelated conditions. Indeed the potential for making a significant impact on morbidity and mortality reduction is such that these innocuous, non-toxic, dietary components could very well emerge as one of the most important disease preventive modalities of the decade. Thus confirmatory prospective, controlled clinical trials should be given the highest priority on the national research agenda.

## REFERENCES

**1.**    Parkin SM, Laara E, Muir CS. Estimates of the worldwide frequency of sixteen major cancers. Int J Cancer (Phila). 1988;41:184-197.
**2.**    Boring CC, Squires TS, Tong T. Cancer statistics, 1993 Cancer J Clin. 1993;43:7-26.
**3.**    Cancer Statistics Review (1973-87), NCI Division of Cancer Prevention and Control Surveillance Program, Publication No. 90-2789 (US Dept of Health and Human Services), PHS, NCI, NIH, Bethesda, MD; 1990.

**4.** Kotwall C, Razack MS, Sako K, Rao U. Multiple primary cancers in squamous cell cancers of the head and neck. J Surg Oncol. 1990;40:97-99.

**5.** Slaughter DP, Douthwich, HW, Smejkal W. Field cancerization in oral stratified squamous epithelium: clinical implications of multicentric origin. Cancer (Phila). 1953;5:963-968.

**6.** Block G, Patterson B, Subar A. Fruit, Vegetables and Cancer Prevention: a review of the epidemiologic evidence. Nutr Cancer. 1992;18, 1-29.

**7.** Barone J, Taioli E, Hebert JR, Wynder EL. Vitamin Supplement Use and Risk for Oral and Esophageal Cancer. Nutr Cancer. 1992;18:31-41.

**8.** Gridley G, McLaughlin JK, Block G, Blot WJ, Gluch M, Fraumeni JF. Vitamin Supplement Use and Reduced Risk of Oral and Pharyngeal Cancer. Am J Epidemiology. 1992;135:1083-1092.

**9.** Stich HF, Hornby AP, Dunn BP: Beta-carotene Levels in Exfoliated Mucosa Cells of Population Groups at Low and Elevated Risk for Oral Cancer. Int J Cancer. 1986;37:389-393.

**10.** Peng YM, Peng Y, Moon T, Roe D. Effect of Multivitamin Supplements and Smoking on Levels of Carotenoids, Retinoids and Tocopherols in Human Plasma, Skin and Buccal Mucosal Cells. Proc Am Assoc Cancer Res; 1993.

**11.** Som S, Chatterjee M, Bannerjee MR. Beta-carotene inhibition of DMBA-induced transformation of murine mammary cells in vitro. Carcinogenesis. 1984;5:937-940.

**12.** Stich HF, Dunn BP. Relationship between cellular levels of beta-carotene and sensitivity to genotoxic agents. Int J Cancer. 1987;38:713-717.

**13.** Schwartz J, Suda D, Light G. Beta-carotene is associated with the regression of hamster buccal pouch carcinoma and induction of tumor necrosis factor in macrophages. Biochem Biophys Res Commun. 1987;136:1130-1135.

**14.** Shklar G. Oral mucosal carcinogenesis in hamsters: inhibition by vitamin E. J Natl Cancer Inst. 1982;68:791-797.

**15.** Stich HF, Rosin MP, Hornby AP. Remission of oral leukoplakias and micronuclei in tobacco/betel quid chewers treated with beta-carotene and with beta-carotene plus vitamin A. Int J Cancer. 1988;42:195-199.

**16.** Stich HF, Stich W, Rosin MP, Vallejera DM. Use of the micronucleus test to monitor the effect of vitamin A, beta-carotene and canthaxanthin on the buccal mucosa of betel nut/tobacco chewers. Int J Cancer. 1990;34:745-750.

**17.** Silverman S, Shillitoe EJ. Etiology and predisposing factors in oral cancer. S Silverman. Ed.: 7-39 3rd Edition. American Cancer Society New York; 1990.

**18.** Hansen LS, Olson JA, Silverman S. Proliferative verrucous leukoplakia. A long-term study of thirty patients. Oral Surg Oral Med Oral Pathol. 1985;60:285-298.

**19.** Silverman S, Eisenberg E, Renstrap G. A study of the effects of high doses of vitamin A on oral leukoplakia (hyperkeratosis), including toxicity, liver function and

skeletal metabolism. J Oral Ther Pharmacol. 1965;2:9.
**20.** Wong R, Epstein J, Millner A. Treatment of oral leukoplakia with topical bleomycin. Cancer (Phila). 1989;64:361-365.
**21.** Koch HF. Biochemical treatment of precancerous oral lesions: the effectiveness of various analogues of retinoic acid. J Maxillofac Surg. 1978;6:59-63.
**22.** Shah JP, Strong EW, DeCosse JJ. Effects of retinoids on oral leukoplakia. Am J Surg. 1983;146:466-470.
**23.** Garewal HS, Meyskens FL, Killen D. Response of oral leuko-plakia to beta-carotene. J Clin Oncol. 1990;8:1715-1720.
**24.** Malaker K, Anderson BJ, Beecroft WA, Hodson DI. Management of oral mucosal dysplasia with beta-carotene retinoic acid: a pilot crossover study. Cancer Det and Prev. 1991;15:335-340.
**25.** Brandt R, Kaugars G, Silverman S, Lovas J, Chan W, Singh V, Dezzutti B Dao Q. Regression of oral lesions with the use of antioxidant vitamins and beta-carotene supplements. Pennington Symposium "Vitamins & Cancer Prevention." Louisiana State University Press. Baton Rouge, Louisiana; 1991.
**26.** Toma S, Benso S, Albanese E, Palumbo R, Nicolo G, Mangiante P. Response of oral leukoplakia to B-carotene treatment. Pennington Symposium "Vitamins and Cancer Prevention." Louisiana State University Press. Baton Rouge, Louisiana; 1991.
**27.** Garewal HS, Pitcock J, Friedman S, Alberts D, Meyskens F, Ramsey L, Peng YM, Girodias K. Beta-carotene in oral leukoplakia. Proceedings of American Society of Clinical Oncology (28th Meeting). 1992;11:141.
**28.** Zaridze D, Evstifeeva T, Boyle P. Chemoprevention of oral leukoplakia and chronic esophagitis in an area of high incidence of oral and esophageal cancer. Ann Epidemiol, 1993;3:225-234.
**29.** Benner SE, Winn RW, Lippman SM, Poland J, Hansen KS, Luna MA, Hong WK. Regression of oral leukoplakia with alpha-tocopherol: a community clinical oncology program chemoprevention study. J Natl Cancer Inst. 1993;85:44-47.
**30.** Hong WK, Endicott J, Itri LM, et al 13-cis-retinoic acid in the treatment of oral leukoplakia. N Eng J Med. 1986;315:1501-1505.
**31.** Shapshay W, Hong WK, Fried M. Simultaneous carcinomas of the esophagus and upper aerodigestive tract. Otolaryngol. Head Neck Surg. 1980;88:373-377.
**32.** Hong WK, Lippman SM, Itri LM, et al. Prevention of second primary tumors with isotretinoin in squamous cell carcinoma of the head and neck. N Engl J Med. 1990;323:795-801.
**33.** Bolla M, Lefur R, Ton Van J, Domange C, Badet JM, Koskas Y, Laplanche A. Prevention of second primary with etretinate in squamous cell carcinoma of oral cavity and oropharynx. A randomized double blind study. Proceedings of Second Interna-tional Cancer Chemoprevention Conference, Berlin, Germany; 1993.

**34.** Gaziano MJ, Manson JE, Ridker PM, Buring JE, Hennekens GH. Beta-carotene therapy and chronic stable angina. Circulation 82 (supplement); 1990, (abstract).

**35.** Rimm EB, Stampfer MJ, Ascherio A, Giovannucci E, Colditz GA, Willett WC. Vit E Consumption and the risk of coronary heart disease in men. N Engl J Med. 1993;328:1450-1456.

**36.** Stampfer MJ, Hennekens CH, Manson JE, Colditz GM, Rosner B, Willett WC. Vit E Consumption and the risk of coronary artery disease in women. N Engl J Med. 1993;328:1444-1449.

NUTRITIONAL PREVENTION TRIALS FOR COLORECTAL NEOPLASIA

E. Robert Greenberg, M.D.

Norris Cotton Cancer Center, DHMC

Hanover, NH


## BACKGROUND

   Colorectal cancer ranks as one of the top
three neoplasms in industrialized countries, both
in numbers of new cases and numbers of deaths (*1*).
In the United States, there are approximately
150,000 new colorectal cancer cases and 60,000
deaths each year (*2*).  Rates of colorectal cancer
are somewhat higher in men than women (*1,3*), but
the numbers of new cases and deaths are roughly
equal for both sexes, due to the larger proportion
of older women in our population.  While
colorectal cancer incidence rates in the United
States tended to increase over the past several
decades, mortality rates remained relatively
stable and, in more recent years, both incidence
and mortality have shown signs of diminishing
(*2,4*).


## PROSPECTS  FOR  PREVENTION

   There is now growing hope that we may be able
to avert the substantial morbidity and mortality
associated with colorectal cancers (*5*).  A higher
proportion of these tumors are being diagnosed at
an earlier stage (*2*), and more effective methods

*249*

for treating advanced disease have been developed
(6). There also are firm data from at least one
randomized, controlled clinical trial showing that
screening by testing for fecal occult blood, can
reduce mortality from this condition (7).
Although there are as yet no results from clinical
trials, non-experimental studies have strongly
suggested that endoscopy using either
sigmoidoscopy (8,9) or colonoscopy (10) is also
effective. The benefits of endoscopy presumably
result from detection and removal of adenomas,
precursors of invasive colorectal cancer.

Perhaps the best hope for reducing colorectal
cancer deaths, however, relates to the possibility
that these tumors may be preventable altogether.
Several lines of data support this notion.
Firstly, there are profound geographic variations
in the occurrence of colorectal cancer, with risks
varying by tenfold or more between low-risk
countries, such as those in Africa, Asia, and
South America, and high-risk countries of North
America and Western Europe (11). Secondly,
migrants to the United States from low-risk
countries such as Japan and China rapidly take on
the rates of their new home, particularly if they
are men (12,13) Thirdly, a plethora of
epidemiological studies indicate that, within a
given population, specific dietary factors are
strongly associated with the risk of developing
colorectal cancer (14). For example,
epidemiological studies indicate that risk of
colorectal cancer is about 50% lower in people who
eat greater amounts of fruits and vegetables,
compared to those who rarely eat these foods (15).
Moreover, there are plausible biological
mechanisms to explain an anti-carcinogenic effect
of many substances that occur in fruits and
vegetables (16). Thus, dietary change on a
population level conceivably could reduce
colorectal cancer deaths by half, or even more.

## ROLE OF CLINICAL TRIALS

Two general approaches have been used to

describe the relationship between diet and colorectal cancer. The first involves identification of specific substances within foods (macro nutrients or micro nutrients) that are associated with increased or decreased risk of cancer. For example, higher consumption of total calories and total fats have been related to higher risk, while intake of fiber, antioxidant vitamins, and folate have been associated with lower risk (*14*). The second approach is to examine the relationship between patterns of intake of various foods and cancer occurrence. Such analyses indicate a higher risk of cancer in people who consume larger quantities of animal products and a lower risk in people whose diets include more plant products (*15*).

Thus far, nearly all of the information supporting a role of specific dietary factors in colorectal cancer has come from non-experimental studies. There is widespread opinion that these types of data are insufficient to serve as a basis for public policy recommendation about dietary change to reduce cancer occurrence. The principal concern is that unidentified confounding factors may underlie any perceived associations between diet and colorectal cancer. Also, there are concerns about the quality of the dietary information generated in epidemiological studies, and it is often not clear form these studies whether findings relate to specific foods (such as vegetables) or to specific ingredients found within these foods (for example, antioxidant vitamins or fiber). In light of this uncertainty, some scientists have reasoned that randomized, controlled clinical trials of nutritional interventions will be necessary to develop evidence that is convincing and capable of supporting recommendations about dietary change and nutritional supplementation (*17*).

## FEASABILITY OF CLINICAL TRIALS

A randomized trial of a dietary strategy that has reduced colorectal cancer incidence as its

goal poses enormous logistical difficulties.
First, colorectal cancer is a relatively rare
occurrence in the United States, with an incidence
or roughly one per 1000 persons per year at age 50
and roughly two per 1000 per year at age 65 (3).
Accordingly, a study with invasive colorectal
cancer as its end point would require enormous
numbers of patients so that it could accrue enough
outcome events to have reasonable statistical
power. Also, colorectal cancer appears to result
from multiple genetic events, which likely occur
over a period of decades (18). An intervention
that acts early in this process may not produce a
measurable decline in invasive cancer incidence
within the time of any feasible clinical trial.
An alternative is to perform clinical trials to
reduce invasive cancer among high-risk groups such
as patients with ulcerative colitis or familial
polyposis. Often such trials will not be feasible
because of ethical concerns about not using
effective preventive measures (such as colectomy
or endoscopy with polypectomy). Furthermore,
there are not many people whose risk of colorectal
cancer is known to be very high.

In contrast to the large numbers of patients
required for studies of colorectal cancer end
points, studies focusing on adenomatous polyps
will require far fewer patients. This is because
the prevalence of adenomas in older subjects is
relatively high: roughly 50% of men over age 50 in
industrialized countries have at least one adenoma
found on examination of the entire large bowel
(19). Also, patients who have had an adenoma  in
the past have a high risk (roughly one in three)
of developing at least one new adenoma within the
next three to five years (20). Lastly, patients
with adenoma, and those at high risk of getting a
new adenoma, can be safely observed with
intermittent endoscopy and  removal of adenoma.
More intensive interventions are not required.

Several groups of investigators have initiated
studies of dietary interventions with recurrence
of sporadic adenomas as the primary end point.
These studies have involved random assignment to

interventions, including vitamins C and E (*21*), reduced fat and increased fiber (*22*), calcium carbonate, and antioxidant vitamins (*23*). In their conduct, these trials have entailed many challenges common to virtually all cancer prevention studies; moreover, the trials pose particular difficulties in their interpretation, since the relationship of adenoma to invasive cancer is not entirely understood.

Our group of investigators has been involved in three large multi-center studies of randomized interventions to reduce adenoma occurrence. Our experience in the first of these studies, a randomized trial of antioxidant vitamins (*23*), provides some illustrations of the major issues posed by these types of trials. Briefly, this was a randomized, double-blind, two-by-two factorial study testing whether beta-carotene (25 milligrams per day) or combinations of these vitamins C (1 gram per day) and E (400 milligrams per day) would be effective in preventing the recurrence of adenomas in the large bowel among patients who previously had one of these polyp tumors resected. The study was conducted at six clinical sites. To be eligible, patients must have had at least one adenomatous polyp removed from the large bowel within three months prior to enrollment and must have had a colonoscopy showing no further polyps. They also had to be in general good health and under age 80 years. The study called for a four-year intervention with the occurrence of at least one adenoma during the last three years of the study as the primary end point.

## RECRUITMENT ISSUES

A particularly important factor in our study was the need to recruit adequate numbers of patients. To have a reasonably good chance (80%) of detecting a moderate (35%) reduction in adenoma recurrence over a three year observation period required that at least 750 patients be randomized. Based on endoscopy and pathology reports we estimated that we would have far more potential subjects than we actually required. In practice, however, once the study started we found that we had to search long and hard to come up with enough enrollees. This was partly because patients were counted more than once in the source records due to there having multiple polypectomies. A more important factor was that many of the patients in these record sources were ineligible for study. For example, patients undergoing polypectomy because of a previous diagnosis of invasive cancer, familial polyposis, or ulcerative colitis would not be good candidates for a study focusing on patients with sporadic adenomas. Overall, roughly half of the patients initially thought to be available for study proved to be ineligible. Of the remaining patients, about half chose not to enter the study for various reasons. These included an unwillingness to stop taking vitamin supplements because of a belief that they were good for overall health, as well as a reluctance to take anymore pills, particularly among patients who already had chronic conditions requiring frequent medication. Sometimes the logistical requirements of the study also posed difficulty and argued against patients taking part. Thus, out of the 2029 potentially eligible patients that we identified from chart-review, only 981 agreed to enter our study.

## ADHERENCE TO THE INTERVENTION

The second major issue we faced was ensuring compliance with the study regimen. The staff at each of the clinical centers carefully interviewed patients to assess their enthusiasm for taking part in a trial that would last four years and required daily consumption of study pills and capsules. However, it is often difficult for patients to foresee how they will react to a change in their daily regimens. For that reason, we first tested each patient's adherence to the study regimen using a three-month period in which they were given placebo pills and capsules only. Of the 981 patients who entered this phase of the study, only 864 were eventually randomized. The

remaining patients either lost interest in the
study or found that they were unable to take their
pills or capsules at least 80% of the time. By
randomizing only patients who had successfully
completed this run-in period, we were able to
substantially reduce the problem of non-compliance
later in the study.

Even with these efforts at careful selection
of patients, compliance still proved to be an
issue. During the course of the study, it became
increasingly difficult to keep all patients on a
regimen of daily consumption of the pills and
capsules. During their first year, well over 90%
of patients took the study agents 6 or 7 times per
week. By their fourth year on the study, this
figure had dropped to 80%. Some of the main
reasons patients gave for stopping the study
agents were related to the onset of new illnesses
or the worsening of pre-existing conditions.
Patients who were seriously ill and taking potent
medications for heart disease or other
debilitating conditions often told us that
participating in the study by taking vitamin
supplements had become a lower priority for them.

## ENDPOINT DETERMINATION

The primary endpoint for our study was the
development of a new colorectal adenoma following
randomization to the nutritional intervention. In
accordance with the usual endoscopy practice at
the time of the trial, we mandated that
colonoscopic examinations should be done 12 months
and 48 months following recognition and removal of
the initial adenoma. We decided at the onset of
the trial not to count adenomas found at the first
(12 month) colonoscopic examination as study
endpoints. Earlier studies had shown that a
substantial proportion (10-15%) of small adenomas
are missed at colonoscopy (24). Also, patients
were on the active intervention for only a portion
of the twelve months between their initial
polypectomy and the first colonoscopic
examination. This was due to the time necessary

to identify and recruit patients as well as the
three month placebo run-in period. Thus, any
polyps found at the year one colonoscopy would, in
part, represent the presence of pre-existing
adenomas as well as the growth of new adenomas
during the period before the start of the
intervention. Counting these polyps as endpoints
would tend to dilute any possible real effect of
the vitamin supplement. For that reason we only
considered adenomas detected after the 12- month
colonoscopy examination.

Uniform assessment of adenomas also proved to
be a challenge in our trials. At the onset of our
study it was crucial to ensure that all of the
participating endoscopists agreed to the common
follow-up schedule and to a policy to biopsy all
raised mucosal lesions. Without this policy,
heterogeneity in clinical practice could have
seriously compromised the interpretability of the
study result. For example, some endoscopists
would routinely biopsy only one of several
suspicious lesions and would remove the others by
fulguration, thus obliterating any possible
adenomas. For this trial, however, endoscopists
agreed not to fulgurate any suspicious lesions and
to submit them all for pathological examination.

Also, they all had to agree to follow the schedule
of repeat colonoscopies one year and four years
after the colonoscopy and polypectomy performed
immediately before the patient entered the study.
At times, endoscopists felt that they would
ordinarily follow a patient more closely, perhaps,
with annual endoscopies. They would have
preferred to observe other patients less closely,
particularly if they had only one small polyp
identified initially. For the purposes of the
study, however, the endoscopists all agreed to
abide by a common protocol. This topic became
particularly difficult during the later years of
the study when evidence began to accrue suggesting
that a less frequent follow-up schedule than the
one we prescribed would likely be safe (20).

## INTERPRETATION OF FINDINGS

The ultimate goal of the nutritional interventions used in adenoma trials is to prevent colorectal cancer deaths. However, the preventive effects seen (or not seen) for recurrent adenomas in a trial will not necessarily translate into an effect on death rates from cancer. This issue has been discussed at length elsewhere (25). Alternative explanations are possible for any of the various results of an adenoma prevention trial, and this issue merits careful attention both in the design of a trial as well as in the interpretation of its findings.

For example, in our first polyp prevention study there was no evidence that the intervention reduced adenoma recurrence. Nonetheless, we could not firmly conclude that vitamin supplements would be ineffective in preventing colorectal cancer deaths. The duration of the intervention and follow-up period in our study was three to four years. A longer period of intervention or observation may be needed before an effect becomes evident. Another possibility is that vitamin supplements may not prevent adenomas from forming, but they could inhibit their progression to invasive cancer. We considered these possibilities in our report. They also were raised frequently in discussions with enthusiasts of vitamin supplementation, who argued that our study did not disprove a beneficial effect of supplements. In fact, it is virtually impossible for a single study to demonstrate conclusively that a nutritional intervention does not prevent cancer. A critic can always posit that the timing of the intervention, the duration of the intervention, or the duration of the follow-up period were inadequate to observe a real effect. Nevertheless, we held that a negative result from an adenoma prevention study does provide some evidence against an effect, and it is up to the proponents of the intervention to show conclusively that it does work.

An adenoma prevention trial that clearly shows

a reduction in recurrence may help establish that there is a likely beneficial effect against cancer. However, the results of a positive study are still open to alternative inferences regarding efficacy in preventing cancer deaths. Only a small proportion of adenomas progress to fatal cancers (*19*). The "effective" intervention may just have activity against the harmless adenomas which would never develop further. Also, in adenoma prevention trials the adenoma endpoints are generally diminutive, having grown over only a three to four year time span. Any intervention that masks recognition of these small adenomas, perhaps by making colonoscopy more difficult or reducing edema in the tumors, would appear to be effective. Thus, a finding of reduced rates of adenoma recurrence following a nutritional intervention provides strong, though not entirely conclusive, evidence for a possible benefit against invasive cancer.

## CONCLUSIONS

Epidemiological studies have provided powerful encouragement, but not convincing proof, that colorectal cancer deaths may be diminished by dietary interventions. It will be extremely difficult to construct a trial that can demonstrate a reduction in colorectal cancer deaths following a nutritional intervention. Clinical trials of adenoma prevention are more practical, and experience to date shows that these studies are feasible. These trials pose challenges, however, in achieving adequate recruitment of participants, promoting their adherence to the intervention, and ensuring completeness of their follow-up and endpoint assessment. Also, interpretation of adenoma prevention trials requires caution. They have a relatively brief duration, and thus they may only test the effects of an intervention on one phase of the multi-step process of colorectal carcinogenesis.

## REFERENCES

(1) Boyle P, Zaridze DG, Smans M: Descriptive epidemiology of colorectal cancer. Int J Cancer 36:9-18, 1985

(2) Chow W-H, Devesa SS, Blot WJ: Colon cancer incidence: recent trends in the United States. Cancer Causes and Control 2:419-425, 1991

(3) Miller BA, Ries LAG, Hankey BF: Cancer Statistics Review: 1973-1989: National Cancer Institute, 1992

(4) Greenwald P: Colon cancer overview. Cancer (Supplement) 70:1206S-1215S, 1992

(5) Greenberg ER, Baron JA: Prospects for preventing colorectal cancer death. JNCI 85:1182-1184, 1993

(6) Moertel CG: Chemotherapy for colorectal cancer. New Engl J Med 330:1136-42, 1994

(7) Mandel JS, Bond JH, Church TR: Reducing mortality from colorectal cancer by screening for fecal occult blood. Minnesota Colon Cancer Control Study. New Engl J Med 328:1365-1371, 1993

(8) Selby JV, Friedman GD, Quesenberry CPJ: A case-control study of screening sigmoidoscopy and mortality from colorectal cancer. NEJM 326:653-657, 1992

(9) Newcomb PA, Norfleet RG, Storer BE, et al: Screening sigmoidoscopy and colorectal cancer mortality. Journal of the National Cancer Institute 84:1572-1575, 1992

(10) Winawer SJ, Zauber AG, Ho MN, et al: Prevention of colorectal cancer by colonoscopic polypectomy. New Engl J Med 329:1977-81, 1993

(11) Boyle P, Zaridze D, Smans M: Descriptive pidemiology of colorectal cancer. Int J Cancer 36:9-18, 1985

(12)Whittemore AS: Colorectal cancer incidence among
Chinese in North America  and the Peoples
Republic of China: variation with sex, age and
anatomical site. Int. J Epidemiol 18:563-568,
1989

(13)Shimizu H, Mack TM, Ross RK, et al: Cancer of
the gastrointestinal tract among Japanese and
White immigrants in Los Angeles county. JNCI
78:223-228, 1987

(14)Willett W: The search for the causes of breast
and colon cancer. Nature  338:389-394, 1989

(15)Steinmetz KA, Potter JD: Vegetables, fruit, and
cancer. I. Epidemiology. Cancer Causes and
Control 2:325-57, 1991

(16)Steinmetz K, Potter J: Vegetables, fruit, and
cancer. II  Mechanisms. Cancer Causes and
Control  2:427-442, 1991

(17)Hennekens CH, Buring JE: Contributions of
observational evidence and clinical trials in
cancer prevention. Cancer 74:2625-2629, 1994

(18)Fearon ER, Vogelstein B: A genetic model for
colorectal tumorigenesis. Cell 61:759-767, 1990

(19)Peipins LA, Sandler RS: Epidemiology of
colorectal adenomas. Epidemiologic Reviews
16:273-297, 1995

(20)Bond JH: Polyp guideline: diagnosis, treatment,
and surveillance for patients with nonfamilial
colorectal polyps. Ann Intern Med 119:836-843,
1993

(21)McKeown-Eyssen G, Holloway C, Jazmaji V, et al:
A randomized trial of vitamins C and E in the
prevention of recurrence of colorectal polyps.
Cancer Res 48:4701-4705, 1988

(22)McKeown-Eyssen GE, Bright-See E, Bruce WR, et
al: A randomized trial of a low fat high fibre
diet in the recurrence of colorectal polyps.
Journal of Clinical Epideimology 47:525-536,
1994

(23) Greenberg ER, Baron JA, Tosteson TD, et al: A clinical trial of antioxidant vitamins to prevent colorectal adenoma. New Engl J Med 331:141-147, 1994

(24) Hixson L, Fennerty M, Sampliner R, et al: Prospective study of the frequency and size distribution of polyps missed by colonoscopy. J Natl Cancer Inst 82:1769-1772, 1990

(25) Schatzkin A, Freedman LS, Dawsey SM, et al: Interpreting precursor studies: what polyp trials tell us about large-bowel cancer. Journal of the National Cancer Institute 86:1053-1057, 1994

# PART IV

# Cancer Treatment Studies: Lab Studies

# VITAMINS INDUCE CELL DIFFERENTIATION, GROWTH INHIBITION AND ENHANCE THE EFFECT OF TUMOR THERAPEUTIC AGENTS ON SOME CANCER CELLS IN VITRO

Kedar N. Prasad

Center for Vitamins and Cancer Research,
Department of Radiology, School of Medicine,
University of Colorado Health Sciences Center,
Denver, CO  80262

## CURRENT CONCEPTS IN CARCINOGENESIS

Several hypotheses for human carcinogenesis have been proposed.  A recent review (1) by Duesberg and Schwartz has critically analyzed the various hypotheses of carcinogenesis which include: (a) chromosomal aberrations (b) activation of proto-oncogenes (c) loss of anti-oncogenes (d) infection with certain viruses and (e) substitution of normal promoters of proto-oncogenes with strong promoters of viruses or cellular genes.  Although structural and functional defects in several oncogenes in some human tumors have been observed, the frequency of their occurrence is seldom more than 50% of the cases.  None of the above hypotheses by themselves is sufficient to explain the cause of the cancer.  We propose a 4-stage model of carcinogenesis (2).

**First Stage:  Chromosomal Damage and Gene Mutation:**  The chromosomal aberrations and/or gene mutations induced by spontaneous errors during cell replication, carcinogen treatment or a combination of these can occur in any dividing cell.  This can lead to mutations due to loss, gain, or rearrangement of genes and chromosomes. Cells may survive or die depending upon the extent and type of chromosomal damage. The surviving cells, which contain chromosomal damage and/or gene mutation may continue to divide, differentiate and die in a normal pattern, similar to those cells which do not have these defects. Neither chromosomal damage nor gene mutation by itself is sufficient for transformation; however, cells carrying these defects are at higher risk for transformation to cancer cells.

**Second Stage: Abnormalities in the Expression of Genes Which Cause Differentiation:** When genes which cause differentiation, become abnormal in one or a few normal cells or cells with pre-existing gene mutations and/or chromosomal damage, the affected cells do not differentiate and consequently, they continue to divide forming hyperplastic lesions. These lesions are considered precancerous. Examples of such lesions are polyps in the colon, adenoma in the parotid gland, and cystic mastitis in the female breast. The genes responsible for causing cell differentiation have not been identified in any cell type as yet.

**Third Stage: Abnormalities in the Expression of a New Set of Genes in Hyperplastic Cells Which Cause Them to Invade Distant Organs:** In humans, the hyperplastic cells may continue to divide for several years and may accumulate additional chromosomal damage and/or gene mutations during that period. This may lead to increased genetic imbalances in all affected cells, but may not be sufficient for transformation to cancer cells. However, when the expression of certain oncogenes and/or cellular genes becomes abnormal in one or a few hyperplastic cells, they could become cancer cells and the remaining hyperplastic cells continue to divide. Examples of such a process are seen in colon polyps where scattered foci of cancer cells among numerous hyperplastic cells are seen. The genes which cause hyperplastic cells to become cancer cells have not been identified in any cell type as yet.

**Fourth Stage: Abnormalities in the Expression of a New Set of Genes in Cancer Cells Which Make Them More Aggressive:**

chromosomal damage and/or gene mutations which may lead to increased genetic imbalances in all cancer cells, but these imbalances may not be sufficient for inducing changes that cause them to invade distant organs. However, when the expression of certain genes becomes abnormal in one or a few cancer cells, they become more aggressive and metastasize to distant organs. These genes have not been identified as yet. The proposed hypothesis will predict the following: (a) Since the location of chromosomal injuries are random events following exposure to carcinogens or mutagens the type of chromosomal damage may vary from one cell to another in the same organ, and from one time to another within the same cell. This may be the primary reason for marked variations in the type of chromosomal damage from one cell to another in the same tumor, and from one individual to another with the same kind of tumor. Indeed, extensive works published on this issue support this prediction. (b) Alterations in gene expression in hyperplastic, cancer, or aggressive cancer cells are random events, and can occur in genes described in the 4 stages of carcinogenesis as well as in genes which are non-specific for carcinogenesis. Although some mutated genes such as the c-ras oncogene, several over-expressed oncogenes such as the c-myc or rearranged oncogenes such as the c-able and c-myc have been reported to occur in several human tumors (3-6), the frequency of these occurrences in any tumor is never more than 50%; therefore, they represent abnormalities in genes that are not sufficient for carcinogenesis; however, they may be considered one of the risk factors. (c) Cancer cells can be converted to normal-like cells with increased differentiated functions in the presence of chromosomal aberrations and structural gene defects, if the defects in the expressions of genes responsible for causing differentiation and/or maintaining cancer phenotype are corrected. The first part of this prediction has already been documented in 1971 when we demonstrated that an elevation of adenosine 3',5'-cyclic monophosphate (cAMP) in neuroblastoma cells, which were polyploid, induced terminal differentiation in many of these cells (7). The differentiated neuroblastoma cells exhibited increased cell-specific differentiated functions (8). An elevation of cAMP also reversed cancer phenotypes in other tumor cells which include murine melanoma (9) and human neuroblastoma (8,10). Other agents such as butyric acid (11-12) and dimethylsulfoxide (13) also induced terminal differentiation in erythroid leukemic cells as shown by the production of hemoglobin in these cells. However, the genes responsible for causing differentiation in any cell type have not been identified. The hybrids generated from fusion of normal and cancer cells become non-tumorigenic (14) suggesting that the chromosomes from normal cells provide sufficient amounts of differentiating gene products which reverse cancer phenotype. The loss of normal chromosomes from the hybrid cells can restore malignant behavior in hybrids. This study also suggests that cancer phenotype is reversible in the presence of chromosomal damage and structural genetic imbalances. In spite of uncertainties about the mechanisms of carcinogenesis, the role of vitamins in cancer prevention is fairly well established in most experimental systems, and several new prevention trials in humans are in progress. However, the role of vitamins in cancer treatment has not drawn scientific enthusiasm as yet. The purpose of this review is to analyze available data on the potential role of vitamins in cancer treatment.

The properties of useful cancer treatment agents should include the following: (a) they induce cell differentiation in cancer cells; (b) they inhibit the growth of tumor cells without significantly affecting normal cells; (c) they enhance the effect of currently used tumor therapeutic agents on tumor cells, but protect normal tissue against their adverse effects; and (d) they stimulate the immune system. Vitamins possess all these properties in varying levels depending upon tumor type and chemotherapeutic agents.

**Vitamins Induce Differentiation and Growth Inhibition in Tumor Cells:** Vitamins also induce differentiation in some tumor cells in culture. The understanding of the processes of differentiation is very important for developing new strategies of cancer prevention and treatment. Multiple differentiating agents having different mechanisms of action can be used for the prevention as well as the treatment of cancer in a highly selective manner. Retinoids (15-17), vitamin D (18), d-alpha tocopheryl succinate (alpha-TS) (19-20), and beta-carotene (21-22) induce cell differentiation and growth inhibition in several transformed cell lines. Vitamin C only inhibits growth of cancer cells (23-24).

Alpha-TS and beta-carotene (BC) also enhance the effect of other differentiating agents (25-26). For example, alpha-TS enhances the effect of other differentiating agents such as cAMP on melanoma cells (25). Similarly BC also enhances the level of cAMP-induced morphological differentiation in neuroblastoma cells in culture (Fig. 1). These results suggest that the gene products which are responsible for maintaining the transformed phenotype and which prevent the expression of differentiated phenotype can be suppressed in some cell types more effectively if BC or alpha-TS is present with cAMP. The mechanisms of vitamin-induced differentiation of cancer cells are unknown. However, this provides a unique opportunity to identify gene products which play a crucial role in maintaining the transformed phenotype as well as in causing differentiation.

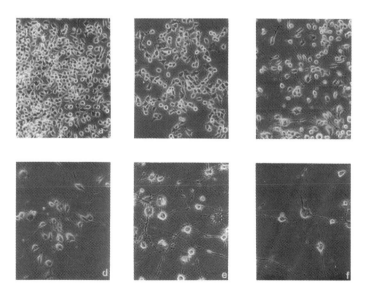

Fig. 1. Photomicrographs of neuroblastoma cells in culture after treatment with RO20-1724 and ß-carotene. Control (a) 4 days after plating (50,000 cells/60 mm dish) showing mostly round cells; ß-carotene (20 μg/mL)-treated cells (b) 4 days after treatment showing no significant change in morphology; RO20-1724 (200 μg/mL)-treated cells (c) 4 days after treatment revealing increased number of cells with neurites; cells treated with RO20-1724 plus ß-carotene (d) for a period of 4 days showing more differentiated cells than those produced by RO20-1724 treatment alone; cells treated with RO20-1724 plus ß-carotene for a period of 8 days (e) and 11 days (f) showing large cells with extensive and multiple neurites (x200). (26)

**Vitamins Enhance the Effect of Tumor Therapeutic Agents:** Vitamin C, alpha-TS, BC, retinyl palmitate, and retinoic acid modify the effect of some chemotherapeutic agents, x-irradiation and hyperthermia on tumor cells (24, 27-32). One clinical study has reported that supplementation with high doses of a vitamin mixture improves the cure rate (33). These studies indicate that supplementation with vitamins during therapy may improve the efficacy of currently used cancer therapeutic agents. However, there are no adequate pre-clinical data available on which clinical protocols can be developed. Therefore, we initiated a new study to evaluate the effectiveness of multiple vitamins, vitamin C, BC, d-alpha-TS and 13 cis-retinoic acid (RA) in modifying the efficacy of the currently used chemotherapeutic agents for the treatment of melanoma which include, cis-platin, tamoxifen, decarbazine (DTIC), and recombinant interferon-alpha 2b on human melanoma (SK-30) cells in culture.

**Effects of Individual Vitamins:** Vitamin C inhibited growth of melanoma cells in a concentration-dependent manner without affecting the morphology (24). Alpha-TS at a high concentration (20 μg/ml), or RA alone (15, 7.5 and 3.8 μg/ml) did not significantly affect the growth of melanoma cells in culture. RA treatment induced morphological changes as evidenced by the formation of multiple short cytoplasmic processes; however, alpha-TS treatment did not (24).

**Effects of a Mixture of Two Vitamins:** Vitamin C, in combination with BC, RA or alpha-TS inhibited the growth of melanoma cells more than that produced by vitamin C treatment alone. BC, in combination with alpha-TS or RA, was ineffective (Table 1).

**Table 1.** Effect of a Mixture of Two Vitamins on Growth of
Melanoma Cells in Culture[a-c]

| Treatments | Growth,<br>% of Untreated Control |
|---|---|
| Vit C (100 $\mu$g/ml) | 64 ± 3* |
| BC (10 $\mu$g/ml) | 96 ± 2 |
| BC (20 $\mu$g/ml) | 99 ± 3 |
| Vit C + BC (10 $\mu$g/ml) | 34 ± 2[d] |
| Vit C + BC (20 $\mu$g/ml) | 29 ± 1[d] |
| $a$-TS (10 $\mu$g/ml) | 102 ± 3 |
| $a$-TS (20 $\mu$g/ml) | 47 ± 3* |
| Vit C + $a$-TS (10 $\mu$g/ml) | 37 ± 2[d] |
| Vit C + $a$-TS (20 $\mu$g/ml) | 39 ± 3 |
| RA (15 $\mu$g/ml) | 95 ± 3 |
| RA (7.5 $\mu$g/ml) | 103 ± 3 |
| Vit C + RA (15 $\mu$g/ml) | 37 ± 2[d] |
| Vit C + RA (7.5 $\mu$g/ml) | 29 ± 1[d] |
| BC (10 $\mu$g/ml) + $a$-TS (10 $\mu$g/ml) | 96 ± 3 |
| BC (10 $\mu$g/ml) + RA (7.5 $\mu$g/ml) | 97 ± 3 |

a:  Values are means ± SE. (24)
b:  Cells (5 x $10^4$ /60-mm dish) were plated in tissue culture dishes, and vitamin C, ß-carotene (BC), d-$a$-tocopheryl succinate ($a$-TS), and 13-cis-retinoic acid (RA) were added in various combinations 24 hours later. Growth was determined 3 days after treatment. Each experiment was repeated 3 times, involving 3 samples/treatment group. Each value represents an average of 9 samples. Average no. of cells per dish in untreated control cultures was 87 ± 3 x $10^4$.
c.  Statistical significance is as follows: *, different from control (p = 0.05).
d.  Synergistic effect.
e.  Less than additive.

**Effects of a Mixture of Three Vitamins:** Vitamin C, in combination with BC and alpha-TS reduced growth of melanoma cells more than that produced by vitamin C treatment alone; BC and alpha-TS by themselves were not effective (Table 2). BC, in combination with alpha-TS and RA, markedly inhibited growth of melanoma cells, although individual vitamins themselves were not effective (Table 2).

When the concentration of BC was increased by 2-fold, the combined treatment further reduced the growth of melanoma cells, although this increased concentration of BC by itself produced no effect on the growth. Increasing the concentration of alpha-TS by 2-fold resulted in reduced growth of melanoma cells in combination studies more than that produced by alpha-TS alone (Table 2). Reducing the concentration of BC, alpha-TS and RA by half produced no significant effect on the growth of melanoma cells (24).

Table 2. Effect of a Mixture of Three Vitamins on Growth of Melanoma Cells in Culture[a-b]

| Treatments | Growth, % of Untreated Control |
|---|---|
| Vit C (100 $\mu$g/ml) + BC (10 $\mu$g/ml) + $a$-TS (10 $\mu$g/ml) | 40 $\pm$ 3[c] |
| BC (10 $\mu$g/ml) + $a$-TS (10 $\mu$g/ml) + RA (7.5 $\mu$g/ml) | 59 $\pm$ 3[c] |
| BC (20 $\mu$g/ml) + $a$-TS (10 $\mu$g/ml) + RA (7.5 $\mu$g/ml) | 31 $\pm$ 3[c] |
| BC (10 $\mu$g/ml) + $a$-TS (20 $\mu$g/ml) + RA (7.5 $\mu$g/ml) | 17 $\pm$ 3[c] |
| BC (5 $\mu$g/ml) + $a$-TS (5 $\mu$g/ml) RA (7.5 $\mu$g/ml) | 90 $\pm$ 1 |

a.  Values are means $\pm$ SE. (24)
b.  Cells (5 x $10^4$/60-mm dish) were plated in tissue culture dishes, and vitamin C, BC $a$-TS, and RA were added in various combinations 24 hrs. later. Growth was determined 3 days after treatment. Each experiment was repeated 3 times, involving 3 samples/treatment group. Each value represents average of 9 samples. Average no. of cells per dish in untreated control cultures was 87 $\pm$ 3 x $10^4$
c.  Synergistic effect.

**Effects of a Mixture of Four Vitamins:** Vitamin C, in combination with BC, alpha-TS, and RA, significantly reduced growth of melanoma cells compared to that produced by vitamin C alone (Table 3). Reducing the concentration of vitamin C by 50% also decreased the level of growth inhibition produced by a mixture of 4 vitamins. Reducing the concentration of each vitamin by 50% produced no significant effect on growth (24).

**Table 3. Effect of a Mixture of Four Vitamins on Growth of Melanoma Cells in Culture[a,b]**

| Treatments | Growth, % of Untreated Control |
|---|---|
| Vit C (100 $\mu$g/ml) + BC (10 $\mu$g/ml) + $\alpha$-TS (10 $\mu$g/ml) + RA (7.5 $\mu$g/ml) | 13 ± 1[c] |
| Vit C (50 $\mu$g/ml) + BC (10 $\mu$g/ml) + $\alpha$-TS (10 $\mu$g/ml) + RA (7.5 $\mu$g/ml) | 56 ± 3[c] |
| Vit C (50 $\mu$g/ml) + BC (5 $\mu$g/ml) + $\alpha$-TS (5 $\mu$g/ml) + RA (3.8 $\mu$g/ml) | 98 ± 4 |

a:      Values are means ± SE. (24)

b:      Cells (5 x 10⁴/60-mm dish) were plated in tissue culture dishes, and vitamin C, BC, $\alpha$-TS, and RA were added in various combinations and at different concentrations 24 hrs later. Growth was determined 3 days after treatment. Each experiment was repeated 3 times, involving 3 samples/treatment group. Each value represents average of 9 samples. Average no. of cells per dish in untreated control cultures was 87 ± 3 x 10⁴.

c.      Synergistic effect.

**Modification of Tamoxifen-Effect by Vitamins:** Tamoxifen inhibited growth of melanoma cells in a concentration-dependent manner (24). Addition of vitamin C(100 $\mu$g/ml) increased the growth inhibitory effect of tamoxifen as did a mixture of three vitamins. A mixture of four vitamins containing 100 $\mu$g/ml of vitamin C did not significantly change the tamoxifen-effect. However, a mixture of four vitamins which contained 50 $\mu$g/ml of vitamin C increased the growth inhibitory effect of tamoxifen (Table 4).

Table 4. Modification of the Effect of Chemotherpeutic Agents by a
Mixture of Four Vitamins on Growth of Melanoma Cells in Culture[a-d]

| Treatments | Growth, % of Untreated Control |
|---|---|
| Solvent | 101 ± 4 |
| *cis*-Plat (1 μg/ml) | 67 ± 4* |
| *cis*-Plat + Vit C + BC + α-TS + RA | 38 ± 2[f] |
| *cis*-Plat (2 μg/ml) | 41 ± 2* |
| *cis*-Plat + Vit C + BC + α-TS+ RA | 34 ± 2[g] |
| Tamox (2 μg/ml) | 81 ± 3* |
| Tamox + Vit C + BC + α-TS + RA | 30 ± 2[e] |
| Tamox (3 μg/ml) | 57 ± 3* |
| Tamox + Vit C + BC + α-TS + RA | 24 ± 3[e] |
| DTIC (30 μg/ml) | 93 ± 4 |
| DTIC + Vit C + BC + α-TS + RA | 53 ± 1 |
| DTIC (100 μg/ml) | 71 ± 2* |
| DTIC + Vit C + BC + α-TS + RA | 38 ± 2[f] |
| Interferon (10,000 IU/ml) | 82 ± 5* |
| Interferon + Vit C + BC + α-TS + RA | 29 ± 1[e] |
| Interferon (20,000 IU/ml) | 66 ± 3* |
| Interferon + Vit C + BC + α-TS + RA | 33 ± 1[f] |

a:    Values are means ± SE. (24)
b:    Abbreviations are as follows: *cis*-Plat, *cis*-platin; Tamox,
      tamoxifen; DTIC, decarbazine; Interferon, intferon-α2b.
c:    Doses for vitamins are as follows: vitamin c, 50 μg/ml; BC, 10
      μg/ml; α-TS, 10 μg/ml; RA (7.5 μg/ml). Cells (5 x 10⁴/60-mm
      dish) were plated in tissue culture dishes, and agents were
      added 24 hrs later. Growth was determined 3 days after
      treatment. Each experiment was repeated 3 times, involving 3
      samples/treatment group. Each value represents average of 9
      samples. Average no. of cells per dish in untreated control
      cultures was 87 ± 3 x 10⁴.
d:    Statistical significance is as follows: *, different from control (p
      = 0.05).
e.    Synergistic effect
f.    Additive effect.
g.    Less than additive.

**Modification of DTIC Effect by Vitamins:** DTIC was not effective in reducing the growth of melanoma cells in culture until a concentration of 100 μg/ml was reached (24). Addition of vitamin C at a concentration of 100 μg/ml enhanced the growth inhibitory effect of DTIC; however, a mixture of 3 or 4 vitamins which contained 100 μg/ml of vitamin C did not result in further suppression of growth (24). A mixture of 4 vitamins which contained 50 μg/ml of vitamin C markedly enhanced the DTIC effect on melanoma cells (Table 4).

**Modification of Interferon Effect by Vitamins:** Interferon by itself decreased growth of melanoma cells in a concentration-dependent manner (24). Addition of vitamin C alone, or a mixture of three vitamins (BC, alpha-TS and RA), enhanced the growth inhibitory effect of interferon on melanoma cells in culture. A mixture of four vitamins which contained 100 μg/ml of vitamin C enhanced the interferon effect at a concentration of 20,000 I.U./ml. A mixture of four vitamins which contained 50 μg/ml of vitamin C also significantly increased the interferon effect on human melanoma cells in culture (Table 4). Their results show that a mixture of 4 vitamins (vitamin C, BC, alpha-TS and RA) or 3 vitamins (BC, alpha-TS and RA) markedly reduced the growth of human melanoma cells in culture.

A mixture of 3 vitamins (BC, alpha-TS and RA) enhanced the growth-inhibitory effects of tamoxifen, cis-platin and interferon, but did not significantly alter the DTIC effect. A mixture of 4 vitamins which contained 50 μg/ml of vitamin C markedly enhanced the growth-inhibitory effect of all chemotherapeutic agents used in this study. Increasing the vitamin C concentration to 100 μg/ml in a mixture of 4 vitamins reduced growth of melanoma cells by about 85%. This vitamin mixture, in combination with cis-platin and interferon, further reduced growth of melanoma cells, but in combination with DTIC or tamoxifen no such effect was observed. These results suggest that the addition of vitamin C, BC, alpha-TS and RA at non-toxic doses of each vitamin may enhance the growth inhibitory effect of currently used therapeutic agents on human melanoma cells in culture.

This study shows that individual vitamins, such as

vitamin C, inhibited growth of human melanoma cells in culture. Likewise, we have shown that alpha-TS can also reduce the growth of human melanoma cells in culture (24). The growth-inhibitory concentrations of alpha-TS for human melanoma cells was four-fold higher than those reported for murine B-16 melanoma cells (21), suggesting that human melanoma cells are more resistant to alpha-TS than murine B-16 melanoma cells. This study also revealed that BC, even at a high concentration of 20 $\mu$g/ml, did not affect the growth or the morphology of human melanoma cells in culture. This is in contrast to a similar study reported with murine melanoma cells in which the same concentration of BC causes growth inhibition and morphological differentiation (21). Finally, we have shown that RA induced morphological differentiation without growth inhibition in human melanoma cells in culture (24). Other studies have reported that RA can induce differentiation and/or growth inhibition in rodent and human melanoma cells in culture (17).

The present study proposes a new concept, namely that individual vitamins at non-toxic concentrations, when combined together, produce growth inhibitory effects on human melanoma cells in culture. Such vitamin mixtures also enhance the growth inhibitory effect of currently used chemotherapeutic agents on melanoma cells. The combination of at least 3 vitamins was essential for the above effect. These findings suggest that such a combination of vitamins and standard chemotherapeutic agents may be useful clinically, by increasing therapeutic efficacy.

Another scientific rationale for using vitamins in combination with chemotherapeutic agents involves the reduction of toxicity of chemotherapeutic agents on normal cells by vitamins. This rationale can not be tested in tissue culture systems. However, several studies using individual vitamins have shown that they can reduce tumor therapeutic agent-induced toxicity in animal models. For example, in normal animals (primarily rat and rabbits), vitamin E reduces bleomycin-induced lung fibrosis (34), adriamycin-induced cardiac toxicity (35-38) and skin necrosis (39). It also reduces adriamycin-induced toxicity in liver, kidney, and intestinal mucosa (40). Several studies have shown that alpha-tocopherol protects normal tissue in-vivo against radiation damage (41-43), whereas others have reported no such effect of vitamin E either on normal or tumor tissue (44-45). The reasons for this discrepancy are unknown. Some studies have reported that BC or retinyl palmitate supplementation enhances the cell-killing effect of X-irradiation and cyclophosphamide on transplanted breast adenocarcinoma in rats, while protecting the normal tissue against the adverse effects of these agents on normal cells in animals (31). Vitamin C also reduces adriamycin-induced toxicity in normal mice and guinea pig (46). Vitamin C, alpha-TS and RA reduce bleomycin-induced chromosomal breakage (47).

The mechanism of action of vitamins on tumor cells is not totally clear. From the results discussed above, one can propose a working hypothesis that a mixture of 4 antioxidant vitamins might enhance the growth-inhibitory effect of cancer therapeutic agents selectively on tumor cells, while protecting normal tissues against their adverse-effects. This hypothesis appears inconsistent with the fact that vitamin C, BC, alpha-TS and RA are known to have antioxidant functions, and one of the actions of most tumor therapeutic agents involves the generation of free radicals. Therefore, these vitamins should protect both normal and tumor tissues. However, in-vitro and in-vivo studies have repeatedly shown that high doses of these vitamins, when used individually, reduce growth and/or induce differentiation of tumor cells, and protect normal tissues against some of the adverse effects of tumor therapeutic agents. We have postulated that tumor cells can pick up excessive amounts of antioxidant vitamins due to a loss of the homeostasis control mechanism for the uptake of these vitamins, whereas normal cells do not pick up excessive amounts of vitamins, because they do not have the above membrane defect. The accumulation of excessive amounts of vitamins in tumor cells can shut off the oxidation reactions responsible for generating energy and may alter other vital cellular functions such as inhibition of protein kinase C activity and oncogene expression, and production of increased amounts of growth inhibitory growth factors. This was demonstrated with alpha-TS. For example, alpha-TS inhibits protein kinase C activity (48) and oncogene expression (49), and causes increased production of transforming growth factor (50). The extent of inhibition of the above cellular functions depends upon the level of intracellular accumulation of vitamins. This can lead to cell death, reduction in rate of cell proliferation and induction of differentiation, depending upon the extent and type of inhibition of cellular functions in tumor cells. These acquired biological features of tumor cells following exposure to high doses of vitamins overrides any protective action of antioxidant vitamins that may be operating on tumor cells.

## CONCLUSIONS

Several hypotheses for human carcinogenesis have been proposed. These include chromosomal aberrations, activation of oncogenes, loss of anti-oncogenes, infection with certain viruses and substitution of normal promoters of proto-oncogenes with strong promoters of viruses or cellular genes. None of these alterations by itself is sufficient to cause cancer. We have proposed a 4-stage model of carcinogenesis in which chromosomal damage and/or gene mutations occur in all stages. The nature of these genes or their abnormality at each step has not been identified. In spite of uncertainties regarding the mechanisms of carcinogenesis, several vitamins such as beta-carotene (BC), vitamins A, C and E have been identified to be of cancer protective value.

The effect of a mixture of vitamins in modifying the efficacy of commonly used drugs in the treatment of human cancer cells has not been adequately studied. Vitamin C and d-alpha-tocopheryl succinate (d-alpha-TS) reduced the growth of human melanoma (SK-30) cells in culture, whereas beta-carotene (BC) and 13-cis-retinoic acid (RA) alone were ineffective. RA did cause morphological changes as evidenced by flattening of cells and formation of short cytoplasmic processes. A mixture of 4 vitamins (vitamin C, BC, alpha-TS and RA) was more effective in reducing growth of human melanoma cells than a mixture of three vitamins. The growth inhibitory effect of cis-platin, DTIC (decarbazine), tamoxifen and recombinant interferon-alpha-2b was enhanced by vitamin C alone, a mixture of three vitamins (BC, alpha-TS and RA), and a mixture of 4 vitamins (vitamin C, BC, alpha-TS and RA) which contained 50 $\mu$g/ml of vitamin C. These data show that a mixture of 3 or 4 vitamins can enhance the growth inhibitory effect of currently used chemotherapeutic agents on human melanoma cells.

**Acknowledgements:**

This work was supported by an NIH grant from the Office of Alternative Medicine R21-RR09566 and Shafroth Memorial Fund.

## REFERENCES

1.   Duesberg, P.H. and Schwartz, J.R.  Latent viruses and mutated oncogenes: no evidence for pathogenicity. Proc. Nuc Acid Res. Mol. Biol. 43: 135-204, 1992.

2.   Prasad, K.N., Edwards-Prasad, J., Kumar, S. and Meyers, A. Vitamins regulate gene expression and induce differentiation and growth inhibition in cancer cells.  Their relevance in cancer prevention." Arch. Otolaryngol. Head and Neck Surg. 119: 1133-1140, 1993.

3.   Bishop, J.M. Cellular oncogenes and retrovirus. Ann. Rev. Biochem. 52: 301-354, 1983

4.   Varmus, H.E.  The molecular genetics of cellular oncogenes, Ann. Rev. Genet-18: 533-612, 1984

5.   Reddy, E.P., Reynolds, R.K., Santos, E. and Barbacid, M. A point mutation is responsible for acquisition of transformed properties by the T24 human bladder carcinoma oncogene. Nature 300: 149-152, 1982.

6.   Ramsay, G.M., Moscovici, G., Moscovici, C., and Bishop, J.M.,  Neoplastic transformation and tumorigenesis by human protooncogene myc. Proc. Natl. Acad. Sci. USA. 87:2102-2106, 1990.

7.   Prasad, K.N., and Hsie, A.W. Morphologic differentiation of mouse neuroblastoma cells induced in vitro by dibutyryl adenosine 3',5'-cyclic monophosphate. Nature New Biol. 233:141-142, 1971.

8.   Prasad, K.N., Differentiation of neuroblastoma cells: A useful model for neurobiology and cancer. Biol. Rev. 66:431-451, 1991.

9.   Johnson, G.S., and Pastan, I. $N^6o^2$-dibutyryl adenosine 3',5'-monophosphate induces pigment production in melanoma cells. Nature New Biol. 237:267-268, 1972.

10.  Helson, L., Helson, C., Peterson, R.F. and Das, S.K.. A rationale for the treatment of metastatic neuroblastoma. J. Natl. Cancer Inst. 57: 727-729, 1976.

11.  Leder, A., and Leder, P., Butyric acid, a potent inducer of erythroid differentiation in cultured erythroid leukemia cells. Cell 5: 319-322, 1975

12. Prasad, K.N. Butyric acid: A small fatty acid with diverse biological functions. Life Sciences 27:1351-1358, 1980.
13. Friend, C., Scher, W., Holland, J.G. and Sato, T. Hemoglobin synthesis in murine virus-induced leukemia cells in vitro. Stimulation of erythroid differentiation by dimethysulfoxide. Proc. Natl. Acad. Sci. USA 68:378-382, 1971.
14. Harris, H., Miller, O.J., Klien, G., Worst, P., and Tachibana, T. Suppression of malignancy by cell fusion. Nature 223:363-368, 1968.
15. Sporn, M.B., and Roberts, A.B. Role of retinoids in differentiation and carcinogenesis. Cancer Res 43: 3034-3040, 1983
16. Griep, A.E., and DeLuca, H.F. Decreased c-myc expression is an early event in retinoic acid-induced differentiation of F-9 teratocarcinoma cells. Proc. Natl. Acad. Sci. USA. 83:5539-5543, 1986.
17. Lippman, S.M., Meyskens, F.L. Jr., Retinoids as anticancer agents. In: Tryfiates, G.P. and Prasad K.N., eds. Nutrition, Growth and Cancer. Alan R. Liss, New York, pp 229-244, 1988.
18. Brelvi, Z.S. and Studzinski, G.P. Inhibition of DNA synthesis by an inducer of differentiation of leukemic cell $1a$-25-hydroxy vitamin $D_3$ precede down regulation of the c-myc gene. J Cell Physiol. 128: 171-179, 1986.
19. Prasad, K.N., Edwards-Prasad, J. Effect of tocopheryl (vitamin E) acid succinate on morphological alterations and growth inhibition in melanoma cells in culture. Cancer Res. 42: 550-555, 1982.
20. Kline K., Cochran, G.S. and Sanders, B.G., Growth inhibitory effects of vitamin E succinate on retrovirus-transformed tumor cells in vitro. Nutr Cancer 14:27-31, 1990.
21. Hazuka, M.B., Edwards-Prasad, J., Newman, F., Kinzie, J., and Prasad, K.N. ß-Carotene induces morphological differentiation and decreases adenylate cyclase activity in melanoma cells in culture. J. AM. Coll. Nutr. 9: 143-149, 1990.

22.  Schwartz, J. and Shklar, G. The selective cytotoxic
     effect of carotenoid and alpha-tocopherol on human
     cancer cell lines in vitro. J. Oral Maxilofac. Surg. 50:
     367-373, 1992.
23.  Cameron, E., Pauling, L., and Leibowitz, B. Ascorbic acid
     and cancer. A review. Cancer Res 39: 663-681, 1979.
24.  Prasad, K.N., Hernandez, C., Edwards-Prasad, Nelson, J.,
     Borus, T., and Robinson, W. Modification of the effect of
     tamoxifen, cis-platin, DTIC, and interferon-*a*-2b on human
     melanoma cells in culture by a mixture of vitamins. Nutr.
     Cancer. 22::233-245, 1994.
25.  Prasad, K.C. Induction of differentiated phenotypes in
     melanoma cells by a combination of an adenosine 3'-5'-
     cyclic monophosphate stimulating agent and d-alpha-
     tocopheryl succinate. Cancer Lett. 44: 17-22, 1989.
26.  Prasad, K.N., Kentroti, S., Edwards-Prasad, J.,
     Vernadakis, A., Imam, M., Carvalho, E. and Kumar, S.
     Modification of the expression of adenosine 3',5'-cyclic
     monophosphate-induced differentiated functions in
     neuroblastoma cells by beta-carotene and d-alpha-
     tocopheryl succinate. J. Am. Coll. Nutr. 13: 298-303,
     1994.
27.  Prasad, K.N., Sinha, P.K., Ramanujam, M. and Sakamoto,
     A. Sodium ascorbate potentiates the growth inhibitory
     effects of certain agents on neuroblastoma cells in
     culture. Proc. Natl. Acad. Sci. USA 76: 829-832, 1979.
28.  Josephy, P.D., Paleic, B., and Skarsgard, L.D. Ascorbate-
     enhanced cytotoxicity of misonidazole. Nature 271: 370-
     372, 1978.
29.  Ripole, E.A.P., Rama, B.N. and Webber, M.M. Vitamin E
     enhances chemotherapeutic effects of adriamycin in
     human prostate carcinoma cells in vitro. J. Urol. 136:
     529-531, 1986
30.  Prasad, K.N. and Rama, B.N., Modification of the effect
     of pharmocological agents, ionizing radiation and
     hyperthermia on tumor cells by vitamin E. In Vitamins,
     Nutrition and Cancer. Prasad, K.N. (ed). Basel: Karger, pp
     76-104, 1984.

31. Seifter, E., Rettura, A., Padawar, J., and Levenson, S.M. Vitamin A and ß-carotene as adjunctive therapy to tumor excision, radiation therapy and chemotherapy. In: Vitamins, Nutrition and Cancer, Prasad, K.N. (ed) Basel: Karger, pp 1-19, 1984.

32. Lippman, S.M., Parkinson, D.R., Itri, L.M., Weber, R.S. and Schantz, S.P. et al. 13 cis-retinoic acid and interferon *a*-2a: Effective combination therapy for advanced squamous cell carcinoma of the skin. JNCI 84: 235-241, 1992.

33. Hoffer, A. Orthomolecular oncology. In: Adjuvant Nutrition in Cancer Treatment. Quillin, P., (ed) Arlington Heights Cancer Treat. Found. pp.361-370, 1993.

34. Yamanaka, N., Fukishima, M., Koizumi, K., Nishida, K., Kato, T., et al: Enhancement of DNA chain breakage by bleomycin and biological free radical producing systems In Tocopherol, Oxygen and Biomembrane, C DeDuve and T Hayashi (eds) New York: North Holland, pp. 59-69, 1978.

35. Myers, CE, McGuire, W., and Young, R: Adriamycin amelioration of Toxicity by alpha-tocopherol. Cancer Treat. Rep 60, 961-962, 1976.

36. Sonnevald, P: Effect of alpha tocopherol on cardiotoxicity of adriamycin in the rat. Cancer Treat Rep 62: 961-962, 1976.

37. VanVleet, J.F., Greenwood, L., Ferands, V.J. and Rebar, A.H. Effect of selenium-vitamin E on adriamycin-induced cardiomyopathy in rabbits. Am. J. Vitamin Res 39: 997-1010, 1978.

38. Wang, Y.M., Madanat, F.F., Kimball, J.C., Gieser, C.A., Ali, M.K., et al Effect of vitamin E against adriamycin-induced toxicity in rabbits. Cancer Res 40: 1022-1027, 1980.

39. Svingen, B.A., Powis, A., Abbel, P.L. and Scott, M. Protection against adriamycin-induced skin necrosis in the rat by dimethylsulfoxide and alpha-tocopherol. Cancer Res. 41: 3395-3399, 1981.

40. Geetha, A., Sankar, R., Marar, T., and Devi, C.S.S. Alpha

tocopherol reduces doxorubicin-induced toxicity in rats—Histological and biochemical evidences. Indian Physiol. Pharmacol 34: 94-98, 1990.

41. Srinivasan, V., Jacobs, A.L., Simpson, S.A., and Weiss, J.F. Radioprotection by vitamin E effect on Hepatic enzymes, delayed type hypoersensitivity and post-irradiation survival in mice. In Modulation and Mediations of Cancer Cells by Vitamins. F.L. Meyskens, Jr., and K.N. Prasad (eds) Basel: Karger pp 119-131, 1983.

42. Malick, M.A., Roy, R.M. and Sternberg, J. Effect of vitamin E on post-irradiation death in mice. Experientia 34: 1216. 1978.

43. Londer, H.M., and Myers, C.E. Radioprotective effects of vitamin E Am. J. Clin. Nutr. 31: 705a, 1978.

44. Rostock, R.A., Stryker, J.A., and Abt, AB. Evaluation of high dose vitamin E as a radioprotective agent. Radiology 126: 763-765, 1980.

45. Ershoff, B.H., and Steers, C.W., Jr. Antioxidants and survival time of mice exposed to multiple sublethal doses of x-irradiation. Proc. Soc. Exp. Biol. Med. 104: 274-276, 1960.

46. Fujita, K., Shinpo, K., Sato, T, Niime, H., Shamoto, M., et al. Reduction of Adriamycin-toxicity by ascorbate in mice and guinea pigs. Cancer Res 42: 309-316, 1982.

47. Trizna, Z., Shantz, S.P., Lee, JJ, Spitz, M.R., Goepfert, H., et al. In Vitro Protective effect of chemopreventive agents against bleomycin-induced genotoxicity in lymphoblastoid cell lines and peripheral lymphocytes of head and neck cancer patients. Cancer Detect. Prev. 17: 575-583, 1993.

48. Gopalakrishna, R., Gundimeda, U. and Chen, Z., Vitamin E succinate inhibits protein kinase C: correlation with its unique inhibitory effects on cell growth and transformation. In: Nutrients in Cancer Prevention and Treatment. Prasad, K.N., Santamaria, L. and Williams, L. (eds), Humana Press: N.J. (In press).

49. Prasad, K.N., Cohrs, R.J., Sharma, O.K. Decreased expression of c-myc and H-ras oncogenes in vitamin E

succinate-induced differentiated murine B-16 melanoma cells in culture. Biochem. Cell. Biol. 68: 1250-1255, 1990.

50.   Kline, K., Yu, W., Zhao, B., Israel, K., Charpentier, A., Simmons-Menchaca, M., and Sanders, B.G. Vitamin E Succinate: Mechanisms of action as tumor cell growth inhibitor. In: Nutrients in Cancer Prevention and Treatment. Prasad, K.N., Santamaria, L., Williams, R.M. (eds) Humana Press: N.J. (In press)

# Molecular and Biochemical Control of Tumor Growth Following Treatment With Carotenoids or Tocopherols

## Joel L. Schwartz

Laboratory for Oral Biomarkers
Molecular Epideminology and Oral Disease
Prevention Program
National Institute of Dental Research

Chemopreventative agents such as retinoids, carotenoids or tocopherols have been shown *in vitro* and in animal models to inhibit, prevent, and regress established malignancies when they are administered in combination. Their mode of action appears to involve oxygen reactivity, which results in either the control or the promotion of tumor cell growth. Recent evidence indicates that there are common mechanisms for the growth inhibitory effects of these different chemopreventative groups. These include the reduction of mutant p53 protein expression with increases in protein expression of wild type p53 and stress protein 70 and 90 kD in treated tumor cells. An accumulation of cells in G1 of the cell cycle, a change in cyclin complex activities, and a reduction in the expression of transcription protein factors in tumors cells was also noted for carotenoids and alpha tocopherol activity. There was also an increase in programmed cell death as determined by the nucleosome formation. At higher concentrations these agents can induce increased growth and mitotic activity dissociated from programmed cell death processes.Oxygen reactive nutrients may inhibit

287

growth but they also may contribute to the triggering of side effects in human populations.

**Introduction:**

In this article we shall review the data which this laboratory has developed in the past few years concerning the molecular and biochemical characteristics of carotenoids and tocopherols. These characteristic biologic cellular changes will be related to the suppression of tumor cell growth or the development of malignant transformation.

In the past decade retinoids, carotenoids and tocopherols have been reported to prevent, inhibit, or regress established oral carcinoma of the hamster buccal pouch. These carcinomas were induced by through a chemical carcinogen. This carcinogen requires an oxidative metabolic activity to be converted to a diol epoxide which could then be incorporated into the hamster genetic material.

The groups of molecules to be discussed here have a general responsive capacity to change in various oxidative cellular states. Particularly, tocopherols, and carotenoids can exhibit either an antioxidant or prooxidant biochemical activity in the cell depending on the partial pressure of oxygen. Retinoids are in general less responsive to these oxygen pressure changes.

It is our hypothesis that this characteristic for response to changes in oxygen cellular states that results in their function as chemopreventative or therapuetic agents. Specifically, the inhibition of oral carcinogenesis that has been reported to be a consequence of this characteristic.

## Pathway for control of cell growth:

To place these oxidative responsive capacities in perspective we have provided figure 1.

**Antioxidant-Prooxidant:**

This figure shows our view that various chemopreventative agents exert biologic influence through changes in their oxidative activity while they act as reducing or oxidizing agents. The beneficial activity for these agents will also be defined by the cellular environment. For example if these agents act as prooxidant or oxidizing agents in normal cells, then damage to normal DNA could occur, resulting in the dysregulation of cell growth and more importantly differentiation could proceed in an abnormal manner. In contrast a prooxidant character produced by carotenoids or tocopherols could in tumor cells inhibit the growth of the premalignant or malignant cells. Carotenoids or tocopherols has not been identified with a genotoxic or mutagentic effect in normal cells. Although both β-carotene and alpha tocopherol can alter sister chromatid exhange (1).

The development of a antioxidant or reducing agent in premalignant of malignant cells could promote the growth and the transformation process. This would occur because there would be a resulting reduction in reactive oxygen intermediates that increase peroxidation and free radical generation resulting in genetic instablity and damage. In normal cells such as inflammatory cells which are directed toward the control of foreign antigen through the production of reactive oxygen intermediates, the control of additional reactive oxygen radicals could enhance the efficiency of immune responsiveness. This laboratory and others have observed that carotenoids and tocopherols could enhance various immune reactions (2,3). Some of these immuine responses are cytotoxic to tumor cells.

**Development of Apoptosis:**

A reactive oxygen state, which was exemplified by the reduction in the activity of superoxide dismutase, gutathione-S-transferase, and lower levels of non protein sulfhydryls, in tumor cells was also tied to the development of programmed cell death (apoptosis) (4).

Apoptosis appears to be an end stage through

which the transforming cell has attempted differentiation. In some cells, such as, oral mucosal cells, differentiation appears to stablize the mucosal tissue reestablishing normal cellular relationships. In the transformed cells, differentiation could be their death knell. In normal cells the recognized biologic prinicpal has been that cells only have a defined number of mitotic divisions. In the mucosal cells as in other epidermal cell types this biologic characteristic is linked in an unknown manner to differentiation, as identified through keratohyolin granular fromation and cytokeratin expression. Transformed cells may exhibit a certain degree of undifferentiation, which could be linked to increased proliferative capacity (proliferating cell nuclear antigen, cyclin and kinase activity, inhibition of growth arrest genes (GADD)), and response to various growth factors such as epidermal growth factor or transforming growth factor alpha. Upon recieving the signal to differentiate the transformed cell may demonstrate increased genetic instability. These signals may also be in conflict and incompatible for the survival of the malignant cell. In association with these confusing and conflicting signals there develops an increased need for DNA repair.    The blocking of DNA repair will have a significant effect on the inhibition of tumor cell growth. In this genetic damaged state previously expressed genes and their products which inhibited apoptosis, for example, bcl-2 are either decreased in expression or complexed with other proteins which block their function. This situation is exemplified by BAX or Bcl-X genes and their products (5).

The growth arrest genes (e.g., GADD) which had in the malignant state been suppressed in their functional activity could in conjunction with tumor suppressor genes such as p53 or possibly p16 modulate the cyclins and their kinases to increased activities. Resulting in the accumulation of tumor cells in $G_1$ of their cell cycle (6).

The tumor cells could also be pushed through mitosis only to stall in a presynthesis limbo. The markers for this process will be the markers for apoptosis and cell cycle rearrangment, such as hsp 70, p53, bcl-2, and the related oxygen protective cellular enzymes. The initators for this process could be prooxidants/oxidizing agents (7).

In normal cells, for example inflammatory cell types, the generation of reactive oxygen products could increase the development of apoptosis and if they reach toxic levels, produce necrosis.

This type of situation has been partly uncovered in oral lichen planus. In this inflammatory keratotic lesion we have observed that the inflammatory infiltrate was proliferative and the primary cell a CD4+ lymphocyte, expressed high levels of Bcl-2. We speculate that the patient was infected originally with a virus, probably a adenovirus or herpes family related virus. This virus then triggered the expression of Bcl-2 or produced a mimic which also suppressed apoptosis. In the oral mucosa we observe the development of apoptosis which was characterized by nucleosome formation in the stratum basal layer. In these cells we also find the expression of stress proteins, which are signals for the development of apoptosis. In conjunction with the enhanced expression of stress proteins was the increased expression for p53. The adjacent supra basaliar layer of cells exhibited a proliferation characterized by an increased expression for proliferating cell nuclear antigen (e.g., cyclin acitivity). The generation of stress proteins (e.g., oxidative stress) such as hsp 60, or 70 could have additional significance because of their abilities to bind to p53, modify the half like of this tumor suppressor protein (wild type form) and binding and stablize the presentation of self histocompatibility antigen. This latter relationship could increase the development of autoimmune reactions (8). In our clinical experience the administration of either /or β-carotene or alpha tocopherol could enhance the development of autoimmune phenomenon in lichen planus. Therefore there is a complex interaction of cellular responses which could trigger the pathogenesis of disease following the administration of antioxidant /reducing agents to apparently normal tissue.

The process of apoptosis has also been connected with the ageing process. The use of antixoidants removing or reducing oxygen free radicals has been considered a method of decreasing the ageing process. During the time span of cellular metabolic activity the cell accumulates degraded glycoproteins, lipoproteins, and nuclear binding proteins. The cell must package and eliminate these proteins. If these proteins are not removed from the cell they could bind aberrantly to other cellular proteins or form non dissociated inorganic protein complexes. The end result is the induction of  cellular stresses such as oxidative stress. Antioxidants could inhibit this process by reducing the oxidative capacity of proteins,  inhibiting the development of apoptosis and perhaps slowing the ageing process. The markers for this process may be decreasing binding of hsp 70 to degrading proteins reducing the formation of stress protein-protein complexes. A decrease level of these protein complexes could reduce binding to a cis acting promotor region for the hsp 70 gene. The hsp factors (1 or 2) and elements could also modify the activity of not only hsp 70 protein complexes but other genes linked to the hsp 70 gene such as  tumor necrosis factor, or histocompatibility genes, extending the biologic effects of reducing nuclear binding (8).

In comparison with necrosis, apoptosis does not develop when there is a genotoxic response that results in the loss of viability and necrosis of the tissue. The development of apoptosis is totally dependent on the expression of various genes or their products.  Necrosis is associated usually with inflammatory responses and the development of necrosis could be related to the level of a toxin  or the time differential between the release of toxin and the ability of the cell to institute repair mehanisms (9).

## Biochemical Relationships Related to Apoptosis:

In figure 2. we detail some of the biochemical relationships which have been associated with the development of apoptosis. The scheme presented is a general outline and an atempt to organize the cellular relationships for the role of chemopreventatives in the development of apoptosis.

### Inflammatory Influence:

Regardless of the origin of the trigger (e.g.,inflammation, pathogenesis of disease) the initial response by a cell is the propagation of reactive oxygen intermediates (ROIs). These ROIs will trigger through Fenton or Haber Weiss reactions the further accumulations of other ROIs.  Some of these ROIs linked to peroxidations reactions, for example hydroxyl radicals, will have half lives that will allow  them to interacte with either cellular receptors, associated proteins, or signal inductive complexes. Other products such as the free radical, superoxide anion, nitric oxide anion, or hydrogen peroxide, will either undergo further peroxidation reactions or become neutralized because of their short half lives. The neutralization process will result through the activity of intracellular antioxidants, such as reduced glutathione and related pathways, or inorganic protein complexes that act as reducing agents. These interactions with the molecular components of the cell are inevitably tied to either electron transfer and the cytochrome system, or the action of kinases related to GTP or cAMP activity (e.g. NAD(P)H oxidase) (10).

Exogenous agents can trigger changes in this cellular response system. These include agents that trigger the T cell receptor (TCRs), the FAS antigen, the tumor necrosis factor antigen (TNF), arachidonic acid metabolites, such as HETE, and stress or heat shock proteins (Hsps). These immune products influence the development of apoptosis by influencing growth arrest, differentiation, and DNA repair (11,12).

The production of ROIs and their derivatives are also controlled indirectly because soluble Fas and possibly other soluble immune products also inhibit the development of apoptosis. Bcl-2 can inhibit the development of apoptosis but this protein also suppresses the apoptotic influence of TNF, FAS, phorbol myrisitic acid, and other immune reactive products. Bcl-2 can be controlled by the activity of the BAX gene. The activity of Bcl-2 may also be influenced by the production of Bcl-2 like proteins derived from the activation of viral genes (e.g., adenovirus, herpes or endogenous retrovirus family) (13,14).

**Antioxidant    Effect:**

Intracellular antioxidants such as thioredoxin, and reduced glutathione or tocopherols, and carotenoids can reduce the expression of Bcl-2. In addition signal inducive complexes such as NF-κB, have also been shown to be effected by antioxidant activity (15).

**NF-κB-Signal   Induction  :**

NF-kB is a signal inductive molecule that compexes with IκBα which undergoes degradation and activation. The control for this system is throught to be through cyclophilin activity. Cyclophilins are charperonin like molecules that facilitate the movement of other proteins in the cell. Cellular antioxidants and inflammatory derived proteins catalyze the transfer between thiol radicals and cysteine containing proteins such as the intracellular proteins thioredoxin and reduced glutathione,or superoxide dismutase. This characteristic also controls NF-κB expression (16).

The oxygen reactive enzymes of the cell such as, superoxide dismutase (SOD), can also influence another signal inductive system which is composed of G proteins, such as p21$^{ras}$ (17).

SOD has been associated with membrane carboxyl methylation altering the conversion of guanine dinucleotide to guanine triphosphate, and the kinase activity of the G proteins.

The chemopreventative agents also effect chaperonin activity by enhancing the expression of stress proteins such as hsp 90, and 70. β-carotene is an example of one of these chemopreventative agents (18).

**Membrane Peroxidation**:

One of the fundalmental concepts related to the action of hydrophobic chemopreventative agents such as,carotenoids, or tocopherols, is the process of prenylation. Prenylation is a chemical process facilitating protein interations between hydrophobic proteins and hydrophobic molecules. This relationship is also important when considering the interactions of hydrophobic molecules to receptors that contain prenyl groups such as a cysteine-aliphatic amino acid-X amino acid arrangement (CaaX,where X= serine, alanine, methionine, leucine) (19). The superfamily of receptors which includes for example epidermal growth factor, retinoid, and thyroxine, contains prenylated transmembrane domains.

Amino acid oxidation developes from the action of oxygen radicals such as carbonyl, hydroxyl or ferrous ion. These radicals have longer half lives than radicals such as superoxide anion, allowing them to form oxidative relationships with cellular proteins. Mixed oxidation systems (MCO) produce the ROIs and ferrous ion that oxidize the amino acids. Using the iron chelator o-phenanthroline (o-PA) we have observed the

inhibition of tumor suppressive activity of β-carotene
(20). o-PA inhibits the inactivation of many membrane
related enzymes except creatine kinase and glucose-6-
phosphate dehydrogenase, which become oxidized. o-PA
in combination with α-tocopherol synergistically
decreased the viability of various tumors cells in culture.
α-tocopherol, presumably inhibited the peroxidation of
the membrane associated proteins and reduced the
binding of ferrous ion or hydroxyl radical to the proteins.

In addition, non-enzymic MCO systems generate
ascorbate-ferric ion -oxide, non protein sulfhydryl-thiol
containing ferric ion oxide complexes, as well as,
hydrogen peroxide and ferrous ion.

These ions and ROIs react in a site specific manner
modifying the metal binding sites of amino acids and
producing fragmentation of their polypeptides. Amino
acids such as, histidine, methionione, and cysteine are
particularly subceptible to the development of oxidized
metal binding sites. Some amino acids are in general
more eaisly oxidized producing their carbonyl radical
these include: proline, arginine, and lysine. Other amino
acids, such as, proline, arginine or lysine, are more
sensitive to oxidation by the MCO producing α amidation,
a carbonyl radical and  fragmentation of their
polypeptide. The oxidation of proteins could also produce
changes in calcium binding, reducing nuclear binding,
kinase activity, or reduce alky hydroxyperoxides altering
cytochrome electron transport. For example levels of
reduced flavoproteins which are associated with the
cytochrome system, undergo autooxidation to form
hydrogen peroxide. To prevent cellular damage from ROIs
(e.g.,further oxidation of proteins, decreased DNA repair)
intracellular antioxidants such as,thioredoxin, reduced
glutathione, and enzymes such as, superoxide dismutase,
or catalases are increased in concentration.

## Experimental Evidence For Apoptosis
**Development.** Defining early neoplastic markers: This laboratory has continued to investigate the development of biochemical and molecular protein markers during the induction of oral carcinogenesis in the hamster buccal pouch tumor model. The treatment with the carcinogen results in early observable changes in the number of cells in synthesis. This was verified by the use of in situ hybridization for histone 3 (figure 3.)

The treatment with the carcinogen 7,12 dimethylbenz(a)anthracene (DMBA) results in the early expression of Bcl-2 in apparently non dysplastic oral mucosa. This expression is coupled with some of the mucosal cells expressing apoptotic (programmed cell death) changes (nucleosome formation) consistent with the normal oral mucosa. Further treatment with DMBA results in the histopathologic appearance of dysplasia, followed by carcinoma-in-situ, then oral squamous cell carcinoma. Through this cascade of malignant change there was observed increasing but localized areas of Bcl-2 expression. This was also coupled with decreasing levels of apoptotic-nucleosome formation. Other potential markers substantiated this modification of apoptosis. For example, increased levels of mutant p53 (tumor promotor) was found in association with identically treated cells expressing high levels of low molecular weight cytokeratins. In contrast, lower levels of wild type p53 (tumor suppressor) and high molecular weight keratins were observed (figure 4, 5).

The results showed that early neoplastic changes could be detected by focusing on the differentiation process of the oral mucosal cells. Distinguished by their loss of programmed cell death, the expression of mutant p53, and low molecular keratins. These features of protein expression could also be correlated with other biomarkers for example, a high proliferative capacity, increased localized level of stress proteins such as, hsp 25 or 70, production of transforming growth factor alpha and epidermal growth factor, and increased association with neovacularization.

These results indicated the close relationship of this carcinogenesis model to human oral cancer and demonstrated a repertoire of biomarkers that could be considered for clinical evaluation.

**Determining a mechanism of action for anticancer chemopreventatives: Biomarkers of their activity.**

1. *In vivo* **studies:**

Several studies were conducted to evaluate the role of chemopreventative agents in the control of malignant growth. These studies included evaluation of the *in vivo* observation of inhibition by chemopreventive agents. This was accomplished using Western immunoblotting, flow cytometry and immunohistochemistry.

**Programmed cell death induction and the inhibition of oral carcinogenesis**

The inhibition of oral carcinogenesis appears to begin in histopathologically normal oral mucosa. This tissue exhibits an apparent shift in the regulation of oral mucosal cells growth in comparison to the oral mucosal cells observed during carcinogen treatment. Therefore treatment with various chemopreventative agents reduced the numbers and size of oral carcinomas formed. Compared to the tissue only treated with the carcinogen DMBA, the buccal pouch treated with β-carotene reduced the number of cells in synthesis (figure 3.) Other cellular changes related to apoptotic change was demonstrated through increases in the number of basal cells in the oral mucosa exhibiting nucleosome formation (DNA fragmentation), increased protein expression of wild type (tumor suppressor) p53, with decreased levels of mutant p53 protein expressed (figure 4.,5,). Increased expression for the stress proteins hsp 70 and 90 were also seen and decreased expressions of Bcl-2 protein, and stress protein hsp 25 was noted. Histopathologic change was not seen after three weeks of treatment with the chemo-preventative agent and/or the carcinogen DMBA or treatment with DMBA by itself. Although the immunohistochemical changes described above were first observed at this stage of oral carcinogenesis. These changes persisted and became more evident as oral carcinogenesis progressed. At six to nine weeks, moderate to severe dysplasia could be found although there were fewer and smaller areas of dysplasias in the chemopreventative treated oral mucosa compared to the DMBA controls. In sections from animals treated nine to twelve weeks, dysplasia, carcinoma-in-situ, and invasive squamous cell carcinoma was present. The differences between the chemopreventative treated oral mucosa and those sections from animals only DMBA treated was more evident because the tissue sections from the DMBA treated controls showed large areas of the sections exhibiting malignant changes. Grossly, the animals exhibited larger and more oral carcinomas in the DMBA controls compared to the chemopreventative agent and DMBA treated groups (21, 22). Microscopic analysis revealed that β-carotene treatment for example, produced marked increases in the number of malignant cells undergoing programmed cell death (e.g. nucleosome formation). This was correlated with increased expressions for the p53 protein, and stress proteins hsp 70 and hsp 90. Bcl-2 and hsp 25 were also significantly reduced in expression. There was also observed an decreased number of basal oral mucosal cells in synthesis phase of cell growth, defined by the expression of proliferating cell nuclear antigen and Ki-67, in the DMBA treated controls. Flow cytometry substantiated this response and further determined that the tumor cells were accumulating in $G_1$ of the cell cycle (a presynthesis phase) (figure 6.).

**Growth   regulation,***in vivo* **transformation**
Cell growth regulatory signals were also noted to be
changed. For example p21$^{ras}$ , protooncogene protein was
found to be increased in expression following treatment
with β-carotene, but mutant derived protein was
decreased in expression (23). Further immunohistochemical analysis showed increased levels of
expression for c-fos, and transforming growth factor-β
(TGF-β), while transforming growth factor-α (TGF–α) and
epidermal growth factor were decreased in expressions
(23). Other studies indicated a change in the expression of
cytokeratins, with increased amounts of high molecular
weight keratins produced instead of the lower molecular
weight keratin found in the DMBA treated controls (24).
Neovacularization was also apparently reduced as
distinguished by fewer factor VIII antigen positive
endothelial cells present in the tissue sections (data not
shown).

The immunohistochemical results indicated that
various kinds of chemopreventative agents could produce
similar protein responses   leading to the suppression of
cell growth   in malignant and premalignant populations
of oral mucosal cells.

*In vitro* **studies:**
The in vitro studies substantiated the in vivo effects
noted above. In general the in vitro studies have been
developed to enhance the details of our knowledge of the
activities of the chemopreventatives such as, retinoids,
carotenoids, tocopherols, reduced glutathione, or ascorbic
acid which were used in the in vivo experiments.

Using human and hamster oral cell lines we have
conducted immunohistochemical, Western
immunoblotting, in situ hybridization, and flow
cytometry assays to detect the following biochemical
changes:

**Programmed cell death and cell cycle analysis:**
Increased numbers of the tumor cells in a dose response
manner exhibited nucleosome formation (DNA
fragmentation) following treatment with various
chemopreventative agents (figure 7.). In contrast to other
agents, β-carotene inhibited calcium flux, indicating a
possible reduction in glutathione synthesis. This was
further substantiated by determining a reduction in the
concentration of total mercaptans and non protein
sulfhydryls in the tumor cells. The protein expression
analysis also disclosed an increased expression for wild
type p53 and stress proteins hsp 90, and 70 (figure 8,9.).
In an immunoprecipitation assay hsp 70 was found to be
bound to mutant p53. The protein expression for mutant
p53 was also found to be decreased in expression. The
cells were also found to be accumulating in the pre
synthesis phase, $G_1$ of the cell cycle (figure 6.). P53 and
hsp 70 have both been shown in other studies to be
expressed in this phase of the cell cycle. Bcl-2 which is
known to suppress apoptosis was also seen to be
decreased in expression following treatment with β-
carotene and other chemopreventative agents.

To further characterize the cell cycle we
determined the levels of expression for various cyclins
and their kinases. The results indicated that cyclins A and
D were increased when β-carotene was used to treat the
oral cancer cells. These cyclins have been associated with
pre synthesis phases of the cell cycle. The cyclin kinases
cdck2 and cdcHs were also found to be increased in
expression. Cdc 2 kinases have been reported to be
connected to the development of programmed cell death.
Recently we have identified in our epidermal cancer cell
lines the increased expression of the FAS antigen. This
antigen has been related to the development of apoptosis
in thymocytes. Another tumor suppressor protooncogene
perhaps complexed to p53 and cyclin proteins is

retinoblastoma. The wild type form of protein was observed to be increased following β–carotene treatment of human oral carcinoma cells. Other protooncogenes associated with tumor promotion are c-neu and c-erbB2. The expression of protein products derived from these genes have both been found to be depressed with β-carotene treatment.

These results demonstrate remarkable protein biochemical changes and subsequent alterations in the growth potential of oral squamous carcinoma cells. The reduction in growth has indirectly been associated with the enhanced activity of tumor suppressor gene products.

**Signal and transcription factor induction:** Many of the chemopreventative agents are also associated with changes in the signal induction processes of the cell. We have documented these changes by observing the proteins and kinases associated with the G proteins. These observed protein changes help explain changes in the expression of various transcription factors. Specifically p21$^{ras}$ mutation derived protein was observed to be decreased in expression while the protooncogene form was observed to be increased in expression (23). Related to the ras type proteins are proteins that bind to the ras G protein complex. One of these proteins is SOS-1, and another is S6. They were found to be decreased in expression when the tumor cells were treated with β-carotene. Another protein which is related to this signal response cascade and is closer to the initiation of transcription factor expression is raf-1. Treatment with carotenoids such as, β-carotene and canthaxanthin depressed raf-1 expression while, retinoid treatment increased the expression of this signal protein. The process of signal induction is controlled by many kinases and enzymes. Carotenoids and retinoids tend to increase the expression of MAP kinase and protein kinase C, while decreasing phosphotyrosine kinase. This set of data indicates that various chemopreventative agents could alter the responsiveness of malignant cells by changing the signal responsive mechanism of these cells.

Other assays using the chemopreventative agent also produced changes in the protein products of various transcription factors. For example, β-carotene consistently increased the protein expression of c-fos and c-jun while the mRNA and the protein expression for c-myb was also increased. c-fos induction may be associated with increased DNA damages and apoptosis.

These studies indicated a series of possible indicators for the anti-tumor activity of β-carotene, other carotenoids, and tocopherols.

## The relationship of β-carotene to EGFR

Oral squamous cell carcinomas experimentally induced and those of unknown etiology presented by human patients, exhibit increased levels of expression for epidermal growth factor (EGF), and the number and affinity of the EGF receptor. EGF therefore is thought to play a major role in the promotion of oral carcinoma growth. Studies were undertaken to observe the relationship and role of EGF between a chemo-preventative agent, β-carotene, and the observed inhibition of oral cancer development.

Evidence that β-carotene could alter the responsiveness of oral squamous carcinoma cells to exogenous growth factors such as epidermal growth factor (EGF) came from binding studies, proliferation assays, Western immunoblotting, ELISA assays, immunohistochemistry, and the in situ hybridization for the mRNA expression of epidermal growth factor receptor(EGFR). These studies utilized oral cancer cell lines and a positive cell line control, A431, which exhibits high levels of EGFR.

The binding studies showed that β-carotene could compete with radiolabelled EGF and reduce the binding of this growth factor. The proliferation assay and the Western immunoblotting and other assays indicated that β-carotene inhibited the growth of the oral cancer cells by reducing the level expression of the EGFR and EGF. Additional Western immunoblotting indicated that the EGF-like protein and possible tumor promoting agent, TGF-a was also reduced following β-carotene treatment. The protooncogene c-erbBb2, which has been linked to EGFR derived protein presentation was also reduced in expression. These studies indicated a suppressive relationship with one or more growth factors that could reduce the growth of oral squamous cell carcinoma.

Changes in EGFR expression appears to be a later event in the development of oral malignancy, therefore consideration of EGFR changes may be indicative of a more aggressive malignant behavior.

**VE study assays:**

Previous *in vivo* studies have shown that alpha tocopherol acid succinate (VE) when administered either systematically or locally to an hamster undergoing oral carcinogenesis exhibited a significant inhibition of tumor development. We have also reported that VE could suppress the expression of mutant p53 protein during oral carcinogenesis (25). To further investigate this phenomenon in vitro studies were conducted. VE (50 μM) was used to treat the hamster oral carcinoma cell line, HCPC-1 for 3, 12, and 24 h. The inhibition of the tumor cell growth was confirmed using $^3$H-thymidine incorporation. This inhibition was reversed using the glutathione synthesis inhibitor butathionine-S,R-sulphoximine (100 μM) (BSO). VE treatment consequently increased the level of non protein sulfhydyls and total mercaptan concentrations. Cell cycle analysis using propidium iodide stained cells demonstrated the accumulation of the tumor cells in G1 of the cell cycle, with fewer cells in S or G2 + Mitosis compared to the untreated cell controls. Identically treated cells were analyzed for mutant and wild type p53 protein expression. Newly synthesized proteins were assessed by depleting the cells of methionine and then incorporating $^{35}$S-methionine for 6 h. VE (50 mM) 24h treatment produced changes in the protein profile. These radiolabelled lysates were used in immunoprecipitations demonstrating the suppression of mutant p53 expression. Analysis with cold HCPC-1 and VE treatment using Western immunoblotting and ELISA assays, confirmed that mutant p53 protein expression was reduced,while wild type expression was increased. Analysis with the confocal microscope also confirmed this pattern of p53 expression during the inhibition of oral carcinogenesis. In addition, Western immunoblotting showed the cyclin kinase cdc2 was increased as well as the formation of nucleosomes, as determined by a terminal transferase tunneling technique. This data appears to indicate that the VE mechanism of inhibition of tumor cell growth may involve the development of programmed cell death(figure 7.). Other comparable studies were conducted with VE acetate. These studies indicated that at the identical dose that VE acid succinate would decrease the growth of the tumor cells (50 µM) VE acetate would increase the growth of these tumor cells. In addition, VE acetate at this concentration would increase the expression of mutant p53, while also increasing wild type p53 expression. There was also a synergistic inhibitory growth effect observed between reduced glutathione and VE (25).

These studies indicated that VE possibly acts through a glutathione associated pathway. The end result is the development of programmed cell death, which was associated with changes in p53 expression and could therefore be considered as markers of VE antitumor activity.

These studies indicate that there are unique and interesting molecular and biochemical realtionships between chemopreventaative agents and their ability to suppress tumor cell growth. Further investigations into these relationships will help us to develop markers for determining the efficacy of their use in a clinical setting.

**Legends to figures:**

1.This figure provides a scheme of the relationships between antioxidants and prooxidants and their biologic effects.

2. The figure shows some biochemical relationships related to the development of apoptosis.

3. In situ hybribization of with antisense mRNA probe for histone 3. (1) normal oral hamster mucosa, (2) treatment with β-carotene and DMBA (6 wk.), (3) DMBA treatment (6wk.). (arrows show positive areas).

4. Scheme of relationship of oral carcinogenesis and apoptosis.

5. (A) Wild type p53 immunohistochemistry (hamster) (1.) normal mucosa, low level. (2.) β-carotene + DMBA treatment (12 wk), high level. (3) DMBA treatment (12 wk), lower levels. (4) β-carotene treatment normal mucosa, increased over normal levels. (B) mutant p53 staining and hsp 70 staining (1) normal oral mucosa, low level (2a) β-carotene +DMBA treatment, high levels of hsp 70 (12 wk), (2b) β-carotene + DMBA treatment (12 wk), low level of mutant p53, (3a) DMBA treatment (12 wk), lower hsp 70 staining, (3b) DMBA treatment (12 wk), high clonal levels of mutant p53.

6. Flow cytometry and Hoechst staining indicating β-carotene did not damage DNA of keratinocyte cell, or change cell cycle.

7. Induction of apotosis following treatment with chemopreventtative agents. Note changes in the morphology of these oral carcinoma cells. β-carotene

compared to heat shocking, both induced apoptosis but appear different.

8. Protein analysis. (A.) Lane 1. untreated oral cancer cells. Lane 2. heat shocking (42°C for 40 min). Lane 3. β-carotene (70 μM) (6h.).

(B) Immunoprecipitation with anti hsp 70. Western blot for p53. Lysate from β-carotene treatment. Hsp 70 binds p53. (m) markers, (1) antibody control, (2) untreated cells.

9. Western blotting for (A) hsp 70. Lane 1, untreated, Lane 2, heat shocking, Lane 3, β-carotene, Lane 4, canthaxanthin (70 μM, 6h), and Lane 5, retinyl palmitate (70 μM, 6h). Treatment increases hsp 70 expression. (B) Lane 2, 3, and 5 increases hsp 72 (constitutive). (C) Lane 2, 3, decreases mutant p53 expression. (D) Lanes 2–5 increases wild type p53 expression.

Figure 1.    **Pathway for Control of Cell Growth**

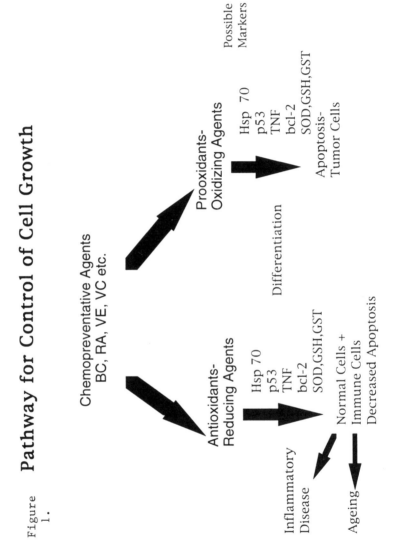

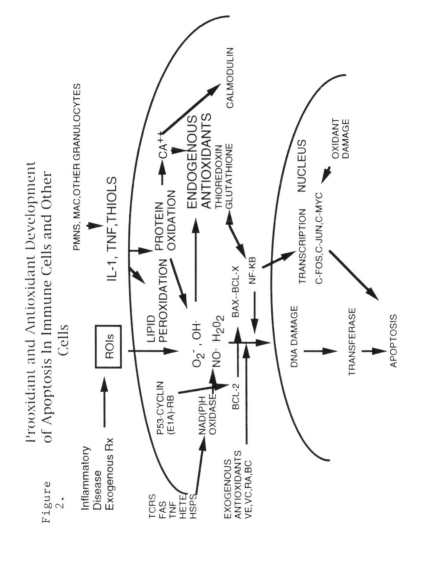

Figure 2. Prooxidant and Antioxidant Development of Apoptosis In Immune Cells and Other Cells

309

FIGURE 3.

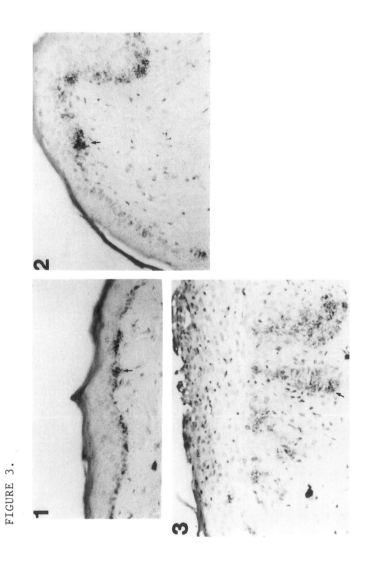

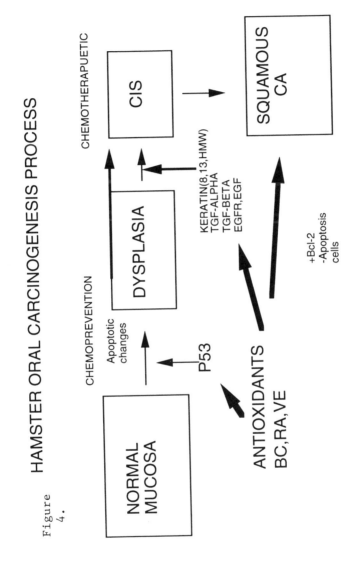

Figure 4. HAMSTER ORAL CARCINOGENESIS PROCESS

FIGURE 5.

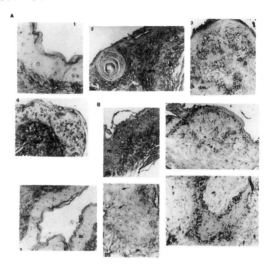

Figure 6.

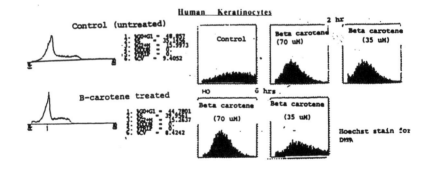

Figure 7.

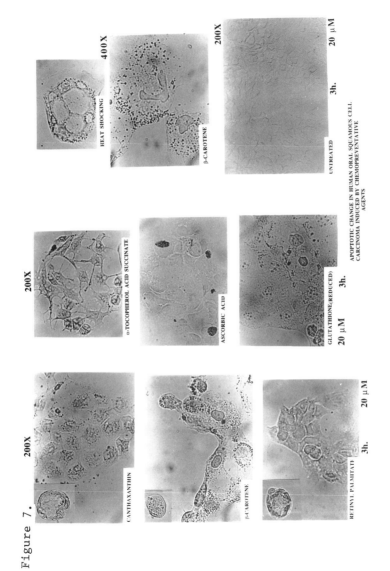

CANTHAXANTHIN

200X

β-CAROTENE

RETINYL PALMITATE

3h.          20 μM

α-TOCOPHEROL ACID SUCCINATE

200X

ASCORBIC ACID

GLUTATHIONE(REDUCED)

3h.

20 μM

HEAT SHOCKING

400X

β-CAROTENE

UNTREATED

200X

3h.          20 μM

APOPTOTIC CHANGE IN HUMAN ORAL SQUAMOUS CELL
CARCINOMA INDUCED BY CHEMOPREVENTATIVE
AGENTS

*313*

Figure 8.

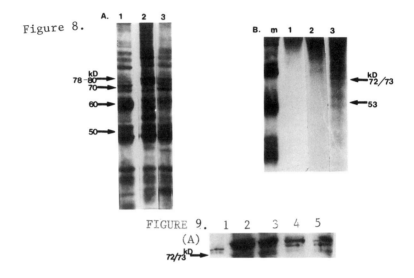

FIGURE 9.

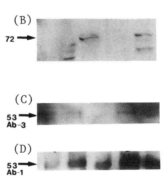

314

**Cited References**

1. Sugiyama M, Ando A, Furano A, et al. Cancer. Lett. 38; 1-7, 1987.

2. Schwartz JL, Sloane D, Shklar G. Tumor Biol. 10; 297-309, 1989.

3. Bendich A, Shapiro SS. J. Nutr. 116; 2259-2264, 1986.

4. Schwartz JL, Tanaka V, Khandekar V, Herman TS, Teicher BA. Cancer Chemother. Pharmacol. 29; 207-213, 1992.

5. Hockenberry D, Ohari ZN, Yin XM, Millman CL, Korsmeyer SJ. Cell 75; 241-251, 1993.

6. Mercer WE, Shields MT, Lin D, Appella E, Ullrich SJ. Proc. Natl. Acad. Sci. USA. 88; 1958-1962, 1991.

7. Reed JC. J. Cell Biol. 124; 1-6, 1994.

8. Welch WJ. Scientific Amer. May: 56-64, 1993.

9. Buttke TM, Sandstrom PA. J. NIH. Res. 6; 27-30, 1994.

10. Hightower LE. Cell 66; 191-197, 1991.

11. Hockenberry D, Nunez G, Milliman C, et. al. Nature. 348; 334-336, 1990.

12. Shi Y, Glynn JM, Guilbertt LJ, et. al. Science 257, 212-214, 1992.

13. Itoh N, Tsujimoto Y, Nagata S. J. Immunol. 151; 621-627, 1993.

14. Jacobson MD, Burne JF, King MP, et. al. Nature 361; 365-369, 1993.

15. Israel N, Gargerot-Pocidalo MA, Aillet F, Virelizier JL. J. Immunol. 149; 3386-3393, 1992.

16. Israel A. Nature. 369; 443-444, 1994.

17. Schwarrtz JL, Antonaides DZ, Zhao S. N. Y. Acad. Sci. 1228; 262-279, 1993.

18. Schwatz JL, Shklar G. J. Oral Maaxilo Fac. Surg. 50; 363-373, 1992.

19. Marshall CJ. Science 259; 1865-1866, 1993.

20. Levine RL, Oliver CN, Fulks RM, Stadtman R. Proc. Natl. Acad. Sci. USA 78; 2120-2124, 1981.

21. Shklar G., Schwartz JL. Oral Oncol. Eur. J. Cancer. 29B; 9-16, 1993.

22. Suda D, Schwartz JL, Shklar G. Carcinogenesis. 7; 7121-715, 1986.

23. Schwartz JL, Chapter 11, Adjuvant Nutrition in Cancer Treatment. 173-233, 1993.

24. Shklar G, West K, Schwartz JL. J. Dent Res. 73; 359, 1994.

25. Schwartz JL, Shklar G, Trickler D. Oral Oncol. Eur. J. Cancer. 29B; 313-318, 1993.

INHIBITION AND REGRESSION OF EXPERIMENTAL ORAL CANCER BY

BETA CAROTENE AND VITAMIN E:    EMERGING CONCEPTS

Gerald Shklar

Harvard School of Dental Medicine

188 Longwood Avenue, Boston, MA    02115

Abstract

The hamster buccal pouch experimental model for oral
cancer has proven to be a superior model for oral mucosal
carcinogenesis and is now receiving wide attention as one
of the better overall experimental models for carcinogenesis.  The malignant tumors are epidermoid carcinomas that
develop slowly, in response to polyaromatic hydrocarbon
carcinogen application, and are preceded by a keratotic
and dysplastic lesion comparable to human precancerous
leukoplakia.  The hamster lesions are indistinguishable
histologically from human oral epidermoid carcinomas of
the well-to-moderately differentiated variety, at both
light microscopic and ultrastructural levels. Both animal
and human lesions have similar metabolic markers, such as
gamma glutamyl transpeptidase (GGT) and lactic dehydrogenase.
The hamster carcinoma develops with the activation and
expression of specific oncogenes, often similar to those
expressed in human oral cancer. These include c-erbB1, H-
ras, K-ras, and mutant p53. The hamster lesions are clearly
visible at all times and can be counted and measured at
different stages of development so that figures can be
obtained for overall tumor burden.  The hamster tumors are
also closely related to immune control, as in humans. The
hamster tumor development is enhanced by immunosuppressive
drugs such as cortisone and methotrexate, and retarded by
immunoenhancing agents such as levamisole or BCG.

In the quest for chemopreventative agents, it was found

that hamster oral carcinogenesis could be retarded by
retinoids such as 13-cis-retinoic acid. However, retinoids
were found to be toxic and to have a co-carcinogenic potential.  Beta carotene and vitamin E were found to be non-
toxic and inhibited oral carcinogenesis when applied
topically, injected in the tumor area, or administered
systemically by mouth.  Regression of established carcinomas was also possible when beta carotene or vitamin E
was injected into the tumor site. Mixtures of beta carotene
and vitamin E were found more effective antitumor agents
than the individual substances, indicating a synergism.
Mixtures of various antioxidants have been studied and
found to be highly effective. Current research is aimed at
an understanding of mechanism. These studies use both
hamster tumors and cell lines in culture from both hamster
carcinomas and human oral carcinomas. A concept has been
established of a common pathway for the destruction of cancer cells.  Beta carotene, vitamin E, and other antioxidants
act as immunostimulators in one branch of the pathway. They
stimulate the migration to tumor site and the antitumor
activity of cytotoxic macrophages, bearing TNF-alpha, and
cytotoxic T lymphocytes, bearing TNF-beta. In the other
branch of the common pathway, the antioxidant nutrients
stimulate enhanced expression of a variety of proteins,
including 70 and 90 kD stress proteins.  There is also a
dramatic reduction in mutant p53 and an increased
expression of the wild type (antioncogene) p53 protein
product. The antioxidant nutrients appear to enhance the
tumor suppressor p53 gene and to dysregulate or inactivate
the mutant p53 oncogene. The cancer cells are selectively
destroyed in a process described as apoptosis. The antioxidants also inhibit angiogenesis, which would also
contribute to the death of cancer cells. Many clinical
applications can be suggested, based on this animal
research.


Introduction

    The relationship of nutrition and nutritional supple-
ments to cancer incidence and development can be studied
by epidemiologic and clinical approaches, but these
investigations must depend upon a proper appreciation of
basic biologic principles underlying tumor development.
These principles are being elucidated from extensive
animal experimentation, studies in the clinical pathology
of cancer patients undergoing therapy, and studies of human
and animal tumors in cell culture. Animal models of cancer

have the major advantage of actually initiating the malignant tumors and following their course of development or natural history. The developing tumors can be observed grossly and examined microscopically. Animals can be autopsied for detailed study of tumor spread, both local and metastatic. Tumor cells can be studied with increasing magnigication through the techniques of electron microscopy. Molecular events can be studied during carcinogenesis, and various growth factors, genes and gene products can be studied with molecular techniques such as in-situ hybridization and immunohistochemistry. A good animal model simulates the human cancer that it is meant to study, and may even be preceded by a precancerous state comparable to that in the human condition. Animal models should also be able to respond to various preventative and therapeutic modalities, suggesting approaches to human cancer.

The hamster cheek pouch carcinoma model is an excellent model for mucosal carcinogenesis. It is the best available model for oral cancer and is currently receiving widespread attention as one of the better animal models for solid tumors (1). This model, originally established by Salley in 1954 (2), and developed by Morris (3) and others (4,5) has many obvious advantages. The tumors are epidermoid (squamous cell) carcinomas, they develop slowly in response to the application of polyaromatic hydrocarbon carcinogen, and are preceded by a keratotic and dysplastic lesion comparable to human oral leukoplakia (6.7). The hamster lesions are indistinguishable from human oral squamous cell carcinomas of the well-to-moderately differentiated variety, at both light microscopic and ultrastructural levels (8,9). Both hamster and human carcinomas have similar metabolic markers, such as gamma glutamyl transpeptidase (10,11), lactic dehydrogenase (12,13), and keratin 19 (14).

The hamster buccal pouch lesions are clearly visible at all times and can be counted and measured at different stages of development so that figures can be obtained for overall tumor burden and these can be demonstrated graphically to illustrate significant differences in tumor yield under various experimental conditions (15). Significant recent findings in this model relate to immune control, gene expression, and molecular markers. The development of tumors in the hamster cheek pouch model was found to be related to immune control, as in humans (16). The tumors were found to develop more rapidly when the animal's

immune system was depressed by cortisone (17), methotrexate
(18), or specific antilymphocyte serum (19). Conversely,
tumor development was inhibited by immunoenhancing agents,
such as bacillus Calmette-Guerin (BCG) (20), or levamisole,
an antihelminthic drug (21). The hamster tumors were also
found to express specific oncogenes, often similar to those
expressed in human oral cancer. The hamster carcinoma was
found to develop with the expression of the c-erbB1
oncogene (22), a specific oncogene expressed in many human
oral cancers (23). Increased expression of mutated Ha-ras
and Ki-ras oncogenes also occurred in both animal and human
oral cancers (24-26). Another important feature of the
hamster buccal pouch model is that it can be studied for
influences that may initiate or promote (1,27). This concept
of initiation and promotion is of major importance in
attempting to evaluate various environmental and infectious
influences in humans, such as tobacco, alcohol, chronic
irritation, or herpes simplex virus. The hamster buccal
pouch has been used to demonstrate the co-carcinogenic or
promoting effect of chronic irritation (28), alcohol (29)
or herpes infections (30). A further advantage of the
hamster cheek pouch model for oral cancer is that cancer
cell lines can be developed from this model (31) and these
can be compared to human oral cancer cell lines for the
study of molecular and genetic markers.

A series of experiments carried out in our laboratory
has utilized the hamster cheek pouch to study the effect of
micronutrients on oral cancer development, separately, and
in various combinations. Based on investigations showing
the effect of retinoids on experimental bladder cancer (32),
we found that 13-cis-retinoic acid inhibited carcinogenesis
of the hamster buccal pouch (33). However, the systemic
dosage required for the significant tumor inhibition produced both renal and hepatotoxicity in many of the animals.
Retinyl acetate was found to be less toxic but also less
effective than 13-cis-retinoic acid as a tumor inhibiter
(34). Vitamin E (alpha tocopherol) was found to be an
extremely effective inhibiter of cancer development in the
hamster model (35), and was free of toxicity. The development of both precancerous leukoplakia and carcinomas was
significantly inhibited.  In subsequent studies, using a
modification of the hamster pouch model with application of
a 0.1 % solution of DMBA three times per week rather than
the standard 0.5% solution, vitamin E was able to totally
prevent the development of precancerous leukoplakia or
cancer (36). Beta carotene was found to inhibit experi-

mental oral carcinogenesis in the hamster (37) and also was
found to be free of toxicity. Schwartz and associates (38,39)
demonstrated that beta carotene not only inhibited the
development of cancer in the hamster buccal pouch, but
could also regress established cancer in this animal model,
when injected close to the tumor site.Vitamin E was also
found to be capable of regressing established cancers, when
injected locally (40). While beta carotene and vitamin E,
administered separately by oral route, could not effect
cancer regression, they were able to do so in combination
by acting synergistically (41). Other antioxidants, such
as reduced glutathione (42), have also been shown to be
capable of inhibiting carcinogenesis of the hamster buccal
pouch, and a mixture of beta carotene, vitamin E, vitamin C
and glutathione has been shown to be the most effective
anticancer or cancer preventative grouping of antioxidants
for the hamster model (43).

Current studies are attempting to elucidate the
mechanisms whereby the antioxidant micronutrients exert
their cancer preventative effect. From these studies has
emerged the concept of a common pathway through which these
agents act (44). Despite their different chemical structures,
these agents appear to act in a similar manner through the
common pathway for anticancer activity. The pathway has two
major functional channels. One wing of the common pathway
is a series of immune reactions, resulting in immunoenhance-
ment and destruction of cancer cells through "immunosurveillance". In the hamster system it has been shown that
there is an increased production of cytotoxic macrophages
carrying tumor necrosis factor alpha, and cytotoxic lymphocytes carrying tumor necrosis factor beta. These cells are
attracted to the tumor site and act to destroy the tumor
cells (45). Even in the experiments where there is a complete prevention of gross tumors, there is microscopic
evidence of tumors being initiated and being destroyed by
the immune cells; and this has been the first clear demonstration of the concept of "immunosurveillance", originally
postulated by Ehrlich in 1909 (46). The nature of the
"signal" coming from the tumor site has not yet been established, but is has been shown that in early cancer development in the hamster model, there is an influx of mast cells
into the tumor site and a deposition of the mast cell
granules at the tumor site (47). This will be a fruitful
area for further research. Eosinophil leukocytes are also
attracted to sites of early carcinogenesis, and have been

found by Wong and associates to be a rich source of transforming growth factor-alpha (TGF $\lambda$) within experimental oral
tumors (48). Whatever the "signal" is, it is effective in
stimulating a series of immune and molecular events that
comprise the common pathway and result in a potent anticancer effect.

The other wing of the common pathway is a stimulation
by the tumor cells of a group of proteins, including heat
shock proteins kD 70 and 90. (49). This appears to exert an
influence on the p53 gene complex in the tumors. Using the
hamster model, it has been shown that there is increased
expression of the natural or "wild type" p53 protein. This
is the tumor suppressor gene product. There is also a
decreased expression of mutant p53, which is recognized as
an oncogene, and appears to be expressed in many different
types of malignancy (50). The p53 wing of the common pathway has been shown to be activated by vitamin E, beta
carotene, and glutathione (51). The cancer cells are shown
to be killed in the process of "apoptosis" or programmed
cell death (52). Another aspect of the common pathway for
tumor inhibition by antioxidant micronutrients is an inhibition of tumor angiogenesis. It can be shown in the hamster
model that there is a notable decrease in vascularity as
the carcinomas are regressing under the influence of micronutrient mixtures, and there are also significantly fewer
capillaries at the tumor margins in the experiments where
tumor inhibition is effected by micronutrients. This may be
further evidence for the concept, originally formulated by
Folkman (53), that tumors are angiogenesis-dependent. The
micronutrients, in some way, are blocking those factors
that stimulate tumor angiogenesis. TGF may be one of these
factors, and this is now being studied.

Clinical applications

There are many clinical applications that are obvious.
Several epidemiologic studies have offered some persuasive
evidence through serum or plasma levels that beta carotene
and vitamin E relate to the incidence of lung cancer (54)
and dysplasia and cancer of uterine cervix (55). Recent
clinical investigations have demonstrated the effectiveness
of various micronutrients in regressing oral precancerous
leukoplakis. (56-58) Well planned long-term prospective
studies, based on the fundamental principles of cancer
biology, will be required to determine whether these
nutritional supplements (probably in combinations for

synergistic effect) will lower the risk for oral cancer and other forms of cancer. Injections or infusions of micronutrients may be successful in regressing tumors if they can reach the tumor site in sufficient quantity. Human cancer cells in culture are easily destroyed by these micronutrients (59). These agents may also be effective in conjunction with various chemotherapeutic drugs, as shown in recent experiments (60).

The future of antioxidants micronutrients, of course, is limitless. They are already being prescribed to lower the risk of heart attacks and they may play a significant role in affecting the aging process generally. The cancer story has been the opening chapter in this fascinating biomedical story, but future research will use micronutrients to attack many problems in medicine and biology.

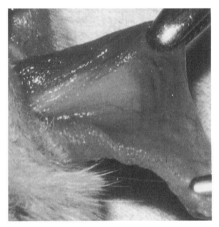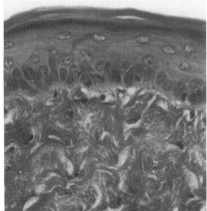

Left buccal pouch in normal untreated hamster. Mucosa is slightly keratinized.

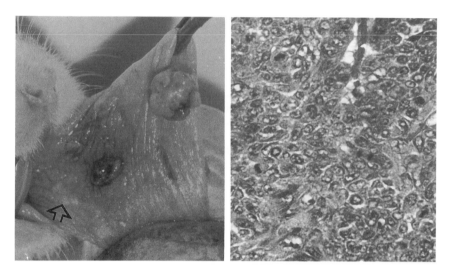

Left buccal pouch in hamster after 12 weeks of thrice
weekly applications of a 0.5 per cent solution of
7,12-dimethylbenz(a)anthracene in heavy mineral oil.  Note
leukoplakic patches (arrow) and epidermoid carcinomas.
Histology is that of carcinoma at right.

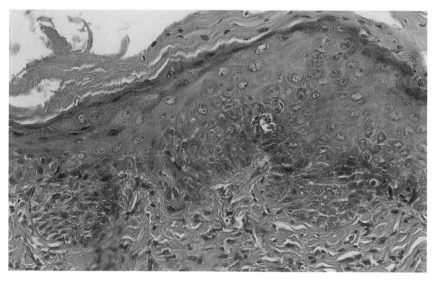

Hyperkeratosis and dysplasia characteristic of the
leukoplakic lesions induced by DMBA application.

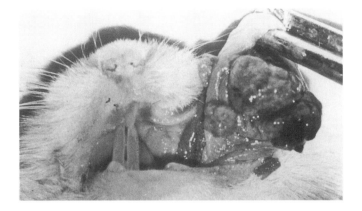

Large mass of tumor in cheek pouch of control animal after 28 weeks of thrice weekly application of a 0.1 per cent DMBA solution in heavy mineral oil.

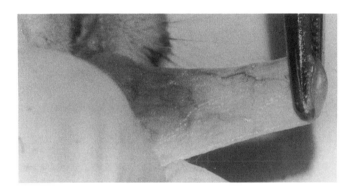

Cheek pouch of experimental animal after 28 weeks of thrice weekly DMBA painting with a 0.1 per cent solution, and given 10 mg vitamin E thrice weekly on days alternate to DMBA painting. No tumors or leukoplakic lesions are apparent. There has been complete prevention of lesions by the systemically administered (by mouth) vitamin E.

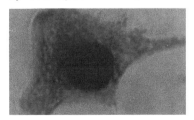

Macrophage stained specifically for tumor necrosis factor alpha.

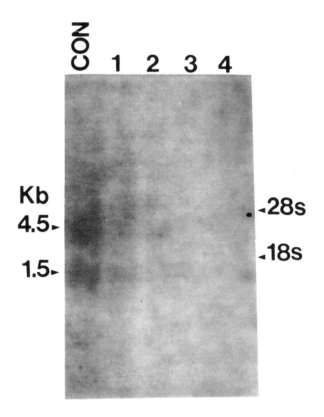

Gel showing expression for c-erbB1 proto-oncogene in HCPC
epidermoid carcinoma cell line derived from a hamster
cheek pouch tumor (control, left lane). The succeeding
lanes show loss of expression of the oncogene with
increasing doses of beta carotene added to the cultures
of the cancer cells.

A Common Pathway For Cancer Inhibition/Prevention/Regression
By Nutrients

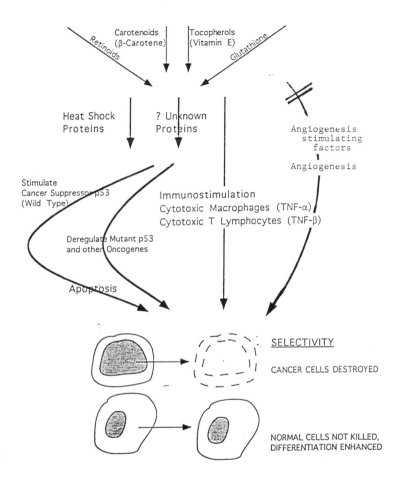

References:

1.  Gimenez-Conti, I. B., and Slaga, T. J. The hamster
    cheek pouch carcinogenesis model. J. Cellular Biochem.,
    17F: 83-90, 1993.
2.  Salley, J. J. Experimental carcinogenesis in the cheek
    pouch of the Syrian hamster. J. Dent. Res., 33: 253-
    258, 1954.
3.  Morris, A. L. Factors influencing experimental car-
    cinogenesis in the hamster cheek pouch. J. Dent. Res.,
    40: 3-10, 1961.
4.  Silberman, S., and Shklar, G. The effect of a carci-
    nogen (DMBA) applied to the hamster's buccal pouch in
    combination with croton oil. Oral Surg., 16: 1344-
    1355, 1963.
5.  Shklar, G. Experimental oral pathology in the Syrian
    hamster. Prog. Exp. Tumor Res., 16: 518-538, 1972.
6.  Santis, H., Shklar, G., and Chauncey, H. The histo-
    chemistry of experimentally induced leukoplakia and
    carcinoma of the hamster buccal pouch. Oral Surg.,
    17: 207-218, 1964.
7.  Shklar, G. Oral leukoplakia. N.E.J. Med., 315: 1544-
    1546, 1986.
8.  Weerapradist, W., and Shklar, G. Vitamin E inhibition
    of hamster buccal pouch carcinogenesis. A gross, his-
    tologic and ultrastructural study. Oral Surg., 54:
    304-312, 1982.
9.  Shklar, G., Eisenberg, E., and Flynn, E. Immuno-
    enhancing agents and experimental leukoplakia and
    carcinoma of the hamster model pouch. Prog. Exp. Tumor
    Res., 24: 269-282, 1979.
10. Solt, D. B. Localization of gamma-glutamyl-transpep-
    tidase in hamster buccal pouch epithelium treated
    with 7,12 dimethylbenz(a)anthracene. J. Natl. Cancer
    Inst., 67: 193-200, 1981.
11. Solt, D. B., and Shklar, G. Rapid induction of gamma-
    glutamyl transpeptidase-rich intraepithelial clones in
    7,12-dimethylbenz(a)-anthracene treated hamster buccal
    pouch. cancer Res., 42: 285-291, 1982.
12. Shklar, G. Lactic dehydrogenase activity in cytologic
    smears of normal oral mucosa and epidermoid carcinoma,
    Acta. Cytol., 9: 437-439, 1965.
13. Shklar, G. Metabolic characteristics of experimental
    hamster pouch carcinomas. Oral Surg., 20: 336-339,
    1965.

14. Lindberg, K., and Rheinwald, J. G. Suprabasal 40 Kd keratin expression as an immunohistological marker of premalignancy in oral epithelium. Am. J. Path., 134: 89-98, 1989.

15. Niukian, K., Schwartz, J., and Shklar, G. Effects of Onion extract on the development of hamster buccal pouch carcinogenesis as expressed in tumor burden. Nutr. Cancer, 9: 171-176, 1987.

16. Woods, D. A. Influence of antilymphocyte serum on DMBA induction of oral carcinomas. Nature, 224: 276-279, 1969.

17. Shklar, G. cortisone and hamster buccal pouch carcinogenesis. Cancer Res., 26: 246-263, 1966.

18. Shklar, G., Cataldo, E., and Fitzgerald, A. The effect of methotrexate on chemical carcinogenesis of hamster buccal pouch. Cancer Res., 26: 2218-2224, 1966.

19. Giunta, J., and Shklar, G. The effect of antilymphocyte serum on experimental hamster buccal pouch carcinogenesis. Oral Surg., 31: 344-355, 1971.

20. Giunta, J., Reif, A. E., and Shklar, G. Bacillus Calmette-Guerin and antilymphocyte serum in carcinogenesis. Arch. Pathol., 98: 237-240, 1974.

21, Eisenberg, E., and Shklar, G. Levamisole and hamster buccal pouch carcinogenesis. Oral Surg., 43: 562-574, 1977.

22. Wong, D. T. W., and Biswas, D. K. Activation of c-erb B oncogene in the hamster cheek pouch during DMBA-induced carcinogenesis. Oncogene, 2: 67-72, 1987.

23. Merlino, G. T., Xu, H. Y., Ishii, S., et al: Elevated epidermal growth factor receptor gene copy number and expression in a squamous carcinoma cell line. Science, 224: 417-491, 1974.

24. Husain, Z., Fei, Y., Roy, S., Solt, D. B., Polverini, P. J., and Biswas, D. K. Sequential expression and co-operative interaction of c-Ha-ras and c-erb B genes in in vivo chemical carcinogenesis. Proc. Natl. Acad. Sci. USA., 86: 1264-1268, 1989.

25. Gimenez-Conti, I. B., Bianchi, A. B., Stockman, S. L., Conti, C. J., and Slaga, T. J. Activating mutation of the Ha-ras gene in chemically induced tumors of the hamster buccal pouch. Mol. Carcinogenesis, 5: 259-263, 1992.

26. Wong, D. T. W., Gertz, R., Chow, P., et al: Detection of Ki-ras mRNA in normal and chemically transformed hamster oral keratinocytes. Cancer Res., 49: 4562-4567, 1989.

27. Odukoya, O., Shklar, G. Initiation and promotion in experimental oral carcinogenesis. Oral Surg., 58: 315-323, 1984.

28. Silberman, S., and Shklar, G. The effect of a carcinogen (DMBA) applied to the hamster buccal pouch in combination with croton oil. Oral Surg., 16: 1344-1360, 1963.

29. Freedman, A., and Shklar, G. Alcohol and hamster buccal pouch carcinogenesis. Oral Surg., 46: 794-810, 1978.

30. Oh, J. S., Paik, D., Christensen, R., Akoto-Amanfo, E., Kim, K., and Park, N-H. Herpes simplex virus enhances the 7,12-dimethylbenz(a)anthracene (DMBA) induced carcinogenesis and amplification and over expression of c-erb-B1 proto-oncogene in hamster buccal pouch. Oral Surg., 68: 428-435, 1989.

31. Okukoya, O., Schwartz, J., Weichselbaum, R., and Shklar, G. An epidermoid carcinoma cell line derived from hamster 7,12 dimethylbenz(a)anthracene induced buccal pouch tumors. J. Natl. Cancer Inst., 71: 1253-1264, 1983.

32. Sporn, M. B., Dunlop, N. M., Newton, D. L., and Smith, J. M. Prevention of chemical carcinogenesis by vitamin A and its synthetic analogs (retinoids). Fed. Proc., 35: 1332-1338, 1976.

33. Shklar, G., Schwartz, J., Grau, D., Trickler, D. P., and Wallace, D. K. Inhibition of hamster buccal pouch carcinogenesis by 13-cis retinoic acid. Oral Surg., 50: 45-53, 1980.

34. Burge-Bottenbley, A., and Shklar, G. Retardation of experimental oral cancer development by retinyl acetate. Nutr. Cancer., 5: 121-129, 1983.

35. Shklar, G. Inhibition of oral mucosal carcinogenesis by vitamin E. J. Natl. Cancer Inst., 68: 791-797, 1982.

36. Trickler, D., Shklar, G. Prevention by vitamin E of oral carcinogenesis. J. Natl, Cancer Inst., 78: 165-169, 1987.

37. Suda, D., Schwartz, J., Shklar, G. Inhibition of experimental oral carcinogenesis by topical beta carotene. Carcinogenesis., 7: 711-715, 1986.

38. Schwartz, J., Suda, D., Light, G. Beta carotene is associated with the regression of hamster buccal pouch carcinoma and the induction of tumor necrosis factor in macrophages. Biochem. Biophys. Res. Commun., 136: 1130-1135, 1986.

39. Schwartz, J., Shklar, G. Regression of experimental oral carcinoma by local injection of beta carotene and canthaxanthin. Nutr. Cancer., 11: 35–40, 1988.
40. Shklar, G., Schwartz, J., Trickler, D. P., Niukian, K. Regression by vitamin E of experimental oral cancer. J. Natl. Cancer Inst., 78: 987–992, 1987.
41. Shklar, G., Schwartz, J., Trickler, D., and Reid, S. Regression of experimental cancer by oral administration of combined alpha tocopherol and beta carotene. Nutr. Cancer., 12: 321–325, 1989.
42. Trickler, D., Shklar, G., and Schwartz, J. Inhibition of oral carcinogenesis by glutathione. Nutr. Cancer., 20: 139–144, 1993.
43. Shklar, G., Schwartz, J., Trickler, D., and Reid-Cheverie, S. The effectiveness of a mixture of beta carotene, alpha tocopherol, glutathione and ascorbic acid for cancer chemoprevention. Nutr. Cancer., 20: 145–151, 1993.
44. Shklar, G., and Schwartz, J. L. A common pathway for the destruction of cancer cells: experimental evidence and clinical implications. Int. J. Oncol., 41: 215–224, 1994.
45. Shklar, G., Schwartz, J. L. Tumor necrosis factor in experimental cancer regression with alpha tocopherol, beta carotene and alga extract. Eur. J. Cancer Clin. Oncol., 24: 839–850, 1988.
46. Shklar, G., Schwartz, J. L., Trickler, D. P., and Reid, S. Prevention of experimental cancer and immunostimulation by vitamin E (Immunosurveillance). J. Oral Pathol. Med., 19: 60–64, 1990.
47. Flynn, E. A., Schwartz, J. L., and Shklar, G. Sequential mast cell infiltration and degranulation during experimental carcinogenesis. J. Cancer Res. Clin. Oncol., 117: 115–122, 1991.
48. Wong, D. T. W. TGF-alpha and oral carcinogenesis. Oral Oncol. Eur. J. Cancer., 29B: 3–7, 1993.
49. Schwartz, J. L., Antoniades, D. Z., and Zhao, S. Molecular and biochemical reprogramming of oncogenesis through the activity of prooxidants or antioxidants. Ann. N.Y. Acad. Sc., 478, 1993.
50. Schwartz, J. L., Shklar, G., and Trickler, D. P. p53 in the anticancer mechanism of vitamin E. Oral Oncol. Eur. J. Cancer., 29B: 313–318, 1993.

51.  Trickler, D. P., West, K., Shklar, G., and Schwartz, J. L. Mutant p 53 decrease during glutathione inhibition of oral carcinogenesis. J. Dent. Res., 73: 264, 1944.

52.  Schwartz, J. L. Beta carotene induced programmed cell death. J. Dent. Res., 72: 283, 1993.

53.  Folkman, J. What is the evidence that tumors are angiogenesis dependent? J. Nat. Cancer Inst., 82: 4-6, 1990.

54.  Menkes, M. S., Comstock, G. W., Vuilleumier, J. P., et al: Serum beta carotene, vitamins A and E, selenium and the risk of lung cancer. N. Engl. J. Med., 315: 1250-1254, 1986.

55.  Palan, P. R., Mikhail, M. S., Basu, J., and Romney, S. L. Plasma levels of antioxidant beta carotene and tocopherol in uterine cervix dysplasia and cancer. Nutr. Cancer., 15: 13-20, 1991.

56.  Hong, W. K., Endicott, J., Itri, L. M. et al: 13-cis retinoic acid in the treatment of oral leukoplakia. N. Engl. J. Med., 315: 1501-1510, 1986.

57.  Brenner, S. E., Winn, R. J., Lippman, S. M., Poland, J., Hansen, K. S. et al: Regression of oral leukoplakia with tocopherol: A community clinical oncology program. Chemopreventative study. J. Natl. Cancer Inst., 85: 44-48, 1993.

58.  Garewal, H. S., Meyskens, F. L., Killen, D., et al: Response of oral leukoplakia to beta carotene. J. Clin. Oncol., 8: 1711-1720, 1990.

59.  Schwartz, J., and Shklar, G. The selective cytotoxic effect of carotenoids and tocopherol on human cancer cell lines in vitro. J. Oral Maxillofac. Surg., 50: 367-373, 1992.

60.  Schwartz, J. L., Tanaka, V., Khandekar, V., Herman, T. S., and Teicher, B. A. Beta carotene and/or vitamin E as modulators of alkylating agents in SCC-25 human squamous carcinoma cells. Cancer Chemother. Pharmacol., 29: 207-214, 1992.

NOVEL APPROACHES TO THE PREVENTION OF CHEMOTHERAPY-INDUCED

ALOPECIA

Joaquin J. Jimenez and Adel A. Yunis

Depts. of Medicine and Biochemistry and Molecular
Biology, University of Miami School of Medicine,
Miami, Florida

## INTRODUCTION

Alopecia is a common and most distressing side effect
of cancer chemotherapy.  Although of no prognostic significance, alopecia can impact heavily on the quality of life in
the cancer patient.  Thus, in a recent study, 35 of 46
patients receiving chemotherapy ranked alopecia as a more
important side effect than vomiting (1).  There are currently no satisfactory methods to prevent it.  Our work using
the young rat model has provided new insight into the problem and has opened new avenues for further investigation.
Furthermore some of the agents we have recently used successfully to prevent chemotherapy-induced alopecia in the young
rat have excellent potential applicability in the clinical
setting.

## THE YOUNG RAT AS A MODEL

Prevention of Cytosine Arabinoside (ARA-C)-Induced Alopecia
by ImuVert and Interleukin 1 (IL-1β)

Our initial discovery was made during attempts to cure
chloroleukemia in the rat by a combination of differentiation
induction and chemotherapy.  We used ImuVert, a biological
response modifier prepared from Serratia marcescens as the
differentiation inducer (2) and ARA-C as the chemotherapeutic agent.  Rats receiving ARA-C alone became totally

alopecic whereas rats receiving a combination of ARA-C plus
ImuVert were completely protected from alopecia (3). Each
of these two observations was important. Thus the fact that
we were able to produce alopecia in the young rat by the injection of ARA-C suggested that the young rat could serve
as an excellent animal model for investigating chemotherapy-
induced alopecia. Furthermore, the prevention of the alopecia by a biological response modifier, ImuVert, could have
both biological as well as clinical implications. Indeed
further studies have corroborated both of these conclusions.

The first question we addressed concerned the mechanism
of protection by ImuVert. Since ImuVert is known to stimulate the secretion of cytokines by macrophages, including
IL-1, TNF we postulated that protection may be mediated by
one or more of these cytokines. In further studies we demonstrated that IL-1β was as effective as ImuVert in protecting young rats from ARA-C-induced alopecia (4). We also
provided evidence that protection by IL-1 was, at least in
part, due to a block in DNA synthesis in the hair follicles
(cell cycle blockade) thus rendering them less sensitive to
ARA-C (5).

Induction of Alopecia by Other Chemotherapeutic Agents

Our observations on ARA-C-induced alopecia and its prevention by ImuVert and IL-1, prompted us to pursue this problem further with the objective of enhancing the translation
of our findings to the clinical setting. We, therefore,
embarked on extensive testing to determine: 1. The relative
ability of some of the known chemotherapeutic drugs to produce alopecia in the young rat and, 2. The possible protection of a variety of agents including growth factors,
cytokines, etc.

Drugs known to be potent in producing alopecia in the
clinical setting, e.g. cytoxan (CTX), etoposide (VP16), and
adriamycin (ADM) were also able to produce severe alopecia
in the young rat.

More recently we have also been able to produce alopecia by Taxol. However, somewhat different conditions were
required. Taxol given intraperitoneally at tolerable doses
did not induce alopecia. After extensive experimentation,
it was found that the intradermal injection of 2 μg Taxol on

day 11 and 12 of age produced alopecia at the site of injection. It thus became possible for us to use the young rat as a suitable model to study Taxol-induced alopecia.

Upon further testing we found that the protective effect of ImuVert or IL-1 on ARA-induced alopecia could not be extended to other chemotherapeutic agents. Thus when used under similar conditions neither ImuVert nor IL-1 protected the rat from Cytoxan-induced alopecia. Since cancer chemotherapy more often involves the use of combination regimens which frequently include alkylating agents as well as ADM, we directed our attention to other possible compounds and ways to prevent alopecia from these agents.

### PREVENTION OF CHEMOTHERAPY-INDUCED ALOPECIA BY N-ACETYLCYSTEINE

We first elected to test N-acetylcysteine (NAC) on the basis of a number of previous observations. NAC has been used to protect against toxicity from a variety of agents including paracetamol (6), doxorubicin (7), bleomycin (8), cyclophosphamide (9), and irradiation (10). The results of our studies clearly demonstrated protection from CTX-induced alopecia by parenteral NAC as well as by a preparation of NAC in liposomes applied topically (11). More recently we have demonstrated that the topical application of NAC dissolved in absolute alcohol protected from alopecia induced by CTX or CTX-ADM combination (Fig. 1).

The mechanism of protection from chemotherapy-induced alopecia by NAC is not completely understood. N-acetyl-cysteine is known to possess strong antioxidant activity both because of its ability to enhance glutathione synthesis as well as act as an oxygen radical scavenger. Since toxicity from both CTX and ADM is at least in part a result of oxygen radical damage, NAC could exert its protective effect through its antioxidant activity. However, it is likely that the mechanism is more complex and deserves further study.

The successful prevention of alopecia from combination chemotherapy by NAC applied topically in the rat may have excellent clinical potential in view of the simplicity of application and the nontoxic nature of NAC. Clinical trials should be possible in the near future.

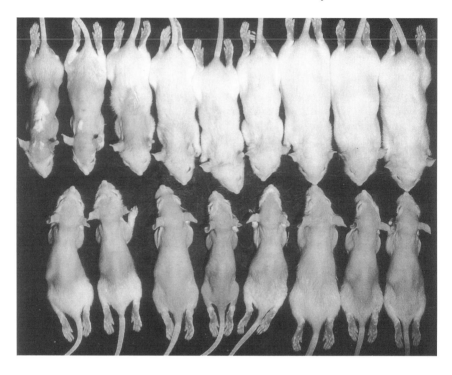

Fig. 1. Protection from (CTX + ADM)-Induced Alopecia by NAC. Two groups of 11 day old rats were given CTX 25 mg/kg i.p. x 1 day and ADM 2.5 mg/kg i.p. x 3 days. In addition, top (experimental) group received NAC (25 mg in 0.25 ml ETOH) applied topically over the head, neck and back one day prior to chemotherapy, followed by daily applications 4 hours prior and 4 hours post chemotherapy and two applications eight hours apart the day after last chemotherapy. Bottom (control) group received ETOH applied topically similarly. After topical treatment with either NAC or ETOH, rats were then kept individually separated for a period of 3 hours, following which the treated area was carefully washed. Photographs were taken on day 10.

PREVENTION OF CHEMOTHERAPY-INDUCED ALOPECIA
BY VITAMIN $D_3$ AND ITS METABOLITES

A very exciting chapter in our work began with the more recent observation that vitamin $D_3$ and its metabolite 1,25-hydroxy vitamin $D_3$ (1,25(OH)2D3) are very effective in preventing chemotherapy-induced alopecia in the young rat model. We began our studies with vitamin $D_3$ itself. In experiments involving over 180 rats, the injection of 25-50 μg vitamin $D_3$ daily for 5 days prior to chemotherapy provided excellent protection from alopecia induced by etoposide, cytoxan and CTX-ADM combination. However, since vitamin $D_3$ itself is biologically inactive and requires a two-step hydroxylation for activity, we designed further experiments to examine the active metabolite 1,25(OH)2D3 (12,13). Again we chose the topical route for its potential applicability to the clinical setting. The pretreatment of rats with 0.2 μg of 1,25(OH)2D3 in absolute ethanol applied topically over the head and neck yielded excellent protection from alopecia induced by VP16, CTX (Fig. 2) or CTX-ADM combination (14). It is of interest that protection was not limited to the treated area but involved the entire body suggesting systemic absorption. When the dose was reduced to 0.1 μg applied to the head area only, protection from VP16 tended to be limited to the site of application.

1,25(OH)2D3 was also effective in protecting rats from Taxol-induced alopecia. The results of one experiment are shown in Fig. 3. Thirteen rats received 0.2 μg 1,25(OH)2D3 topically over the head in 0.1 ml ETOH daily starting on day 5 and ending on 10. Thirteen control rats received ETOH similarly. On day 11 and 12 all rats received Taxol 2 μg intradermally over the head. All control rats developed alopecia at the site of Taxol injection. In contrast, 8 of 13 rats pretreated with 1,25(OH)2D3 were fully protected from alopecia.

The mechanism of protection by 1,25(OH)2D3 remains uncertain at present. It could act indirectly through other factors or directly on the hair follicles. Thus in addition to its primary metabolic action in bone and mineral metabolism, 1,25(OH)2D3 exerts a wide spectrum of biological effect in several tissues (12,13). Among these, the skin appears to be a target (15), with specific receptors for 1,25(OH)2D3 (16-18). Human keratinocytes when incubated with 1,25(OH)2D3 exhibit a time and dose dependent stimu-

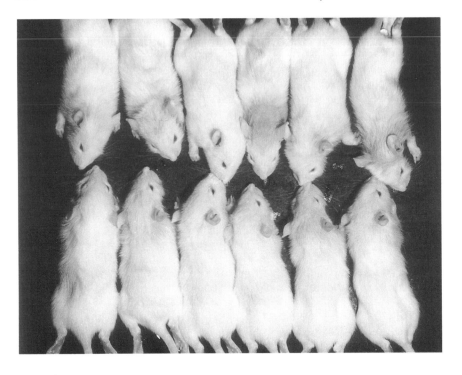

Fig. 2A

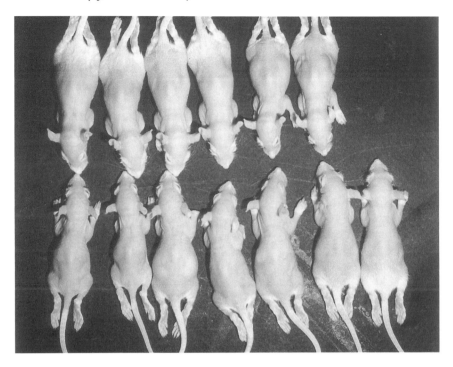

Fig. 2B

Fig. 2. Protection from (CTX + ADM)-Indiced Alopecia by Pretreatment with 1,25(OH)2D$_3$. Five-day old rats were randomly divided in two groups. A (experimental) group, received 0.2 µg of 1,25(OH)2D$_3$ in 0.1 ml ETOH topically over the head and neck daily starting on day five and continuing through day 10. B (control group, received 0.1 ml ETOH similarly. Rats were kept individually separated for a period of 3 hours, following which the treated area was carefully washed. On day 11 all rats received CTX 35 mg/kg i.p. Photographs were taken on day 10.

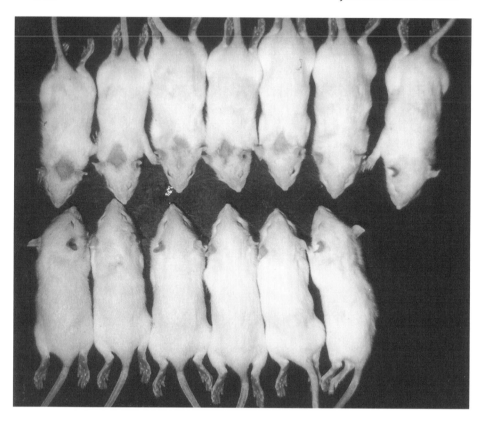

Fig. 3A

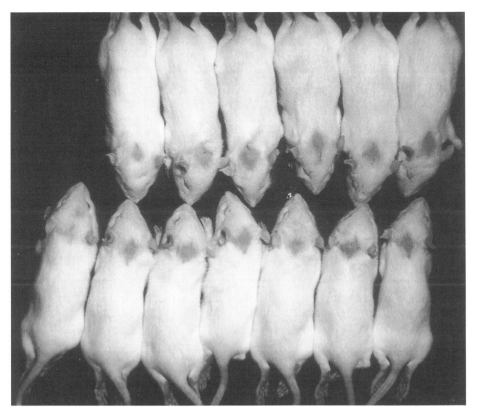

Fig. 3B

Fig. 3. Protection from Taxol-Induced Alopecia by
1,25(OH)2D$_3$. A. Thirteen rats received 0.2 µg of 1,25(OH)
2D$_3$ topically over the head in 0.1 ml ETOH daily starting on
day five and ending on day 10. B. Thirteen control rats
received ETOH similarly. On day 11 and 12 all rats received
Taxol 2 µg i.d. over the head. Photographs were taken on
day 22.

lation of differentiation and inhibition of DNA synthesis
(19). This observation provided the rationale for clinical
trials of topical 1,25(OH)2D$_3$ in psoriasis (15,20,21).

It would appear from these studies that protection
from chemotherapy-induced alopecia by 1,25(OH)2D$_3$ is related to its ability to stimulate differentiation of hair
follicles somehow rendering them resistant to injury by
chemotherapeutic drugs. Further studies are needed to
elucidate the exact mechanism(s).

Does 1,25(OH)2D$_3$ Protect Cancer Cells From Chemotherapy?

The protective effect of topical 1,25(OH)2D$_3$ on hair
follicles observed in our studies and its recent successful
use in the treatment of psoriasis suggest that it may have
excellent potential in the prevention of chemotherapy-
induced alopecia in the clinical setting. However, an important consideration is that 1,25(OH)2D$_3$ may also offer
protection to cancer cells. To examine this questions we
used transplantable rat chloroleukemia as a model (22). C51
is a well characterized cell line established from rat
myelogenous leukemia by Yunis et al (23). The injection of
10$^5$ cells intraperitoneally in 7 day old rats results in
100% mortality from leukemia within 35 days. Leukemia can
be aborted in over 80% of animals by treatment with one
injection of 35 mg/kg Cytoxan i.p. on day 11. We examined
the interaction of 1,25(OH)2D$_3$ with CTX both in vitro and in
vivo. In vitro, the active metabolite of CTX, 4-hydro-
peroxicyclophosphamide was cytotoxic to C51 cells in a dose
dependent manner. The addition of 1,25(OH)2D$_3$ did not protect C51 cells from the cytotoxic effect of 4-HC. In vivo
there was no statistical difference in survival between
C51-injected CTX-treated rats and similar rats pretreated
with topical 1,25(OH)2D$_3$ (90% survival). In addition, rats
pretreated with topical 1,25(OH)2D$_3$ were protected from
CTX-induced alopecia. These results indicated that 1,25(OH)
2D$_3$ did not protect C51 cells from CTX while protecting the
hair follicles.

CONCLUDING REMARKS

Although chemotherapy-induced alopecia has been known
for many decades, little progress has been made in its

treatment or prevention. This is no doubt in part because of lack of a suitable reproducible experimental model. It appears from our studies that the young rat is such a model. Thus severe alopecia can be readily induced in the young rat by all chemotherapeutic agents known to produce alopecia in the clinical setting. The discovery that a number of agents such as cytokines, growth factors, NAC and vitamin D3 can be used to prevent chemotherapy-induced alopecia in the rat has both biological as well as potential clinical significance. In depth studies on the interaction between these agents, chemotherapeutic drugs and the hair follicle should lead to further understanding of the biology of hair growth and the impact of chemotherapy.

Regarding potential clinical applicability, the observations with $1,25(OH)2D_3$ appear to be most exciting. Thus $1,25(OH)2D_3$ used topically is effective in protecting from alopecia induced by all the clinically important chemotherapeutic agents which are known to be potent in producing alopecia, e.g. Cytoxan, Adriamycin, CTX-ADM combination, VP-16, and Taxol. Furthermore, $1,25(OH)2D_3$ appears to exert its protection on the hair follicle without protecting cancer cells from the toxic effect of chemotherapy. These observations, added to the successful clinical use of topical $1,25(OH)2D_3$ for the treatment of psoriasis, strongly suggest that $1,25(OH)2D_3$ has excellent potential for the prevention of chemotherapy-induced alopecia in the clinical setting. Clinical trials are currently in progress.

### REFERENCES

1. Tierney, A., Taylor, J., Closs, S.J., Chetty, U., Rodger, A., and Leonard, R.C.F. Hair loss due to cytotoxic chemotherapy: a prospective descriptive study. Br. J. Cancer 62:527-528, 1990.
2. Urban R.W., U.S. Patent Application No. 057344.
3. Hussein, A.M., Jimenez, J.J., McCall, C.A., and Yunis, A.A. Protection from chemotherapy-induced alopecia in a rat model. Science 249:1564-1566, 1990.
4. Jimenez, J.J., Wong G.H.W., and Yunis, A.A. Interleukin 1 protects from ARA-C-induced alopecia in the rat model. FASEB J. 5:2456-2458, 1991.
5. Jimenez, J.J., Sawaya, M.E., and Yunis, A.A. Interleukin 1 protects hair follicles from cytarabine (ARA-C)-induced toxicity in vivo and in vitro. FASEB J. 6: 911-913, 1992.

6.   Prescott, L.F., Illingworth, R.N., Critchley, J.A.J.H. et al. Intravenous N-acetylcysteine: the treatment of choice for paracetamol poisoning. Br. Med. J. 2:1097–1100, 1979.

7.   Schmiff-Graff, A., and Scheulen, M.E. Prevention of adriamycin cardiotoxicity by niacin, isocitrate or N-acetylcysteine in mice. A morphological study. Pathol. Res. Pract. 181:168–174, 1986.

8.   Giri, S.N., Hyde, D.M., Schiedt, M.J. Effects of repeated administration of N-acetylcysteine on sulfhydryl levels of different tissues and bleomycin-induced lung fibrosis in hamsters. J. Lab. Clin. Med. 111:715–724, 1988.

9.   Botta, J.A., Nelson, L.W., Wieker, J.H., Jr. Acetyl-cysteine in the prevention of cyclophosphamide-induced cystitis in rats. J. Natl. Cancer Inst. 51:1051–1058, 1973.

10.  Blank, E.C.M., Haveman, J., van Zandvijk, N. The radio-protective effect of N-acetylcysteine in thorax irradiation of mice. Radiother. Oncol. 10:67–69, 1987.

11.  Jimenez, J.J., Sheng, H.S., and Yunis, A.A. Treatment with ImuVert/N-acetylcysteine protects rats from cyclophosphamide/cytarabine-induced alopecia. Cancer Inv. 10(4) 271–276, 1992.

12.  Henry, H.L., and Norman, A.W. Vitamin D: metabolism and biological actions. Annu. Rev. Nutr. 4:493–520, 1984.

13.  Reichel, H., Koeffler, H.P., and Norman, A.W. The role of the vitamin D endocrine system in health and disease. N. Engl. J. Med. 320:980–991, 1989.

14.  Jimenez, J.J., and Yunis, A.A. Protection from chemotherapy-induced alopecia by 1,25-dihydroxyvitamin $D_3$. Cancer Res. 52:5123–5125, 1992.

15.  Holick, M.F., Smith, E., and Pincus, S. Skin as the site of vitamin D synthesis and target tissue for 1,25-dihydroxyvitamin $D_3$: use of calcitriol (1,25-dihydroxyvitamin $D_3$) for treatment of psoriasis. Arch. Dermatol. 123:1677–1683a, 1987.

16.  Simpson, R.U., and Deluca, H.F. Characterization of a receptor-like protein for 1,25-dihydroxyvitamin $D_3$ in rat skin. Proc. Natl. Acad. Sci. USA 77:5822–5826, 1980.

17.  Clemens, T.L., Horiuchi, N., Nguyen, M., and Holick, M.F. Binding of 1,15-dihydroxy-[$^3$H] vitamin $D_3$ in nuclear and cytosol fractions of whole mouse skin in vivo and in vitro. FEBS Lett. 134:203–206, 1981.

18. Fledman, D., Chen, T., Hirst, M., Colston, K., Karasek, M., and Cone, C. Demonstration of 1,25-dihydroxyvitamin $D_3$ receptors in human skin biopsies. J. Clin. Endocrinol. Metab. 51:1463-1465, 1980.

19. Smith, E.L., Walworth, N.C., and Holick, M.F. Effect of $1\alpha$, 1,25-dihydroxyvitamin $D_3$ on the morphologic and biochemical differentiation of cultured human epidermal keratinocytes grown in serum-free conditions. J. Invest. Dermatol. 86:709-714, 1986.

20. Morimoto, S., Ouishi, T., Imanaka, S., Yukawa, H., Kozuka, T., Kitano, Y., Yoshikawa, K., and Kumahara, Y. Topical administration of 1,25-dihydroxyvitamin $D_3$ for psoriasis: report of five cases. Calcif. Tissue Int., 38:119-122, 1986.

21. Smith, E.L., Pincus, S.H., Donovan, L., and Holick, M.F.A. A novel approach for the evaluation and treatment of psoriasis. J. Am. Acad. Dermatol. 19:516-528, 1988.

22. Jimenez, J.J., and Yunis, A.A. Tumor cell rejection through terminal cell differentiation. Science 238: 1278-1280, 1987.

23. Yunis, A.A., Arimura, G.K., Haines, H.G., Ratzan, R.J., Gross, M.A. Characteristics of rat chloroma in culture. Cancer Res. 35:337-345, 1975.

# PART V

# Cancer Treatment Studies: Human Studies

# ROLE OF VITAMIN A AND ITS DERIVATIVES IN THE TREATMENT

# OF HUMAN CANCER

Frank L. Meyskens Jr., M.D.

Cancer Center and Department of Medicine
University of California Irvine
101 The City Drive, Building 23, Route 81
Orange, California 92668

Vitamin A and its natural and synthetic derivatives have gained attention in the last five years as promising agents for the management of human cancer. The interest in their preventive role has been intense-although the number of completed trials have been few (see 24)-and this experience will not be repeated here. This current manuscript will summarize the progress that retinoids have demonstrated as potential therapeutic agents, since the first large report of their potential efficacy appeared-a phase II trial of 13-cis retinoic acid (13cRA) in advanced cancers (31).

## SKIN CANCERS

Activity of retinoids against both non-melanoma and melanoma cutaneous malignancies has been sought (Tables 1, 2). Moriarity et al. (1980) first demonstrated in a randomized trial that the retinoid Etretinate could cause sustained regression of the precancerous skin condition actinic keratoses. The first report on the use of oral 13cRA for the treatment of advanced cutaneous squamous cell carcinoma suggested significant activity of the retinoid (23) and a subsequent study in which recombinant interferon-alpha (IFN-$\alpha$) has been added extended these results (29). Of interest is that the retinoid and the combination appeared to produce more activity in advanced regional compared to metastatic disease.

Topical use of trans-retinoic acid (Tretinoin, tRA) has produced substantial clinical and histological regression of dysplastic nevi, a result first reported by us (33) and subsequently confirmed by others (44). However, a randomized trial of oral 13-cRA showed no such benefit (10). Whether

Table I

MAJOR TREATMENT TRIALS OF RETINOIDS IN CUTANEOUS
NON-MELANOMA MALIGNANCIES

| Eligibility | Design | Agent(s) | No. Pt | Result | References |
|---|---|---|---|---|---|
| Actinic keratoses | phase III randomized | Etretinate | 50 | 84% vs. 5% | Moriarity, 1980 |
| Advanced sq cell CA | phase II | 13cRA | 4 | 50% CR | Lippman & Meyskens, 1987 |
| Advanced sq cell CA | phase II | 13cRA + IFN-α | 28 | 80% RR | Lippman, 1992 |

Table II

MAJOR TRIALS OF RETINOIDS IN CUTANEOUS MELANOMA

| Eligibility | Design | Agent(s) | No. Pt | Result | References |
|---|---|---|---|---|---|
| Dysplastic nevi | phase II | topical tRA | 3 | Regression | Meyskens, 1986 |
|  |  |  | 5 | Regression | Schuchter, 1993 |
| Dysplastic nevi | phase II randomized | 13cRA (oral) | 11 | No difference in pre/post biopsies | Edwards, 1989 |
| Stage I melanoma | phase III | Retinol (oral) | 386 | No difference in relapse free or overall survival | Meyskens, 1994 |
| Cutaneous met. nodules | phase II | topical tRA | 3 | Two responded | Levine & Meyskens, 1980 |
| Metastatic melanoma | phase II | 13cRA | 29 | 10% response | Meyskens, 1988 (review) |
| Metastatic melanoma | phase II | 13cRA + IFN-α | 11 | 10% response, short duration | Meyskens, 1992 (unpublished data) |
| Metastatic melanoma | phase II | 13cRA + IFN-α | 28 | 0% response | Dhingra, 1993 |

these results represent the differences between modes of administration
(topical vs oral) or the type of retinoid (13-cRA vs tRA) awaits a direct
comparison of the two in a topical mode and/or a randomized trial of oral
tRA.

Based on promising preclinical observations, activity of retinoids as potential adjuvant or treatment modalities in malignant melanoma has been explored. High doses of retinol (vitamin A) were found to be ineffective in altering the natural history of surgically resected primary melanoma (34). Although topical tRA has been shown to cause regression of metastatic melanoma nodules (20b), systemic oral 13cRA either alone or in combination has produced minimal responses in patients with advanced or metastatic melanoma (9).

In contrast to these results, retinoids have produced substantial responses of the cutaneous T-cell lymphoma, mycosis fungoides, (Table III). 13cRA alone has demonstrated a 50% response rate (20), although an attempt to enhance this activity with IFN-$\alpha$ was unsuccessful (F. Meyskens, unpublished data). The retinoid Etretinate is also quite an effective agent as well and appears synergistic with interferon (8).

### Table III

**MAJOR TRIALS OF RETINOIDS FOR TREATMENT OF MYCOSIS FUNGOIDES**

| Disease | No. | Agent | Response Rate | Reference |
|---------|-----|-------|---------------|-----------|
| Mycosis Fungoides | 78 | 13 cRA | 61% | Meyskens (review), 1988 |
| Mycosis Fungoides | 25 | 13 cRA + IFN-$\alpha$ | 20% | Meyskens (SWOG), unpublished |
| Mycosis Fungoides | 45 | Etretinate + IFN-$\alpha$ | 60% | Dreno, 1991 |

## AERODIGESTIVE TUMORS

Preclinical data suggests that retinoids might have activity against altered aerodigestive epithelium. An early report demonstrated that oral 13cRA produced significant responses against laryngeal papillomatosis (1), an effect which seemingly was enhanced by the addition of IFN-$\alpha$ (25). Both oral $\beta$-carotene and 13-cRA have produced significant regression of oral leukoplakia (14, 17). A recent study to compare the relative efficacy of the two agents to maintain established regressions was inconclusive, largely due to design issues (30). The synthetic retinoid fenretinide also seems active against oral leukoplakia as well (7). A non-randomized phase II trail of Etretinate against bronchial metaplasia suggests reversal  (or suppression) of the preneoplastic process as assessed by a decrease in the metaplastic index (15), an important result which needs to be confirmed. However, using 13cRA Lee et al. (1993) was unable to demonstrate a change in the metaplastic index in a carefully done randomized trial (22).

Two striking results are those emanating from two large randomized trials of retinoids in which the development of secondary malignancies was apparently blocked (18, 40). In the first, a high dose of 13-cRA was used and a significant decrease in the development of second aerodigestive malignancies demonstrated (18). The result has been particularly striking since long-term follow up has demonstrated permanent suppression of lesion development, even after the retinoid was stopped (5). Using high doses of retinyl palmitate similar results were obtained in patients with low stage non-small cell lung cancer by Pastorino et al (40). Particularly relevant in this trial was the lack of vitamin A toxicity, despite the high doses of drug used, and the decrease in metastatic disease as well. However, several trials to demonstrate the activity of 13cRA in advanced NSCL and head and neck cancer (23b) have been negative, even after IFN-$\alpha$ was added (3). tRA was also found to be ineffective against head and neck cancer and NSCL as well (12,19).

## CERVICAL CANCER

Retinoids appear to have activity against cervical precancers and cancers (Table V). We have demonstrated in a series of studies that topical tRA can cause sustained regression of cervical intraepithelial neoplasia or CIN (16, 35). In a large placebo-controlled randomized trial topical tRA produced significant regression in CIN II but not CIN III compared to the placebo cream. In non-randomized trials significant activity of systemic 13-cRA + IFN-$\alpha$ (46) and oral retinamide + riboflavin (Riu, personal communication) against CIN has been demonstrated. Of considerable interest is the impressive 50% major response rate of oral 13 cRA plus subcutaneous IFN-α against advanced/regional cervical cancer (26, 27). Further follow up suggests that these beneficial effects are seen only in previously untreated patients (S. Lippman, personal communication), but the responses are impressive nevertheless. Of related interest is a case report of a dramatic response of a patient with endometrial carcinoma to this combination as well (21).

## GENITOURINARY CANCER

The activity of retinoids against bladder tumors is inconclusive. Two phase II studies with Etretinate suggested a decreased recurrence of bladder patients with prior resection of their bladder cancer while two other studies, one using Etretinate and the other 13-cRA, have demonstrated no effects (2, 41, 42, 45). This disease is very difficult to assess and a carefully-designed randomized phase III trial is needed. A small phase II trial of oral 13-cRA in advanced prostate cancer has suggested no activity (47). In contrast the combination of 13-cRA + IFN-α may produce significant responses in patients with renal cell cancers; in a phase II trial in 24 patients seven attained a partial or completed response (38). Several groups are now attempting to confirm these preliminary results.

We and others have examined 13-cRA for activity in other solid malignancies as well (Table VII) and no responses have been seen in breast, ovarian, and GI malignancies (6, 28, 31) as well as childhood neuroblastoma (11). Modiano et al. has demonstrated that oral 4-hydroxyretinamide is inactive against both melanoma and breast cancer (36).

## HEMATOPOIETIC DISEASES

The activity of retinoids in nonsolid tumors has also been explored (Table VIII). The major activity for retinoids in human malignancies has been the striking clinical effect of oral tRA on acute promyelocytic leukemia (review, 39). Over 85% of patients achieve a clinical complete recission, and although the responses are short, this activity has changed the management of this disease as well as changed the perception of the feasibility of differentiation therapy.

The results of a large randomized trial of high doses of vitamin A in patients with CML has suggested that the natural history of this disease may be altered by the retinoid, with a delay of onset of blast crisis and increased survival (32). In contrast oral 13-cRA and oral tRA have produced minimal benefit in patients with myelodysplasia (16b, 21b) and in a disturbing report 4 hydroxy retinamide may have accelerated leukemia (13). An interesting case report suggests that β-carotene may affect CLL (4), a result which needs to be confirmed.

## CONCLUSION

The use of retinoids as therapeutic anticancer agents has been of interest to a few investigators for nearly 20 years. Only recently has favorable clinical results led to a widespread revival of interest in these compounds. The results with other retinoids as well as trials with various combinations is eagerly anticipated.

### Table IVa

**MAJOR TRIALS OF RETINOIDS IN AERODIGESTIVE CANCERS**

| Eligibility | Design | Agent(s) | No. Pt | Result | References |
|---|---|---|---|---|---|
| Laryngeal papillomatosis | phase II | 13cRA + IFN-α | 3 | major responses | Lippman, 1994 |
| Laryngeal papillomatosis | phase II | 13cRA (high dose) | 6 | 4 of 6 excellent response | Alberts, 1986 |
| Oral leukoplakia | phase II | β-carotene (intermediate dose) | 24 | 71% response rate | Garewal, 1990 |
| Oral leukoplakia | phase III randomized | 13cRA (high dose) | 44 | Marked regression of lesions | Hong, 1986* |
| Bronchial metaplasia | phase II time | Etretinate (high dose) | 36 | Metaplastic index decreased | Gouveia, 1982 |
| Bronchial metaplasia | phase III randomized | 13cRA (high dose) | 307 | No difference in index | Lee, 1993 |

*In a subsequent large study, randomization of responders to lower doses of 13-cRA kept lesions in remission as well.

## Table IVb

### MAJOR TRIALS OF RETINOIDS IN AERODIGESTIVE CANCERS

| Eligibility | Design | Agent(s) | No. Pt | Result | References |
|---|---|---|---|---|---|
| Prior oropharyngeal CA | phase III randomized | 13cRA (high dose) | 103 | Decrease of $2^0$ oropharyngeal cancers | Hong, 1990* |
| Recurrent head & neck | phase II | 13cRA + IFN-$\alpha$ | 21 | 5% PR | Voravud, 1993 |
| Prior stage I, non-small cell lung cancer | phase III randomized | Retinyl palmitate (very high dose) | 307 | Decrease of $2^0$ cancers and distant mets | Pastorino, 1993 |
| NSCL** | phase II | 13cRA + IFN-$\alpha$ | 33 | <5% PR | Arnold, 1994 |
| NSCL | phase II | tRA | 28 | 3/28 RR | Friedland, 1994 |
| NSCL | phase II | 13cRA + IFN-$\alpha$ | 21 | 10% PR | Rinaldi, 1993 |

*A subsequent long-term follow-up (Lee et al., 1993) suggested that patients remained free of disease after initial reduction; even when maintenance 13 cRA was stopped.
**NSCL-non-small cell lung cancer

## Table Va

### MAJOR TRIALS OF RETINOIDS IN CERVICAL CANCERS

| Eligibility | Design | Agent(s) | No. Pt | Result | References |
|---|---|---|---|---|---|
| CIN II or III* | phase II | tRA (topical) | 20 | 50% CR | Meyskens, 1986 |
| CIN II or III | phase III randomized | tRA (topical) | 301 | Increased regression of CIN II but not CIN III | Meyskens, 1993 |
| CIN II-III | phase II | 13cRA + IFN-$\alpha$ | 23 | 53% CR | Toma, 1994 |
| Advanced cervical squamous cancer | phase II | 13 cRA (oral) + IFN-$\alpha$ | 26 | 50 % major response rate | Lippman, 1992 |

*CIN-cervical intraepithelial neoplasia (cervical dysplasia)

**Table VI**

**MAJOR TRIALS OF RETINOIDS IN GU TUMORS**

| Eligibility | Design | Agent(s) | No. Pt | Result | References |
|---|---|---|---|---|---|
| Superficial bladder tumors (resected) | phase II | Etretinate (intermediate dose) | 32 | Decreased recurrence | Alfthan, 1983 |
| Superficial bladder tumors (resected) | phase II | Etretinate (intermediate dose) | 73 | No difference | Pederson, 1984 |
| Superficial bladder tumors (resected) | phase II | Etretinate (intermediate dose) | 86 | Decreased recurrence | Studer, 1984 |
| Superficial bladder tumors | phase II | 13 cRA | 30 | No effect | Prout & Barton, 1992 |
| Advanced RCC* | phase II | 13cRA + IFN-α | 24 | 7/24 PR + CR | Motzer, 1994 |
| Prostate | phase II | 13cRA | 17 | No response | Trump, 1994 |

*RCC-renal cell carcinoma

**Table VII**

**MAJOR TRIALS OF RETINOIDS IN MISCELLANEOUS CANCERS**

| Eligibility | Design | Agent(s) | No. Pt | Result | References |
|---|---|---|---|---|---|
| Breast | phase III | 13cRA | 18 | No response | Cassidy, 1983 |
| Breast, melanoma | phase II | 4HPR | 15 18 | No response | Modiano, 1990 |
| Solid tumors (miscellaneous) | phase II | 13 cRA | 108 | No response breast, ovarian, GI cancers | Meyskens, 1982 |
| Neuroblastoma | phase II | 13cRA | 28 | No response | Finkelstein, 1992 |

## Table VIII

### MAJOR TRIALS OF RETINOIDS IN HEMATOPOIETIC DISEASES

| Disease | No. | Agent | Response Rate | Reference |
|---|---|---|---|---|
| APL | 1500+ | tRA | 85% CR, short duration | Many* |
| Myelodysplasia | 15 | 13cRA | Minimal | Greenberg, 1985 |
| Myelodysplasia | 15 | 4HPR | None, possible disease acceleration | Garewal, 1989 |
| Myelodysplasia | 39 | tRA | Minimal | Kurzrock, 1993 |
| CML (chronic phase) | 151 | Vitamin A | Increased chronic phase & survival by 8 months | Meyskens, 1993 |
| CLL | 1 | β-carotene | Fall in lymphocyte amount | Baranowitz, 1994 |

*See Parkinson and Smith, 1992 for recent review

## References

1.  Alberts DS, Coulthard SW, Meyskens FL Jr (1986). Regression of aggressive laryngeal papillomatosis with 13-cis retinoic acid (accutane). J Biol Resp Mod 5:124-128

2.  Alfthan O, Tarkkanen J, Grohn P, et al. (1983) Tigason (etretinate) in prevention of recurrence of superficial bladder tumors. Eur Urol 9:6-9.

3.  Arnold A, Ayoub J, Douglas L, et al. (1994) Phase II trial of 13-cis-retinoic acid plus interferon alpha in non-small-cell lung cancer. J Nat Canc Inst 86(4):306-309.

4.  Baranowitz S, (1994). Treatment of cutaneous T-cell lymphoma with beta-carotene. New Eng J Med 330(25):1830.

5.  Benner SE, Pajak TF, Lippman SE, et al. (1994). Prevention of second primary tumors with isotretinoin in patients with squamous cell carcinoma of the head and neck: long term follow-up. J Natl Cancer Inst 86:140-141.

6.  Cassidy J, Lippman M, Lacroix A, Peck G. Phase II trial of 13 cis-retinoic acid in metastatic breast cancer. Investigational New Drugs. 925-929.

7.  Chiesa F, Traditi N, Marazza M, et al. (1992) Prevention of local relapses and new localisations of oral leukoplakias with the synthetic retinoid fenretinide (4-HPR): preliminary results. Eur J Cancer 28:97-102.

8.  Dreno B, Claudy A, Reynadier, et al., (1991). The treatment of 45 patients with cutaneous T-cell lymphoma with low doses of interferon-alpha 2a and etretinate. Br J Derm 125 (5):456-459.

9.  Dhingra K, Papadopoulos N, Lippman S, Lotan R, Legha SS (1993). Phase II study of alpha-interferon and 13-cis-retinoic acid in metastatic melanoma. Invest New Drugs 11(1)39-43.

10. Edwards L, Meyskens FL Jr, Levine N (1989). The effect of oral isotretinoin on dysplastic nevi. J. Am Acad Derm 20:257-260.

11. Finklestein JZ, Krailo MD, Lenarsky C, et al., (1992) 13-cis-retinoic acid (NSC 122758) in the treatment of children with metastatic neuroblastoma unresponsive to conventional chemotherapy: Report from the Childrens Cancer Study Group. Medical and Pediatric Oncology 20:307-311.

12. Friedland D, Luginbuhl W, Meehan L, et al. (1994). Phase II trial of all-trans retinoic acid in metastatic non-small cell lung cancer. University of Pennsylvania Cancer Center. Proc Am Soc Clin Oncology 13:1086 abs.

13. Garewal H, Meyskens FL Jr, Buzaid A, et al., (1989) Phase II trial of N-(4 hydroxyphenyl) retinamide [4-HPR] in myelodysplasia: possible retinoid-induced disease acceleration. Leukemia Research 13(4):339-343.

14. Garewal H, Meyskens FL Jr, Killen D, et al., (1990) Response of oral leukoplakia to beta-carotene. J Clin Oncology 8(10):1715-20.

15 Gouveia J, Mathe G, Heranand T, et al. (1982). Degree of bronchial metaplasia in heavy smokers and its regression after treatment with a retinoid. Lancet 2:710-712.

16. Graham V, Surwit ES, Weiner S, Meyskens FL Jr, (1986). Phase II Trial of b-all-trans retinoic acid for cervical intraepithelial neoplasia delivered via a collagen sponge and cervical cap. West J Med 145:192-195.

16b. Greenberg BK, Durie BGM, Barnett TC, Meyskens FL Jr (1985). Phase I-II study of 13-cis retinoic acid in myelodysplastic syndrome. Cancer Treat Rep 69:1369-1374.

17. Hong WK, Endicott J, Itri LM, et al. (1986) 13-cis retinoic acid in the treatment of oral leukoplakia. N Eng J Med 315:1501-1505.

18. Hong WK, Lippman SM, Itri LM, et al. (1990) Prevention of second primary tumors with isotretinoin in squamous-cell carcinoma of the head and neck. N Eng J Med 323:795-801.

19. Jacob HE, Smith DC, Branch RA, et al. (1994). A phase II trial of all-trans retinoic acid (ATRA) in advanced squamous cell carcinoma of the head and neck (SCCHN). Proc Am Soc Clin Oncology 13:930 abs.

20. Kessler JF, Jones SE, Levine NE, et al. (1987) Isotretinoin and cutaneous helper T-cell lymphoma (mycosis fungoides). Arch Dermatol 123:201-204.

20b. Levine N, Meyskens FL Jr (1980). Topical vitamin A-acid therapy for cutaneous metastatic melanoma. The Lancet 2:224-226.

21. Kudelka AP, Freedman RS, Edwards CL, et al., (1993) Metastatic adenocarcinoma of the endometrium treated with 13-cis-retinoic acid plus interferon-alpha. Anti-Cancer Drugs 4(3):335-7.

21b. Kurzrock R, Estey E, Talpaz M (1993). All-trans retinoic acid: tolerance and biologic effects in myelodysplasti syndrome. J Clin Oncology 11(8)1489-1495.

22 Lee JS, Benner SE, Lippman SM, et al. (1993). A randomized placebo-controlled chemoprevention trial of 13-cis retinoic acid in bronchial metaplasia. Proc Am Soc Clin Oncol 12:335 abs.

23 Lippman SM, Meyskens FL Jr (1987). Treatment of advanced squamous cell cancer of the skin with isotretinoin. Ann Int Med 107:499-501.

23b. Lippman SM, Kessler JF, Al-Sarraff M, et al. (1988). Treatment of advanced squamous cell carcinoma of the head and neck with isotretinoin: a phase II randomized trial. Invest New Drugs 6:51-56.

24. Lippman S, Benner SE, Hong WK, (1994). Cancer chemoprevention. J Clin Oncol 12:851-873.

25. Lippman SM, Donovan DT, Frankelthaler RA, et al., (1994) 13-cis-retinoic acid plus interferon-alpha 2a in recurrent respiratory papillomatosis. J Nat Canc Inst 86(11):859-861.

26. Lippman SM, Kavanaugh JJ, Pavedes-Espinoza, et al. (1993). 13-cis-retinoic acid plus interferon-α-2a in locally advanced squamous cell carcinoma of the cervix. J Natl Cancer Inst 85:499-500.

27. Lippman SM, Kavanaugh JJ, Pavedes-Espinoza, (1992). 13-cis retinoic acid plus interferon α-2a: highly active systemic therapy for squamous cell carcinoma of the cervix. J Natl Cancer Inst 84(4):241-245.

28. Lippman S, Kessler J, Meyskens FL Jr, (1987). Retinoids as preventive and therapeutic anticancer agents. Cancer Treat Rep 71:391-405, 493-515

29. Lippman SM, Parkinson OR, Itri LM, et al., (1992). 13-cis-retinoic and intereron α-2a: effective combination therapy for advanced squamous cell carcinoma of the skin. J Natl Cancer Inst 84:235-241.

30      Lippman SM, Batsakis JG, Toth BB, et al. (1993). Comparison of low-dose isotretinoin with beta carotene to prevent oral carcinogenesis. N Eng J Med 328(1):15-20.

31.     Meyskens FL Jr, Gilmartin E, Alberts DS, et al., (1982) Activity of isotretinoin against squamous cell cancers and preneoplastic lesions. Cancer Treat Rep 66:1315-1319.

32.     Meyskens FL Jr, Kopecky K for SWOG (1993)  Vitamin A prolongs relapse free survival and survival of patients with CML treated with bisulfan:  a randomized trial.  Proceedings of the Seventh International Conference on the Adjuvant Therapy of Cancer, Tucson.

33.     Meyskens FL Jr, Edwards SL, Levine NS (1986).  Role of topical tretinoin in melanoma and dysplastic nevi.  J Am Acad Review 15(4):822-825

34      Meyskens FL Jr, Liu PY, Tuthill RJ, et al. (1994).  A randomized trial of vitamin A versus observation as adjuvant therapy in high risk stage I malignant melanoma.  J. Clin Oncol (in press).

35.     Meyskens FL, Surwit ES, Moon TE, et al. (1994)  Enhancement of regression of cervical intraepithelial neoplasia II (moderate dysplasia) with topically applied all-trans retinoic acid:  a randomized trial.  J Natl Can Inst 86(7):539-543.

36.     Modiano MR, Dalton WS, Lippman SM, et al., (1990)  Phase II study of fenretinide (N-[4-hydroxyphenyl] retinamide) in breast cancer and melanoma.  Inv New Drugs 8:317-319.

37      Moriarity M, Dunn J, Darragh A, et al. (1982).  Etretinate in treatment of actinic keratosis:  a double blind crossover study.  Lancet 1:364-366.

38.     Motzer RJ, Murray-Law T, Schwartz L, et al., (1994).  Antitumor activity of interferon alpha-2A and 13cRA in patients with advanced renal cell cancer.  Proc Am Soc Clin Oncology 13:713 abs.

39.     Parkinson OR, Smith MA (1992).  Retinoid therapy for acute promyelocytic leukemia: A coming of age for the differentiation therapy of malignancy.  Ann Int Med 117(4):338-339.

40.     Pastorino U, Infante M, Maioli M, et al., (1993)  Adjuvant treatment of stage I lung cancer with high-dose vitamin A.  J Clin Oncol 11(7):1216-1222.

41.  Pederson H, Wolf H, Jensen SK, et al. (1984) Administration of retinoid as prophylaxis of recurrent non-invasive bladder tumors. Scand J Urol Nephrol 18:121-123

42.  Prout GR Jr, Barton BA (1992). 13-cis-retinoic acid in chemoprevention of superficial bladder cancer. The National Bladder Cancer Group. J Cell Biochem 161:148-52

43.  Rinaldi DA, Lippman SM, Burris HA 3d, Chau C, Von Hoff DD, Hong WK (Feb 1993). Phase II study of 13-cis-retinoic acid and interferon-alpha 2a in patients with advanced squamous cell lung cancer. Anti-Cancer Drugs 4(1):33-6.

44.  Schuchter L, Elder D, Elenitsas R (1993). A pilot study of retin A in patients with dysplastic nevus syndrome. Proc Am Soc Clin Oncol 169:474 abs

45.  Studer UE, Biedermann C, Chollet D, et al. (1984) Prevention of recurrent superficial bladder tumors by oral etretinate: preliminary results of a randomized, double-blind, multicenter trial in Switzerland. J Urol 131:1469-1472.

46.  Toma S, Palumbo R, Gustavino C, et al. (1994). Efficacy of the association of 13-cis-retinoic acid (13cRA) and interferon-$\alpha$2a (IFN $\alpha$2a) in cervical intraepithelial neoplasia (CIN II-III): A pilot study. Pro Am Soc Clin Oncology 13:815 abs.

47   Trump D, Smith D, Stiff D, et al. (1994). All-trans retinoic acid (ATRA) in hormone refractory prostate cancer (HRPC): ineffectiveness due to failure of drug delivery? Proc Am Soc Clin Oncology 13:751 abs.

48.  Voravud N, Lippman SM, Weber RS, et al. (1993) Phase II trial of 13-cis-retinoic acid plus interferon-alpha in recurrent head and neck cancer. Invest New Drugs 11(1):57-60.

# USE OF VITAMINS AS ADJUNCT TO CONVENTIONAL CANCER THERAPY

Jae Ho Kim, M.D. Ph.D., Sang Hie Kim,

Ph.D., Shao-Qin He, M.D.*, Jadranka

Dragovic, M.D., Stephen Brown, Ph.D.

Department of Radiation Oncology

Henry Ford Hospital

2799 W. Grand Boulevard

Detroit, MI 48202 U.S.A.

*Department of Radiation Oncology, Cancer Hospital

Shanghai Medical University

Shanghai, People's Republic of China

## INTRODUCTION

Although the combined use of cytotoxic agents and radiation therapy has given promising results in selected human tumors, increased injury to normal tissues produced by the combined regimen has been a major limiting factor. In an effort to improve the therapeutic effectiveness of radiation therapy in combination with noncytotoxic chemicals, we investigated three well known vitamins as adjunct to radiotherapy and/or hyperthermia.

## Retinoids

Vitamin A and synthetic retinoids have been shown to modulate the growth and differentiation of normal, premalignant, and malignant cells *in vitro* and *in vivo*. Clinical studies have shown that retinoids have antitumor activity in the following clinical settings: 1) inhibition of the conversion of the premalignant oral leukoplakia to cancer; 2) chemoprevention of second aerodigestive tract tumors after treatment of the early stages of head and neck cancers; 3) induction of remission of acute promyelocytic leukemia; and 4) more recently, significant antitumor activity of 13 cis-retinoic acid in combination with recombinant human interferon α-2a in squamous cell cancers of the cervix and skin (1, 2). In each trial, 50% or more of the treated patients have had excellent clinical responses.

We have undertaken cellular radiobiological studies of retinoids alone and in combination with interferon α-2a to determine whether the radiation response of human cancer cells would be enhanced. We used human lung adenocarcinoma cells, A-549, to determine cell survival curves following exposure of cells to 13 cis-retinoic acid (RA), interferon α-2a (INF-α), and the combination of RA and INF-α.

When cells were exposed to RA for up to five days, there was no change in the radiation survival curve, as compared with radiation alone. On the other hand, there was consistently detectable radiation enhancement when cells were exposed to INF-α for 24 hours before irradiation. When cells were treated to the combined RA and INF-α, there was a remarkable enhancement of the radiation response. At a single dose of 8 Gy, there was an additional one log cell kill for the combined regimen (Figure 1).

**FIGURE 1**

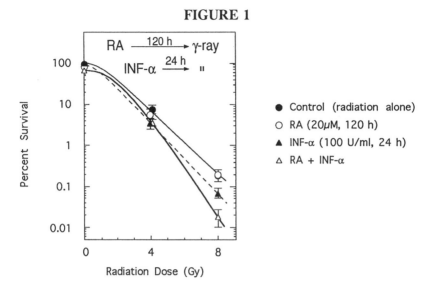

**Figure 1**: Radiation cell survival curves of A-549 (human lung adenocarcinoma cells). Cells were exposed to retinoic acid for five days and to INF-α for one day before radiation.

In our previous study of RA in HeLa cells, cells treated with RA for four days exhibited a resistance to thermal injury (3). No increase in the radiosensitivity of cells exposed to RA was seen in A-549 lung cancer cells. Cells exposed to INF-α exhibited a modest degree of radiation response (4). This phenomenon appears cell line dependent (unpublished data). However, the combined regimen of RA and INF-α is an impressive radioenhancing agent in human lung carcinoma cells. Further studies are in progress with other established human carcinoma cells.

## Vitamin K₃

Vitamin $K_3$, also known as menadione, and its analogue, menadiol sodium diphosphate (MSD), seem to be good candidates for clinical radiosensitizers and hyperthermic sensitizers. Menadiol sodium diphosphate has received some evaluation as a radiation sensitizer in the treatment of head and neck cancers (5). Further, there is some evidence showing that MSD is preferentially localized in human cancers (6).

We carried out a cell culture study to determine whether the cytotoxic effects of menadione could be enhanced by heat, since certain naphthoguinone interfere with energy metabolism. Energy deprivation of cancer cells increases sensitivity to killing by hyperthermia. The cell culture data show that the cytotoxicity is markedly increased in cells deprived of glucose in the medium at 37°C, after exposure to menadione. When cells were exposed to menadione (20 - 40 $\mu$M) and hyperthermia (41 - 42°C), there was a dramatic potentiation of heat induced cytotoxicity in cells deprived of glucose in the medium (7). Evidence has been obtained in our cell culture study showing that the cytotoxicity of menadione is principally mediated by an activated oxygen species, such as superoxide and hydrogen peroxide. Table I shows the magnitude of heat induced cytotoxicity of HeLa cells, with and without menadione.

**Table I -**    **Percent Cell Survival After Exposure of Cells to Menadione( 20 $\mu$M) at 41°C and 42°C for Two Hours**

| Temperature | % Cell Survival | |
| :---: | :---: | :---: |
| | **With Glucose** | **Without Glucose** |
| 37°C | 100% | 50% |
| 41°C | 50% | 20% |
| 42°C | 15% | 0.8% |

A combination of radiation therapy and hyperthermia has been shown to increase the tumor control probability in the treatment of locally advanced superficial cancers of malignant melanoma, breast cancer, and head and neck tumors (8). The cell culture data presented suggest that cancer cells can be selectively killed by the combined treatment of menadione and mild hyperthermia; in particular, those tumor cells existing in a glucose deficient milieu. The conditions of this combined regimen can be readily achievable in humans with currently available heating technology.

## Nicotinamide

Heterogeneous blood flow, large transport distances in the interstitium, and increased interstitial pressure characterize many solid tumors and may be the reason for the decreased effectiveness of various treatment modalities. Drugs that increase blood flow may improve radiation response by delivering oxygen to tumors because oxygen is a potent radiation sensitizer. Nicotinamide, the amide of vitamin $B_3$, has been shown to enhance the radiation response of solid tumors containing an acutely induced hypoxic tumor cell population (9, 10). The drug is totally ineffective as a radiation sensitizer, when tested in an *in vitro* cell culture system. Hence, the drug is thought to regulate intermittent blood flow and to decrease the extent of acute hypoxia.

Our pre-clinical studies with nicotinamide (NA) consist of combining agents to modify either acute or chronic hypoxia of tumor microcirculation. The first approach was an experiment designed to determine the degree of tumor tissue reoxygenation with NA and pentoxifylline, a derivative of methylxanthine, using a murine tumor system (11). The degree of improved tumor oxygenation as a consequence of the two drugs was quite impressive. Based on this finding, we initiated a Phase II clinical study of NA and pentoxifylline, in combination with radiation therapy in locally advanced head and neck cancers and lung cancers. The second approach was an experiment of trimodality therapy, wherein, radiation, heat, and NA were administered in sequence, in order to reduce radioresistant hypoxic tumor cells. Figure 2 shows the percent of local tumor control of MCa mammary carcinoma in C3H mice as a function of a single dose of radiation. NA (500 mg/kg) was administered by intraperitoneal injection one hour before radiation. Hyperthermia (41°C) was also applied for one hour before radiation. There was substantial enhancement of the radiation response of tumor tissue following trimodality therapy, relative to a single treatment modality.

**FIGURE 2**

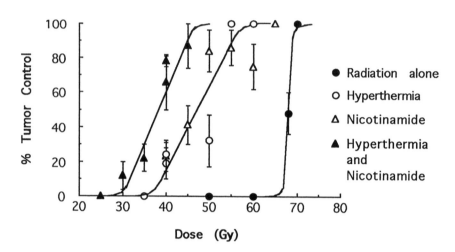

**Figure 2**:  Percent local tumor control of the C3H-MCa mammary carcinoma as a function of a single dose of x-irradiation. Nicotinamide was administered by intraperitoneal injection one hour before irradiation.  Localized mild hyperthermia (41°C) was applied for one hour immediately before irradiation.

Based on the pre-clinical data demonstrating synergism with the trimodality therapy, we carried out a Phase II study of combined nicotinamide, hyperthermia, and radiation therapy in patients with locally advanced breast cancers, head and neck cancers, and malignant melanoma.  NA, up to 9 g per patient, was administered p.o. one hour prior to radiation therapy, was well tolerated in most patients. The peak plasma level of NA following the oral ingestion of 6 - 9 g has been in the range of 1-2 mM at one hour, the drug level of which has been sufficient to enhance the radiation response in murine tumor systems (9, 12).

**Table II - Tumor Response Following Treatment with Nicotinamide, Hyperthermia, and Radiation Therapy**

| Tumor Response | No. of Patients (%) |
|---|---|
| Complete Response | 18  (72) |
| Partial Response | 4  (16) |
| No Response | 2  (8) |
| Unevaluable | 1  (4) |

Breast Cancer (7 patients); Head & Neck Cancers (8 patients); Malignant Melanoma (5 patients); Others (5 patients)

As shown in Table II, the complete response rate following trimodality therapy was 72%, with an overall response (CR + PR) of 88%. The number of patients in this trial is too small for a meaningful comparison with historical controls treated with radiation therapy and hyperthermia.

It should be noted that all patients tolerated the trimodality therapy very well and, to date, no patient has had a recurrence at the treatment site, once they achieved a complete response. Using the method of Tc-99m pertechnetate clearance rate as a measure of the microcirculatory function of the tumor, we have obtained data showing the NA plus hyperthermia significantly increases the efficiency of microcirculation of tumor tissues (Figure 3). It is also

**FIGURE 3**

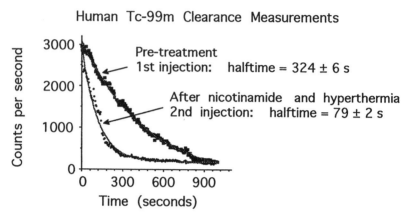

Human Tc-99m Clearance Measurements

**Figure 3**: Radioactive counts per second decrease as a function of time following an injection of isotope directly into the tumor. The rate of washout gives a measure of changes in blood flow. Following the administration of nicotinamide and heat, the clearance rate is increased by a factor of four.

interesting to note that patients who exhibit a significant change in clearance rate following NA and hyperthermia before radiation therapy had a high likelihood of achieving a complete response after the trimodality therapy (i.e., 8 out of 10 patients with CR). Accrual of more data is necessary to confirm the foregoing results, but this clinical experience has been highly encouraging.

# REFERENCES

1. Lippman, S.A., Parkinson, D.R., Itri, L.M., Weber, R.S., Stinson, P., *et al.* 13-cis-retinoic acid and interferon α-2a: Effective therapy for advanced squamous cell carcinoma of the skin. *J. Natl. Cancer Inst.*, 84:235-241, 1992

2. Lippman, S.A., Kavanagy, J.J., Paredes-Espinoza, M., *et al.* 13-cis-retinoic acid plus interferon α-2a: Highly active systemic therapy for squamous cell carcinoma of the cervix. *J. Natl. Cancer Inst.*, 84: 241-245, 1992.

3. Kim, S.H., He, S.Q., Kim, J.H. Modification of thermosensitivity of HeLa cells by sodium butyrate, dibutyryl cyclic adenosine 3':5'-monophosphate, and retinoic acid. *Cancer Res.*, 44: 697-702, 1984.

4. Bonner, J.A., Christianson, T.J.H., Spain, J.A., Shaw, E.G, Koval, T.M. The radiosensitizing properties of gamma interferon in human lung adenocarcinoma cells (A549) and fibroblast cells (CCL 210). *14th Ann. Meet. of Radiat. Res. Soc. Abs.*, pg. 45, 1992.

5. Krishanamurthi, S., Shanta, V., and Sistri, N. Combined therapy in buccal mucosal cancers. *Radiology*, 99: 409-415, 1971.

6. Mitchell, J.S., Brown, I., Carpenter, R.N. Attempts to develop radioactive anticancer drugs. *Intl. J. Radiat. Oncol. Biol. Phys.*, 9: 57-59, 1983.

7. Kim, J.H., Kim, S.H., Dutta, P., and Pinto, J. Preferential killing of glucose-depleted HeLa cells by menadione and hyperthermia. *Int. J. Hypertherm.*, 8: 139-146, 1992.

8. Kim, J.H., Dewhirst, M., Young, C.W. Hyperthermia: Current status. In: DeVita, V., Rosenberg, S.A. (Eds.), *Principles and Practice of Oncology Updates*, Vol. 3: 1-9, 1989.

9.   Horsman, M.R., Chaplin, D.J., and Brown, D.M.
     Radiosensitization by nicotinamide *in vivo*: A greater
     enhancement of tumor damage compared to that of normal
     tissues. *Radiat. Res.*, 109: 479-489, 1987.

10.  Chaplin, D.J., Horsman, M.R., and Trotter, M.J. Effects of
     nicotinamide in microregional heterogeneity of oxygen delivery
     within a murine tumor. *J. Natl. Cancer Inst.*, 82: 672-676,
     1990.

11.  Lee, I., Kim, J.H., Levitt, S.H., and Song, C.W. Increases
     in tumor response by pentoxifylline alone or in combination
     with nicotinamide. *Int. J. Radiat. Oncol. Biol. Phys.*, 22:
     425-429, 1992.

12.  Dragovic, J., Kim, J.H., Brown, S.L., Young, C.W.
     Evaluation of nicotinamide in combination with radiation
     therapy and hyperthermia in human tumors. Phase I/II study.
     In: *Proc. 6th Int. Congress Hypertherm. Oncol.* Taylor &
     Francis (Pub.), pg. 136, 1992.

# ORTHOMOLECULAR TREATMENT OF CANCER

A. HOFFER, M.D., Ph.D.

3A-2727 Quadra St., Victoria, Canada
V8T 4E5

## INTRODUCTION

My interest in schizophrenia and the therapeutic use of vitamin B-3 and vitamin C sensitized me to the use of these two vitamins in treating cancer. Dr. Ewan Cameron and Linus Pauling's[1] book on the treatment of cancer with vitamin C re-awakened my interest, and when the first pancreatic cancer patient was referred to me in Victoria, even though I am a psychiatrist in private practice, I agreed to see her.

In 1960, a retired professor was admitted to a psychiatric ward in a total organic confusional state. His lung cancer had been treated with cobalt bomb radiation, he did not respond and he was declared terminal. My research group was then searching the body for kryptopyrrole, then called the mauve factor. This patient excreted huge quantities. As I had been giving vitamin B-3 and vitamin C to psychiatric patients with this substance in their urine, I had this psychotic patient start on nicotinic acid, 1 gram three times daily, with the same amount of ascorbic acid. In three days he was mentally normal. He remained on the program for 30 months, when he died of a non-cancer death. His x-ray had been normal one year after I started him on the vitamins. The shadow had been getting smaller each quarter year.

A few months later a woman brought her 16 year old daughter to see me. She was to have her arm amputated to treat her Ewing's Sarcoma. I suggested to her physician they delay surgery for one month while she took nicotinamide and ascorbic acid 3 grams daily. She recovered without surgery. She is still well today. These two cases prepared me for the Cameron and Pauling studies.

In 1978 a woman with untreatable pancreatic cancer began to take vitamin C. She was then referred to me and I increased the dose to 40 grams daily plus the B vitamins. Six months later the mass was gone. She is alive and well today. She was working in a book store and began to tell her friends and customers about her recovery. This changed the nature of my practice from a purely psychiatric practice to one which includes about 20 percent of patients where the psychiatric component is relatively small. The number of referrals increased steadily and by mid-1994 I had seen over 600 patients.

## ORTHOMOLECULAR TREATMENT

Pauling[2] was intrigued by the fact that very large doses of vitamin C and vitamin B-3 were useful in treating a number of different conditions. After his analysis he showed how the need to synthesize ascorbic acid could be given up, provided that there was an ample amount of the vitamin in the diet. But when humankind moved from a diet rich in vitamin C to one which is poor in vitamin C, like our present modern diet, the fatal consequences of not being able to make vitamin C became apparent.

The term 'orthomolecular' was designed to draw attention to the use in therapy of optimum amounts of nutrients normally found in the body. I have described in detail the clinical practice of orthomolecular medicine[3]. In orthomolecular medicine we pay attention to the diet, to the use of optimum amounts of nutrients, to the elimination of toxic minerals and organic compounds, and we combine this with the use of essential elements of standard medicine. The program I follow is not meant to represent the program followed by other physicians. This new way of treating patients has not yet become a standard treatment which everyone follows. There are variations between physicians.

## Nutrition

I advise my patients to eliminate processed foods which contain added simple sugars, and to increase their intake of whole, fresh vegetables, fruit, seeds and nuts, but not necessarily to become vegetarians. I have seen too many patients become sick on a vegetarian diet. Human needs vary between those who are more carnivorous to those who are healthier with a herbivorous diet. I also advise them to decrease their fat intake, which may include avoiding dairy products and the margarines containing trans fatty acids. A simple rule is to follow the no junk diet. Processed foods containing added sugars usually contain other additives as well. The no junk diet probably eliminates 80% of all food additives. My second principle is to eliminate any foods to which the patient is allergic. The common foods which cause allergic reactions are dairy products, sugar, eggs, wheat and corn - in short, staples. In most cases a simple history followed by any one of a number of elimination diets will reveal which foods must be eliminated.

## Vitamin Supplements

For the treatment of cancer, the main vitamins are ascorbic acid, vitamin B-3, beta carotene and folic acid. But following the principle that it is better for any person to be as healthy as possible when fighting any disease, I also use the B complex mixtures which are readily available[4].

**A. Vitamin C.**  I start with oral ascorbic
acid, 4 grams three times daily. One teaspoon of
crystalline ascorbic acid dissolved in juice is
given afer each of three meals. A few patients
prefer the 500 or 1000 mg tablets. The dose is
increased until a laxative dose is reached, or
higher doses become  difficult to take for other
reasons. This varies enormously with patients and
ranges from less than 12 to over 50 grams daily.
According to Robert Cathcart, if patients can not
take at least 12 grams they should start on
intravenous ascorbate. The I.V. dose can vary from
50 to 100 grams daily. It does not cause diarrhea
and is remarkably free of side effects. Vitamin C
does not interfere with xenobiotic therapy
(surgery, radiation and chemotherapy). On the
contrary, it increases the efficacy of the
radiation and chemotherapy, and decreases the
toxicity. When surgery is used it increases the
rate of healing. Many patients find the ascorbates
more palatable than the pure ascorbic acid.


**B.  Vitamin B-3.**  Nicotinamide or nicotinic
acid, 500 mg one to three times daily. I use this
vitamin because of its general healing properties
and wide range of therapeutic activity[5], including
its anti cancer properties[6].

**C.  B-Complex.**  Containing either 50 mg to
100 mg each of the major B vitamins. This provides
some balance to the program.

**D.  Beta Carotene.**  25,000 I.U. daily,
occasionally 50,000 I.U.

**E.  Folic Acid.**  5 to 15 mg daily.

**F.  Vitamin E.**  D-alpha tocopherol, 800 IU
daily.


### Mineral Supplements

**A.  Selenium.**  200 to 600 mcg daily, usually
200 mcg.

B. Zinc. Usually 50 mg daily[7].

## XENOBIOTIC THERAPY

Medication considered essential by the family physician or oncologist is continued. If they are depressed I will use antidepressant drugs.

## THE PATIENT POPULATION

Every patient was referred to me by their physician. At first I would not know why they were being referred until I had seen them, but latterly physicians have been advising me and I usually arrange to see them within four days after they have been referred. I have had nothing whatever to do with the selection of these patients. At first the majority were patient-generated but over the past years a larger percentage have been physician generated. Perhaps 90% of the patients seen between 1978 and 1988 had already failed to respond to xenobiotic treatment. Out of 134 seen during that time period 33 would not or could not follow the vitamin regimen for at least two months. This included a small number who died within that period, but a larger group were discouraged from following the program by their family or their physicians, or were too sick from concurrent chemotherapy to be able to retain the vitamins. They survived on average less than 6 months.

Diagnosis was made by the physician in charge, in consultation with the oncologists from the Cancer Clinic. I had nothing to do with diagnosis. Nor did I have any part to play in determining what type of xenobiotic therapy they would receive. They were given standard treatment including surgery, radiation, and chemotherapy in various combinations depending on the diagnosis, the stage of their disease, and the previous treatment. After the first two visits they were followed by the referring physician. If they

wished to see me again they would obtain another
referral.

## THE FOLLOW-UP

Fortunately most of the patients came from
the local area around Victoria, with a smaller
number coming from Vancouver and from the rest of
Vancouver Island. Each year I would contact them
or a member of their family, if I had not already
gotten information about them. If this was not
possible, I would contact their family physicians
and also the Cancer Clinic which kept good
records. Fewer than ten patients have been lost to
follow-up out of over 600 I have seen. I was
interested primarily in their survival after they
had first seen me, and secondarily in their state
of emotional and physical health. Longevity
provided the hard data for these studies.

## REVIEW OF PREVIOUS REPORTS

In our first two reports[8] we provided the
data which led to our conclusion that longevity
was significantly increased when vitamin C and
other vitamins and minerals were added to the
xenobiotic program. In our first report on 134
patients seen between August 1977 and March 1988,
followed until December 31, 1989 we showed that
patients with female-related cancers had improved
their life expectancy about 20 times compared to
our non random control, and 12 times for patients
with other cancers. In our second paper with an
entirely new, more recent cohort of 170 patients
seen between April 1988 and December 1989,
evaluated December 1992, the results were very
similar. We concluded that vitamin C alone might
lead to 10% excellent responders, and that the
addition of the other nutrients increased this to
about 40%.

In order to obtain a comparison group we used
the 33 patients from the original series of 134
who had not followed the program for at last two

months. I have divided the group previously used as a control, into two: (1) the group who did not live for two months after they first saw me - there were 14 and they lived an average 51 days; (2) the group who lived longer than 2 months and did not start on the vitamin program, of whom there were 19. They were alive an average 458 days or 15 months.

The first group represents a terminal group who had failed to respond to standard treatment, or who had suffered a relapse after an initial response to previous treatment, and who may have been compromised by the treatment they had already received. It would have been desirable for patients who had decided for personal reasons never to accept any xenobiotic therapy to become a control group, but this was simply not possible in this study, nor would I recommend this to my patients for ethical reasons. As well, it is quite likely that some of the 101 patients in the treated group would also have died within that two month interval had they not been started on orthomolecular therapy, but this can not be determined for these patients. Perhaps an equal number lived longer than two months as did not make it for the two months after they first saw me. Taking all these factors into account, I think it is fair and reasonable to use the second control group as another valid comparison group, a concurrent group. This should also satisfy critics who maintain that every patient entered into the study must be retained in it, even if they did not follow the treatment protocal.

Using this comparison group there were 101 patients who were able to follow the program, although some of them did not live very long after I first saw them. None were excluded from this group. The results of the treatment on the 101 can be compared with the results of the xenobiotic treatment on the 19. I now have over 600 patients in my series. With this enlarged sample it will be possible to examine these issues more thoroughly.

I found that the difference between the vitamin treated patients and those who were not on the program was sustained. Survival of the two groups, the treated group of 101 and the pseudocontrol group of 19 treated only with xenobiotic therapy, are shown in the following diagram.

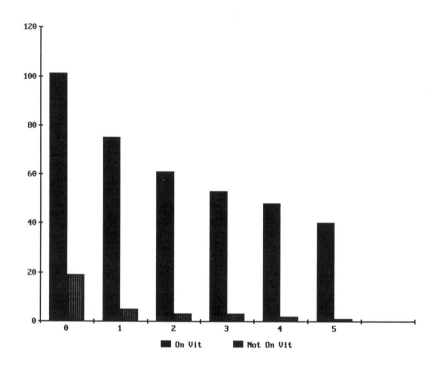

Figure 1.   Effect of Orthomolecular Treatment on Survival of Cancer Patients.

The difference in outcome between these two groups remained large. In the first year, 75% of the group not on the orthomolecular program died, and at the end of five years 5% were alive. From the orthomolecular group 25% died by the end of the first year, and at the end of the 5th year 39% were alive. By January 1, 1992, 41 patients were still alive. The average duration of life from the time I first saw them until this date was 49 months, compared to 15 months for the group treated with xenobiotic therapy only. Pauling[9] as reported by J. Challem stated, "Based on the results so far, I predict that they will live five to seven years. So many are still alive that it's hard to predict how long they'll live." The mean survival time estimate for both groups is about 80 months. The survival of the xenobiotic group resembled much more closely our original group of 33. Therefore, even with this control group which contains all the patients who followed the program for as little as a few days, the outcome of treatment was still supportive of our conclusion that orthomolecular treatment combined with xenobiotic treatment is much superior to xenobiotic therapy alone. As a clinician working with patients for 42 years, I still think the original control group is the sounder one to use scientifically.

Twenty patients out of 59 (34%) survived 8 years. They were first seen between 1978 and 1984. From the remaining 75, seen between 1985 and 1988, 22 (29%) survived 4 years. This suggests that over the next four years this group will also yield a 25%, 8 year survival. The first group included the following types of cancers: pancreas 1, lung 2, sarcoma 2, lymphoma 3, throat 2, uterus 2, ovary 1, breast 5, cervix 1 and colon 1.

Another way to compare the effect of orthomolecular against the standard therapy is to eliminate every patient I have seen who did not survive two months after I first saw them. Following this method I have examined the survival by years of 562 patients, all seen from 1978 to Feb 24, 1994. From this group there were 457 who were on orthomolecular treatment and 52 who were not. The latter is the control group and represents the results of standard treatment they had been getting from the time they first were diagnosed. This data is to be used only to compare these two treatments. It can not be used to predict the outcome of treatment since many of the

SOME DATA FROM THE PRESENT REVIEW

Outcome of all patients with breast and prostate cancer seen between 1978 and the end of 1991, as of December 31, 1993.

I have examined the outcome of all the breast and prostate cancer patients from the first 385 cases seen.

Table 1.  Outcome of Treatment for Cancer

|  | On Regimen | | Not on Regimen | |
|---|---|---|---|---|
|  | N at Start | N Alive | N at Start | N Alive |
| Breast |  |  |  |  |
| Ten years | 8 | 3 | 13 | 0 |
| Five years | 37 | 20 | 13 | 1 |
| Two years | 84 | 63 | 13 | 2 |
| Prostate |  |  |  |  |
| Five years | 11 | 5 | 0 |  |
| Three years | 18 | 10 | 0 |  |
| Two years | 25 | 72 | 0 |  |
| Surgery | 13 | 7 |  |  |
| Radiation | 17 | 15 |  |  |

Every prostate cancer patient followed the regimen. The number of cases is small and the only conclusion is that radiation, in this series, was more helpful than surgery. The breast cancer series is more substantial. The results are significantly better than for the control. The series of patients were mostly grade three and four tumors. This is indicated in the very poor response of the patients not on the program.

The following two case histories will illustrate the treatment response.

## Patient #105. Born 1910

Beginning in June 1983 he noted decreased urinary stream and force, and nocturia. In January 1985 he began to bleed. His prostate was found to be large and fragile. Biopsy showed benign hypertrophy. In December 1985 he had a transurethral resection. He had a poorly differentiated adenocarcinoma, grade C. One nodule about 3 cm in diameter was outside the capsule. After surgery he received 18 irradiation sessions.

On May 11, 1987, I started him on vitamin C 12 G, niacin 1.5 G, B-complex 50's, selenium 500 mcg, beta carotene 60,000 iu and zinc sulfate 220 mg, daily. He was not able to tolerate the niacin flush and I changed it to niacinamide 1.5 G. By May 1989 he was in remission. July 13, 1987, I increased his vitamin C to 16 G. November 1990 he was still well but was informed he had occluded carotid arteries from arteriosclerosis with well developed collaterals. I then started him on niacin 3 G daily. December 30, 1991, he was well. He died October 10, 1993 from a coronary occlusion. His wife told me how grateful she was at the extra years of high quality life he had gained. Two days before he died he was found to have metastases into his bones but he remained active until he died.

## Patient # 44, Born 1916

In May 1984 she noticed a lump in the left breast just below the nipple which was tender and attached to the skin over it. She was diagnosed infiltrating ductal carcinoma, with 1 of 6 nodes positive. After mastectomy the surgeon suspected

deep extension of the tumor to the underlying
muscle. She was given 13 irradiation treatments.
Excessive erythema prevented completing the
series. Before her surgery I started her on
ascorbic acid 12 G, niacinamide 3 G, pyridoxine
250 mg, selenium 600 mcg, folic acid 10 mg,
Vitamin E 800 iu, thyroid 60 mg, beta carotene
30,000 iu and vitamin A 10,000 iu, daily. In May a
lump formed in the right breast and she had a
mastectomy in June, 1988. In January 1990 she was
getting on well. In March 1990 she was started on
tamoxifen which later caused severe side effects
and she was then switched to megace. In August of
1990 she became very weak and short of breath due
to a massive pleural effusion in the left side.
The effusion was aspirated and tetracycline was
injected. With this effusion she also had a very
edematous left arm. This also cleared after
treatment. She then began to develop a large
number of small lumps on her back and front. These
were biopsied and were found malignant. There were
no internal metastases evident. During the last
three months before she died July 2, 1992, she was
very ill. Her vertebra had collapsed causing
severe pain and nausea with fluid in the thoracic
cavity. She died of penumonia probably due to the
massive collapse of her vertebra and difficulty
in breathing. The last six months of her life were
made miserable by her weakness, pain, the
excessive hair growth all over her body so that
she had to shave regularly and the masculinization
which was occurring.

Of the seven 1992 deaths, four were caused by
physical disease and not by their cancer. If they
had not been suffering from these other conditions
they would undoubtedly still be alive today. Two
died directly because of their cancer, and in one
of these severe osteoporosis was a major
complicating factor. The best results were
obtained when the patients remained on the total
regimen.

Since there were no deaths in 1993 it is
likely that most of the survivors, thirty-three,

are cured of their cancer and that their deaths will be determined by other factors associated with aging. The longer the series is followed, the fewer deaths will ensue from cancer, and the greater number will come from other factors such as cardiovascular disease, osteoporosis, accidents and so on. I suspect that these severe cases of osteoporosis arising from hormone blockers are not seen frequently when megavitamin therapy is not used because they do not live long enough for this complication to express itself.

## Coenzyme Q10 (CoQ10 or Ubiquinone)[11]

Q10 is present in the highest concentration in heart muscle. Generally it is present in the greatest concentration where it is needed the most. It is a major antioxidant, as are vitamins E, C and selenium. Vitamin E and selenium help to regenerate Q10. It is not classed as a vitamin due to inconsistencies in vitamin terminology. A vitamin is defined as a natural substance which is required in tiny amounts and can not be made in the body. Using this rule vitamin C is not a vitamin since it is required in large doses, and vitamin B-3 is not a vitamin since some can be made in the body from tryptophan. However, these are by tradition classical vitamins. Q10 can be made in ample quantities in healthy young people, but when anyone is sick, or as we age, it becomes more difficult to make enough. Thus, for the chronic diseases such as cancer, senility, and arthritis it is really a vitamin and ought to be called vitamin Q10. This is Dr. Karl Folkers' view. It is possible the high relation between aging and chronic disease may be due to the increasing difficulty in making and getting enough Q10.

In experimental animals it has been found to decrease the toxicity of chemotherapy, especially adriamycin, and to markedly suppress the growth of induced cancers. Folkers and his colleagues reported eight new cases of cancer plus two

earlier ones where Q10 allowed the survival of 5
to 15 years with no side effects.[12]

In a second report (not yet published),
Lockwood K, Moesgaard S & Folkers K, entitled
Partial and Complete Remission of Breast Cancer in
Patients in Relation to Dosage of Coenzyme Q10 in
Nutritional Therapy, the authors reported, "...an
open trial of 18 months on 32 women with breast
cancer of "high risk". They were treated with 1.2
grams of gamma linolenic acid, 3.5 G of omega 3
essential fatty acids and 90 mg of Q10 daily. No
patient died and all expressed a feeling of well
being. They would have expected three to have
died. In six there was a complete remission, less
morphine was needed and distant metastases were
not seen. In one patient they increased the Q10 to
300 mg daily after being on it for one year at 90
mg daily. Her tumor had stabilized at 1.5 to 2.0
cm.  After three weeks on the higher dose it was
gone.  K.L. stated that in practicing oncology for
20 years and having treated countless cases of
breast cancer, he had never seen a spontanious
remission of this size and had never seen a
comparable regression of any conventional anti
tumor therapy."

Based upon these observations I concluded
that Coenzyme Q10 should be an integral component
of all cancer therapy at the higher dose levels.
If the cancer is entirely gone a lower maintenance
dose probably would be adequate, perhaps 100 to
150 mg daily. It should be taken with the other
vitamins and minerals.

Between Nov. 1, 1993, and May 31, 1994, I
started 49 patients on 300 mg of Q10 in addition
to their usual nutrient program. During that same
interval one patient died. During the same
interval fifteen patients were not started on Q10.
Five died. For comparison I examined the same
statistics for patients seen between Nov. 1, 1992,
and May 31, 1993. None of this group were
receiving Q10. They were on the same program as
were the group given Q10 one year later. Every
patient seen during these intervals was included.

From the earlier group of 41, 6 died within the same interval. Chi Sq for this distribution is 6.4 i.e. P < .01.

This is not a comparison of patients all seen after six months of treatment. The mean follow-up was only three months but both groups are treated equally. It is rare in biological, especially human studies, to achieve such a respectable probability of around one percent. It suggests that Coenzyme Q10 has in reality added to the curative properties of the previous vitamin-mineral regimen.

July 31, 1994, I re-examined the survival data. From the group placed on Q10 between Nov. 1, 1993, and July 31, 1994, 2 out of 70 died. From the group not on Q10 the previous year over the same time interval 6 out of 50 died. Chi Sq is 3.7. P is about 5%. This suggests the effect of Q10 is still being maintained. I also compared the breast and prostate cancers against all the remaining ones. From the P and B group 1 died out of 44. From the other group 9 died out of 76. P about 6%.

## QUALITY OF LIFE

It is difficult to measure quality of life quantitatively, but it is relatively easy to find out whether the patients and their families were more comfortable, suffered less pain, and remained more functional. Almost all of the patients told me they were more comfortable, more functional and suffered less pain. Frequently they were able to decrease the amount of narcotic. Even when they lived for a short time after they saw me they felt they had benefitted, and often after death their families would let me know how grateful they were that they had suffered so much less. I have not had a single complaint from my patients that they suffered more pain and discomfort. This contrasts strongly with xenobiotic therapy which is characterized by severe discomfort of many kinds, nausea, fatigue of long duration, loss of hair, etc. Orthomolecular therapy tends to decrease the discomfort caused by xenobiotic therapy. This is also difficult to quantify, but I believe my patients were telling me what really happened when they reported that they were able to tolerate radiation and chemotherapy better. Their surgeons often were surprised by their rapid recovery from surgery. They were discharged very quickly from hospital.

### SUMMARY

The optimum treatment for cancer is a combination of xenobiotic and orthomolecular combined started as soon as the diagnosis is established. Patients will live longer and feel better. Orthomolecular oncologists can thus offer more hope to their patients than can oncologists who do not use nutrition and supplements. This provides an additional benefit to their patients.

August 5, 1994                          A. Hoffer, M.D., Ph.D.

### FOOTNOTES

[1] Cameron E & Pauling L: Cancer and Vitamin C. W.W. Norton & Co., New York, 1979.

[2] Pauling L: Orthomolecular Medicine. Science 160:265, 1968.

[3] Hoffer A: Orthomolecular Medicine. In, Molecules In Natural Science and Medicine, An Encomium for Linus Pauling. Eds. Z.B. Maksic

& M. Eckert-Maksic, Ellis Horwood Ltd, Chichester, West Sussex, England, 1991.

Hoffer A:  Some Theoretical Principles Basic to Orthomolecular Psychiatric Treatment. In, Ecologic-Biochemical Approaches to Treatment of Delinquents and Criminals. Ed. L.J. Hippchen. Van Nostrand-Reinhold Co., New York, 31-55, 1978.

Hoffer A: Orthomolecular Medicine for Physicians. Keats Publishing, New Canaan, CT, 1989.

4      Hoffer A: Orthomolecular Oncology. In, Adjuvant Nutrition in Cancer Treatment. Eds. P. Quillin & R. M. Williams. 1992 Symposium Proceedings, Sponsored by Cancer Treatment Research Foundation and American College of Nutrition. Cancer Treatment Research Foundation, 3455 Salt Creek Lane, Suite 200, Arlington Heights, IL 60005-1090, 331-362, 1994.

5      Hoffer A: Vitamin B-3 (Niacin) Update. New Roles For a Key Nutrient in Diabetes, Cancer, Heart Disease and Other Major Health Problems Keats Publishing, Inc., New Canaan, CT, 1990.

6      Jacobson M & Jacobson E: Niacin, nutrition, ADP-ribosylation and cancer. The 8th International Symposium on ADP-Ribosylation, Texas College of Osteopathic Medicine, Fort Worth, TX, 1987.

Titus K: Scientists link niacin and cancer prevention. The D.O. 28:93-97, 1987.

7      Woodward B: Zinc, a pharmacologically potent essential nutrient: focus on immunity. Can Med Ass J 145:1469 only, 1991.

Trivers ER: Zinc, An Essential Trace Element. Committee for World Health, P.O. Box 6180, Buena Park, CA 90622, 1991.

Gupta SK, Shukla VK, Vaidya MP, Roy SKI &
Gupta S: Serum trace elements and Cu/Zn ratio
in breast cancer patients. J. of Surgical
Oncology 46:178-81, 1991.

Gal D, Lischinsky S, Friedman M & Zinder O:
Prediction of the presence of ovarian cancer
at surgery by an immunochemical panel: CA 125
and copper-to-zinc ratio. Gynecologic
Oncology 35:246-50, 1989.

Wahrendorf J, Munoz N, Lu JB, Thurnham DI,
Crespi M & Bosch FX: Blood, retinal and
zinc riboflavin status in relation to
precancerous lesions of the eophagus:
findings from a vitamin intervention trial in
the Peoples' Republic of China. Cancer
Research 48, 2280-3, 1988.

8       Hoffer A & Pauling L:  Hardin Jones
Biostatistical Analysis of Mortality Data for
Cohorts of Cancer Patients with a Large
Fraction Surviving at the Termination of the
Study and a Comparison of Survival Times of
Cancer Patients Receiving Large Regular Oral
Doses of Vitamin C and Other Nutrients with
Similar Patients not Receiving those Doses.
J Orthomolecular Medicine 5:143-154, 1990.
Reprinted in Cancer and Vitamin C,  E.
Cameron and L. Pauling, Camino Books, Inc.
P.O. Box 59026, Phila., PA 19102, 1993.

Hoffer A & Pauling L: Hardin Jones
Biostatistical Analysis of Mortality Data for
a Second Set of Cohorts of Cancer Patients
with a Large Fraction Surviving at the
Termination of the Study and a Comparison of
Survival  Times of Cancer Patients Receiving
Large Regular Oral Doses of Vitamin C and
Other Nutrients with Similar Patients Not
Receiving These Doses. Journal of
Orthomolecular Medicine 8:1547-167, 1993.

9       Pauling L. Quoted in The Nutrition Reporter,
Challem, J. Vol 3, page 8, 1992.

10  Hoffer A: Orthomolecular Oncology and S Survival. Adjuvant Nutrition in Cancer Treatment Symposium. San Diego, CA, March 17-19, 1994.

11  Bliznakov EG & Hunt GL: The Miracle Nutrient Coenzyme Q 10. Bantam Books, Toronto, 1987.

12  Folkers K, Brown R, Judy WV & Morita M: Survival of Cancer Patients on Therapy with Coenzyme Q10. Biochemical and Biophysical Research Communications 192:241-245, 1993.

# Subject Index